The New Arab Man

The New Arab Man

EMERGENT MASCULINITIES, TECHNOLOGIES, AND ISLAM IN THE MIDDLE EAST

Marcia C. Inhorn

PRINCETON UNIVERSITY PRESS
PRINCETON AND OXFORD

Copyright © 2012 by Princeton University Press

Published by Princeton University Press, 41 William Street,
Princeton, New Jersey 08540

In the United Kingdom: Princeton University Press, 6 Oxford Street,
Woodstock, Oxfordshire OX20 1TW

press.princeton.edu

Library of Congress Cataloging-in-Publication Data

Inhorn, Marcia Claire, 1957–

The new Arab man : emergent masculinities, technologies, and Islam in
the Middle East / Marcia C. Inhorn.

p. cm.

Includes bibliographical references and index.

ISBN 978-0-691-14888-5 (hardcover : alk. paper)—ISBN 978-0-691-
14889-2 (pbk. : alk. paper) 1. Masculinity—Middle East. 2. Masculinity—Religious aspects—Islam. 3. Men—Middle East. 4. Infertility—Middle
East—Psychological aspects. 5. Fertilization in vitro, Human.
6. Man-woman relationships—Middle East. I. Title.

BF692.5.I54 2012

155.3'32089927—dc23

2011033539

British Library Cataloging-in-Publication Data is available

This book has been composed in Palatino

Printed on acid-free paper. ∞

Printed in the United States of America

10 9 8 7 6 5 4 3 2 1

To my parents,
Shirley and Stanley Inhorn,
for their love and support

Contents

Figures

Tables

Prologue: Hamza, My Infertile Driver

I was sitting in the back seat of a Mercedes sedan on a major highway heading south from Beirut, Lebanon. All of a sudden, my driver, Hamza,[1] put the car in reverse, literally backing up on the busy highway. "What are you doing, Hamza?!" I exclaimed in panic. "Don't worry, Mrs. Marshella. I am just keeping us out of trouble."

I am an anthropologist, whose research career has been devoted to the study of the Middle East. Since September 11, 2001, I have traveled extensively to nine Middle Eastern countries, living in two of them, Lebanon and the United Arab Emirates (UAE), for more than a year. My life in Lebanon was deeply affected by one man, Hamza, with whom I spent hundreds of hours. Hamza was my driver, whom I hired to take me to my field sites in a country where road conditions are dangerous, driving is reckless and unlawful, and many people lose their lives in "RTCs" (road traffic crashes). Hamza cared for me, making sure that I arrived safely at my destinations—despite, in some cases, sitting in traffic for hours and driving off road or backwards in order to bypass obstructions.

My relationship to Hamza was very much affected by our respective positionalities. Hamza is a working-class, high-school-educated, married, Shia Muslim man. I am a white American, middle-class, middle-aged, married woman with a PhD and a long career as a professor. I am not Muslim, although I study and appreciate the complexities of Islam. I was raised as a secular humanist Unitarian (on the far left end of Christianity) and am decidedly agnostic. I am a politically liberal, feminist pacifist and have always opposed the war in Iraq. I went to Lebanon in late 2002 with my young family—husband Kirk, seven-year-old son Carl, and four-year-old daughter Justine—knowing full well that a U.S.-led war in Iraq was likely to begin. I was deemed crazy—an unfit mother perhaps—by many American friends, family members, and colleagues, who seriously questioned my judgment about putting my children in harm's way. And, indeed, opposition to the invasion of March 2003 reverberated throughout Lebanon, as many Lebanese protested what they viewed as an unjust, oil-driven war. I contemplated leaving, as U.S. embassies and American scholarly programs around the Middle Eastern region evacuated all personnel. But, quite amazingly, war-scarred Lebanon remained open for Americans throughout the year. As a Fulbright scholar, I was not required to leave the country. And so Hamza continued to drive me and my small family across Lebanon, keeping us safe.

Through Hamza, I learned much about what it means to be an ordinary man in a Middle Eastern country wracked by political violence. I had come to Lebanon to study male infertility, a condition that affects a disproportionate number of Middle Eastern men and may be attributable in part to the physical stresses of war. As it so happened, Hamza was seriously infertile. He and his wife had been longing for a child for more than a decade. Perhaps this was the reason for his tenderness toward my children, as he held their hands across the street or carried them sleepily from the back seat of his car.

Hamza was born in southern Lebanon to a lower-middle-class Shia Muslim family. There were five sons and five daughters, with Hamza the middle son. Hamza's father, also a driver, was a member of Amal, the Shia Lebanese political party led by Speaker of the Lebanese Parliament Nabih Berri. Not a prosperous man, Hamza's father relied on the social services supplied by Amal. This meant educating his sons in Amal-controlled schools and hoping for a better future for his children.

However, the Lebanese civil war broke out in 1975, and like so many other Lebanese Shia Muslims, Hamza's family began to suffer. As Hamza recalls, "Amal did nothing to help us at that time. My father had done so much for the party. But, when we needed them, they disappointed us." As fighting swept over the southern half of the country, the family fled north to Beirut, finding only a small apartment in the Shia-dominant southern suburbs. Hamza's younger brother, still a teenager, suffered his first psychotic episode, perhaps triggered by the stress of violence, and had to be hospitalized in a psychiatric ward (where he remains today). As forty thousand Syrian troops entered the country, Hamza also had his first run-in with Syrian soldiers, who, without provocation, beat him up "to show him a lesson." Meanwhile, Hamza's father was dragged from his taxi while attempting to flee an episode of crossfire and was shot in cold blood on the side of a road. He died, leaving an illiterate widow and ten children, the oldest in his early twenties.

Having to help support his family and fearing for his own life, Hamza, then only seventeen, did what many young Lebanese men did at the time: he fled the country. Whereas many Lebanese Shia men headed for western and central Africa to try their luck as entrepreneurs and diamond traders, Hamza headed for the Arab Gulf, where he took a waiter's job in a restaurant in Sharjah, United Arab Emirates. Sharjah is the emirate next to Dubai, the latter of which was just beginning its Las Vegas–like boom. But neighboring Sharjah was nothing like Dubai. As the emirate housing Dubai's laboring class, Sharjah was known for its devout religiosity—a form of ardent Sunni Muslim Islam called Wahhabism, emanating from neighboring Saudi Arabia. Wisely, Hamza dissimulated about being Shia, and, in so doing, he eventually came to manage the restaurant where he worked for nearly twenty years.

Hamza described his life in Sharjah as a mostly happy time. He worked hard, earned enough money to remit much of it to his struggling Lebanese family, and still saved enough money for his own wedding. Like many Middle Eastern men, Hamza chose to marry his first cousin, Janna, a pretty, veiled teenager who was the daughter of his paternal aunt. Although Hamza could not be described as a handsome man by Lebanese standards (he wore glasses, had round cheeks, and had grown a paunch), Janna liked his cheerful countenance. Like many other young women who were stuck in Lebanon while their brothers fled, she also had her own desires to leave the war-torn country. Thus, she agreed to marry Hamza and move with him to Sharjah, where she quickly learned to speak English and took a position in a retail cosmetics store.

Like most Middle Eastern–born couples, Hamza and Janna wished to have children immediately following their marriage. However, when this did not happen, the lack of pregnancy was justified to others as an "adjustment period," as they established themselves in the Gulf and worked hard to save money for themselves and their families. Yet, secretly, Hamza and Janna began to worry about why she was not getting pregnant. In Sharjah, she had begun taking days off work to go to doctors, none of whom could find any fault with her reproductive system. Thus, Hamza agreed to get tested and learned that his sperm were "weak." Although his body produced sperm, only 10 percent were active. Sperm tests were repeated, and each time, Hamza learned that he suffered from severe asthenozoospermia (i.e., poor sperm motility), for which there was no real treatment. Although he was prescribed vitamins and hormones, they did little to improve his sperm profile. So, he eventually gave up his search for medicine, hoping that a miraculous pregnancy might happen with the small amount of sperm "still swimming."

Janna was discouraged, but she had grown to love Hamza dearly. Even though divorcing an infertile husband is considered a woman's right under Islamic law, Janna considered such an act to be shameful and unjust. She preferred to leave their case to God, seeing their pregnancy struggle as a test of their patience and faith. But Janna also began to make a plan, as the civil war in Lebanon receded. She hoped to return to southern Lebanon with Hamza, building a home on the hills overlooking the Mediterranean. She also hoped that Lebanese physicians, once renowned across the region for their excellence, would be able to help them make a baby.

By the late 1990s, after years of postwar economic stagnation, Lebanon was coming alive again as émigrés like Hamza and Janna were beginning to return home. With only a high school diploma, Hamza's employment opportunities in Lebanon were relatively limited. But, with money saved from Sharjah, he purchased a used Mercedes sedan, and began working as a for-hire driver at a foreigners' hotel near the American University of Beirut (AUB) campus. With his English skills somewhat developed by his employment in the Gulf, Hamza was able to cater to the scholars, journalists, and European tourists who began flowing back into a country that was being reborn.

In December 2002 I was one of those foreigners who found Hamza. I had just arrived in Beirut with my family, staying at the hotel where Hamza worked with his older brother, Ali. Upon arrival in the country, my family needed to register at the American Embassy, and so Hamza took us on our very first trip across what was known during the war years as the "green line"—from Muslim West Beirut where we were staying, to the heavily fortified American Embassy in the far suburbs of Christian East Beirut. Hamza navigated skillfully through the shell-pocked roads and congested traffic, chatting amiably with my husband in the front passenger seat. Attired in Lebanese *chic*—jeans, black leather jacket, wire-rim glasses, neatly trimmed mustache, and stylishly cut black hair—Hamza nonetheless had a certain "softness" that was reassuring. By the end of the trip, I asked Hamza if he could become my regular driver. He quickly agreed, quoting me a fair price by Lebanese standards. And so it began: Hamza became my driver, but also my interlocutor and protector. We were separated by vastly different social worlds and experiences but were eventually bonded by feelings of respect and friendship. And, as it turned out, I would become a major instrumental figure in Hamza's life, helping him to overcome the secret infertility problem that had plagued him for so many years.

Learning that Hamza had no children after more than ten years of marriage, I suspected that he might be infertile. Middle Eastern couples rarely if ever choose to remain childless. And long-term, intractable infertility problems in the Middle East are often of male origin. When I told Hamza that I had come to Lebanon to study male infertility, he could not believe his good fortune: here he was, driving an "expert" on male infertility, one who might be able to help him with his sperm motility problem. His male infertility story came tumbling out, a kind of catharsis after years of suffering.

After hearing Hamza's story, I told him about intracytoplasmic sperm injection (ICSI), a variant of in vitro fertilization (IVF) designed to overcome male infertility problems. With ICSI, men with very poor sperm profiles— even total absence of sperm in the ejaculate—can become fathers. As long as one viable spermatozoon can be retrieved from a man's body— including through painful testicular biopsies and aspirations—this spermatozoon can be injected directly into an oocyte under a high-powered microscope, effectively forcing fertilization to occur. Since its introduction in Belgium in 1992, ICSI has helped thousands of once hopelessly infertile men to father healthy biogenetic offspring. In Hamza's case, ICSI might be his only hope.

Hamza was excited by this news, quickly reporting our conversation to Janna. Shortly thereafter, I was invited to their home in southern Lebanon, where I met Janna and her family. I saw the impressive home that she and Hamza had built in hopes of starting a family. There, Jana showed me the results of various medical tests she had undertaken, including painful and invasive uterine x-rays and diagnostic laparoscopies that had proved her fertility. However, Hamza's repeated semen analyses pointed to the problem: although he produced adequate numbers of sperm, 90 percent of them were immotile, showing no signs of necessary forward movement under the microscope.

Confirming in my own mind that Hamza truly suffered from a serious male infertility problem, I told Janna about ICSI, which was now being performed successfully at IVF clinics in Beirut. Janna had become quite attached to a local Shia Muslim infertility specialist; however, she agreed to visit a Beirut IVF center with me, even though this one was run entirely by Christian Lebanese IVF physicians.

In May 2003 I arranged an appointment for Hamza and Janna. They met with a senior IVF physician, who reviewed their tests and deemed them candidates for ICSI. After their appointment, I showed Hamza and Janna the IVF ward and introduced them to Najwa, the unit's head nurse, who was also a southern Lebanese Shia Muslim woman. Najwa had invited me and my family to visit her natal home in southern Lebanon, and I explained to her that Hamza would be driving us there.

In late May 2003 Hamza drove us to Tibneen, a town in southern Lebanon, where we met Najwa's elderly parents, toured some local Roman ruins, and ate a sumptuous lunch in a nearby village once occupied by Israelis. Both Najwa and Hamza wanted us to see the political realities of life in southern Lebanon, which had only recently been vacated after nearly twenty years of Israeli occupation (1982–2000). Entire villages had been destroyed, but they were slowly being replaced by cement villas, some of them quite large, to showcase the wealth of returning Lebanese war émigrés. These homes dotted the rolling hillsides, along with the barracks of the United Nations peacekeepers, who patrolled in their jeeps with the telltale blue-and-white UN logo.

Najwa and Hamza asked us if we wanted to see the Lebanese-Israeli border, a no man's land between the two countries. Replying that we were interested, we took a brief journey along the border, which was marked by a shallow gulley and two rows of impenetrable barbed-wire fences. Whereas prefabricated villages on the Israeli side were surrounded by meticulously cultivated fields and orchards reaching right up to the barbed-wire wall, the Lebanese side was comparatively barren. The only signs of human activity on either side of the wire border were the military outposts—concrete bunker pillboxes on the Israeli side and open-air Hizbullah checkpoints on the Lebanese side—where the Israeli soldiers and Hizbullah militia men sat with their heavy weapons trained on each other.

Reflecting on the day's journey, I realized that I knew relatively little about Hamza's own politics. He was a Shia Muslim man, who had escaped most of the ravages of the civil war and the indignities of the ensuing occupation. Perhaps because his job was to transport foreigners, he kept his political convictions to himself. However, on that day, when we traveled back to Beirut, I decided to ask Hamza about his political sympathies. Because I had interviewed so many Lebanese Shia Muslim men as part of my study, I knew that Hizbullah sympathizers at that time generally followed the teachings of the Iranian ayatollah, Ali Hussein al-Khamene'i. Lebanese Shia who did not favor Hizbullah generally followed the leadership of the local Lebanese Shia ayatollah, Muhammad Husayn Fadlallah. After five months of riding with Hamza, I had never asked Hamza the simple question, "Do you follow Shaykh Fadlallah or Shaykh Khamene'i?" It seemed high time for me to ask.

Hamza replied hesitantly, "I follow Shaykh Khamene'i."

"So, you support Hizbullah?"

Rattled, Hamza held up his hands, palms facing toward my husband in a conciliatory "hands up" gesture. "Yes, but I am not a terrorist!"

Desiring to further contextualize his response, Hamza went on to explain how his father, a loyal member of the opposing Shia political party, Amal, had been brutally murdered in the war. Yet, Amal did little if anything to help Hamza's struggling family. Hizbullah, on the other hand, provided poor Shia Muslim families with the social services that had been neglected by the Lebanese government and denied by the Israeli occupiers. In the wake of his father's death, Hamza had switched his allegiances to Hizbullah, attempting to follow its guidance and to lead a respectable and religiously inspired life.

My husband and I reassured Hamza that we understood that Hizbullah provided many social services in southern Lebanon. Nonetheless, I joked with Hamza that I could not tell my nearly-eighty-year-old parents that we were being driven by a member of Hizbullah! They would worry too much.

Then my husband asked Hamza a critical follow-up question: "Would you take up arms if Lebanon were attacked again by the Israelis?"

Hamza replied forcefully and without hesitation, "I would fight for my country, even if it meant losing my own life."

When we arrived home, Kirk and I discussed the meaning of Hamza's revelation. The preceding two months had been a tense period in Lebanon, with several acts of violence toward British and American interests in reaction to the war in Iraq. We had contemplated leaving Lebanon for Cyprus but decided to stay at the urging of Lebanese friends and colleagues. Hamza's paternalistic role in our lives as a knowledgeable Lebanese man and trusted driver had also made us feel secure and protected. After five months of trips across Lebanon, shared meals, help with our children, involvement with Hamza's family, and intervention in his infertility problem, I—we—simply could not see Hamza in any other way than as a good man, a friend and ally. Our children loved him, and I had learned so much about Lebanon from him. We reasoned that having a driver sympathetic to Hizbullah might even be good for our future safety, should the situation deteriorate suddenly in Lebanon.

Fortunately, local reactions to the war in Iraq soon waned, and so we stayed in Lebanon, with Hamza driving us for the entirety of our planned stay. And I did not tell my parents, and particularly my worried mother, about Hamza's political loyalties until *after* we returned home to the United States in August 2003.

As I left Lebanon, I told Hamza that I wanted to stay in touch with him from afar and to learn about the outcome of his ICSI procedure. At the point of my departure, Hamza and Janna had yet to undertake their first cycle of ICSI. They were still completing a series of fertility tests and were putting together the requisite money (U.S. $2,000–3,000 for one cycle of ICSI), in a country where few citizens have any form of health insurance.

I sent Hamza a holiday card that year through the address of the hotel where he worked. Months passed without reply, and I wondered whether I would ever hear from Hamza again—although he had "sworn by God" that he would call me in the United States if he and Janna ever achieved an ICSI pregnancy. Then, at about five o'clock on a cold spring morning in 2004, the phone rang at our home in Ann Arbor, Michigan. Awakened and alarmed by the early morning call, I answered to hear Hamza's voice on the line:

"Mrs. Marshella. It's me, Hamza."

"Hamza! I can't believe it's you. How are you?"

"*Hamdu-lillah* [praise be to God]! Everything is good. And I have some great news to tell you!"

"Is Janna pregnant?"

"Yes! She's pregnant, fourteen weeks. The 'operation' [i.e., ICSI] succeeded!"

"*Alf alf mabruk! Mash Allah!* [A million congratulations! What God wills!] I am *so* happy for you, Hamza. Please tell Janna how happy I am for *both* of you."

Hamza asked about "Mr. Kirk," Carl and Justine, and how we were settling back in Michigan. I told Hamza that all was well, and I made him promise that he would call me once the baby arrived.

But then I heard nothing from Hamza for more than a year, and I worried about two possibilities: either Janna had miscarried, one of the risks of an ICSI pregnancy, or my prominent role in Hamza's life had receded into the past, and he had forgotten to call. I had also lost Hamza's new phone number, scrawled while half-awake on that early spring morning. I had no formal plans to return to Lebanon, and so I realized that I might never see Hamza again, or find out the end of his ICSI story.

Meanwhile, my own career in Middle Eastern reproductive anthropology was moving forward with great rapidity. I was invited as a keynote speaker to a conference at the University of Tehran on "Embryo and Gamete Donation." Specifically, I was asked by the Iranian Shia conference organizers to represent the "Sunni Muslim position" on this subject vis-à-vis my earlier scholarly work in Sunni Egypt. I was also setting up a new research project on "reproductive tourism" in the UAE—led there, in part, by Hamza's positive views of that country. With a trip planned to Iran via Dubai in February–March 2006, I was invited by my colleagues at the American University of Beirut to stop in Lebanon on the way, where I delivered a lecture on "The Public Health Costs of War in Iraq: Lessons from Post-War Lebanon" to a packed auditorium. Although I had only two days to spend in Beirut, I went to the hotel to find Hamza, leaving a message for him with the concierge. Hamza soon called, delighted that I had returned. He said that he would travel to southern Lebanon to pick up Janna, so that they might both see me at the hotel the following afternoon.

But it was not just Janna who Hamza retrieved in southern Lebanon. As he entered the hotel lobby, I could see that Hamza was carrying a baby in his arms—a thirteen-month-old girl with black ringlets for hair, tiny gold earrings, pink overalls, and the same face as her radiant father. As Hamza told me during our brief, joyful reunion, his daughter Heba (her name meaning "gift from God") was the result of their third ICSI attempt. The first two ICSIs had failed at the busy IVF clinic where I had introduced them to the Christian infertility physicians. And so they had returned to their favorite Shia Muslim infertility specialist in southern Lebanon, who had developed his own IVF unit in the city of Saida (a.k.a. Sidon), near their home village. It was there that Heba was conceived—after a total expenditure of nearly U.S. $8,000 for the three ICSI cycles. Hamza joked that in the old days, people had many children without having enough money to pay for them all. But nowadays, people paid great sums of money to have even one child! Yet, Hamza was clearly grateful for ICSI, and for my role in leading him to this revolutionary technology. He and Janna thanked me profusely, bestowing upon me gifts of candy and other Middle Eastern delicacies to take back to my family in America.

I left Beirut feeling exceedingly happy: I had seen Hamza, Janna, and their beautiful baby; my colleagues and friends were doing well, despite the political instability created by the 2004 assassination of former Lebanese prime minister Rafik Hariri; and I was embarking on a new Middle Eastern adventure. Little did I realize that a tragedy was about to unfold.

In the summer of 2006, during a booming tourist season in Lebanon, Hizbullah militia men cut through the impenetrable barbed-wire fence to capture several Israeli soldiers. Israeli prime minister Ehud Ohlmert retaliated with attacks by air, land, and sea. In the blink of an eye, Israel and Lebanon were back at war. Southern Lebanon, the home of Hizbullah, was the site of the most intense fighting and destruction.

Frantically, I emailed my graduate students, colleagues, and friends in both Beirut and Haifa, Israel. All of them were safe, although several relayed harrowing stories of escape from Lebanon. Furthermore, thousands of southern Lebanese refugees were pouring into Beirut to flee the fighting in the south. Hamza's home was in the south, and I could not reach him there. Fearing the worst, I eventually contacted the hotel in Beirut where he worked as a driver. Although Lebanon's telecommunications infrastructure was severely damaged by the Israeli bombing campaign, the hotel concierge urged me to try Hamza's cell phone number, as some cell phone calls were continuing to get through. Sure enough, I reached Hamza. The first thing he said was, "I knew you would not forget me, Mrs. Marshella." He then proceeded to tell me his story.

When the fighting broke out, Hamza feared first and foremost for the life of his wife and daughter. They hurriedly packed a few belongings, locked up their beautiful house in southern Lebanon, collected some money, and drove with Janna's elderly mother into the Chouf Mountains to the north and east. Through his work as a driver, Hamza was acquainted with a number of Druze families in the vicinity. (Druze are a minority religious sect in Lebanon, loosely related to the Shia but with their own communities and religious practices.) He was able to rent a Druze-owned house, where he deposited his immediate family members. Then, he began days of harrowing driving through the Lebanese back roads, collecting his elderly mother and two unmarried sisters, Janna's sisters, and other extended family members. As one of the only senior men in his family still in Lebanon and as the only professional driver, his goal was to get as many of his family members as possible out of harm's way, without losing his own life in the process. Somehow, he managed the feat of bringing his family into the safe haven of the Druze-controlled Chouf Mountains. There, they all waited for six weeks, wondering what had become of their homes, their property, their communities, and the rest of Lebanon.

I talked to Hamza several times during this period. He worried about what would become of his family if the fighting spread throughout the country. He feared that his immaculate, marble-tiled home was already destroyed. He also regretted leaving Sharjah for his godforsaken country where the horrific violence never seemed to end. He lamented the violence, the decisions that had led to the violence. He wanted the violence to end. There was no bravado, only sadness in his voice.

I could not help but think that fatherhood had changed everything for Hamza. Hamza had once proudly professed to me and my husband that he was willing to die for his country as a Hizbullah patriot. But when his country was plunged into war, it was his family—not his country—that he sought to defend. His tiny pink bundle of joy—the little girl whose face was a reflection of her father's—had given Hamza the single-most compelling reason to live.

EPILOGUE

As of this writing, Hamza, Janna, and Heba are alive and well. Quite amazingly, their village was mostly spared from the destruction of the so-called Six-Week Summer War between Israel and Hizbullah, and they returned to their bolted-but-still-beautiful marble dream house in the fall of 2006 after the war ended. Hamza continued to drive the foreign journalists and aid workers who flooded into the country in the war's aftermath. In one of our phone conversations during that period, Hamza attempted to convince me that "Everything is back to normal, Mrs. Marshella. I hope you will come back to Lebanon some time soon." His resilience—and that of the other Lebanese, Palestinian, Syrian, and Iraqi men whose stories will be recounted in this volume—has never ceased to amaze me. At Hamza's urging, I have been back to Lebanon twice since the war, and I have seen Hamza beam over his pride and joy, little Heba, who has already entered elementary school. As of this writing, no other ICSI babies have been born to Hamza and Janna, but they thank God for their ICSI daughter.

The New Arab Man

Reconceiving Middle Eastern Manhood

This book is a tribute to Middle Eastern men such as Hamza, my driver in Lebanon, whose stories never make it to the front pages of the *New York Times*, to flashing news bulletins on CNN, or to Academy Award–winning movies such as *The Hurt Locker*. Hamza is an ordinary man, living through a millennial moment of political violence within the Middle East and between the Middle East and the West. That Hamza was willing to drive me, an American female anthropologist, through a post-9/11 world marked by increasing tension and bloodshed—much of it perpetrated by my own country in the region—seems to me now quite extraordinary. With courage and conviction, Hamza shared his life story, his inner thoughts, his deep sorrows, and his eventual profound happiness with me. Although I came to know Hamza best, he is but one of the hundreds of Middle Eastern men who told me their stories. *The New Arab Man* is my testament to their suffering, their resilience, and their humanity.

Hamza's story reveals many of the themes to be taken up in the chapters that follow. First and foremost, Hamza is infertile; infertility impedes reproduction among a disproportionate percentage of Middle Eastern men. This epidemic of male infertility—which many men attribute to their unrelenting life stresses, including war—has led to a recalibration of manhood in ways to be described at length in this volume. As I argue, reproduction, fatherhood, and manhood are in a state of flux—or what I shall call "emergence"—in the Middle Eastern region as a whole. "Emergent masculinities" bespeak not only the new treatment options available for male infertility but also men's changing desires for a happy life. As seen in Hamza's story, becoming a father was but one of several life goals. Most important to him was the achievement of a loving and understanding relationship with his wife, Janna, his younger cousin. Consanguineous or cousin marriage is widespread across the Middle Eastern region and may be tied to the high rates of male infertility there. However, cousin marriage may also be companionate, marked by romantic love, deep affection, and abiding commitments.

I argue that Hamza and Janna's loving marriage was facilitated by being childless. This finding is counterintuitive, for infertility is widely considered *within* the Middle Eastern region to be an inevitable source of marital duress and eventual divorce. Many men's and women's stories suggest otherwise, and male infertility is no longer the major crisis of masculinity that it was once perceived to be. The notions of a "childless couple" or "child-free living" have yet to enter the cultural lexicon. Nonetheless, Hamza and Janna lived happily for more than a decade as a childless Middle Eastern couple. As dual-income migrants, Hamza and Janna were able to enjoy life together, experiencing the attractions of the booming Arab Gulf economy and saving enough money to realize another major dream when they built a rather palatial, marble-tiled, single-family home back in Lebanon.

Such diasporic dreams are profoundly different from a generation ago. Migration and remittances, nuclear residence, dual careers, companionate marriage, romantic love, being a happily married couple, and a childless couple at that—all of these are new patterns that are definitely emerging across the region but have barely been noticed by scholars and media commentators. In part I of this book, "Emergent Masculinities," this phenomenon of happily married but childless Middle Eastern couples is explored at some length from Middle Eastern men's own perspectives. Many men do not want to be perceived as domineering patriarchs; they do not view fatherhood as the be-all and end-all of masculinity; they value conjugal intimacy and privacy, sometimes at the expense of larger familial commitments; and they often adore their wives as friends and lovers, having learned sexuality together in the context of dual premarital virginity. Hamza's story represents these emerging forms of masculinity and conjugality.

Hamza's story also highlights the emergence of changing moral commitments over the course of a man's lifetime. We see in Hamza's tale the moral quest to be a good Muslim man in a religiously complex, even fractured, environment. Men's religious commitments are the subject of part II, "Islamic Masculinities." We still know too little about Middle Eastern men *as practicing Muslims,* or how Islam shapes men's identities.[1] Although Islam is the dominant regional religion, the Middle East is home to many faiths, with eighteen registered religious sects in the country of Lebanon alone. Hamza was born into the minority Shia branch of Islam, which is the single largest religious group in southern Lebanon, in the southern suburbs of Beirut, and perhaps in the country as a whole. But among the Shia, there are major divergences in levels of religiosity, clerical authority, political affiliation, and attitudes toward modernity, including the use of high-tech reproductive medicine. Hamza considered himself to be a pious Shia Muslim. However, he interacted continuously with foreigners and, like most other Lebanese, did not make his religiosity publicly manifest in a country where sectarian rivalries have been the source of tragic violence. Had I not pursued an anthropological line of questioning with Hamza, I might never have known of his religious allegiances.

Hamza's religious and political convictions also changed over the years and were influenced by the tragedy of his father's wartime death. Hamza eventually sided with Hizbullah, during the local power struggle between two rival Shia political factions. However, Hamza's own piety and comportment could only be described as moderate. Although sympathetic to Hizbullah, Hamza worked vociferously to distance himself from the terrorist label. Despite his patriotic rhetoric, Hamza decidedly did *not* take up arms with Hizbullah against Israel in the 2006 war, instead seeking protection for his young family with the Druze, another minority religious sect.

Like many other Middle Eastern men whose lives are explored in the pages that follow, Hamza did not always agree with religious authorities. For example, Hamza did not view sperm donation as a solution to his male infertility, even though he followed the teachings of Iran's Ayatollah Khamene'i, who had issued a *fatwa*, or religious decree, allowing donor technologies. As shown in part II of this volume, religion has shaped the very contours of the assisted reproductive technology industry in the Middle East, with attitudes toward in vitro fertilization (IVF), intracytoplasmic sperm injection (ICSI), gamete donation, embryo disposition and storage, multifetal pregnancy reduction (a form of abortion), and the possibility of adoption heavily infused with local moral sensibilities. Most Muslim men are keen to follow authoritative Islamic *fatwa*s and bioethical statements, all of which have allowed IVF and ICSI as solutions to infertility. However, Sunni Islamic authorities continue to ban both gamete donation and surrogacy.[2] This Sunni ban on third-party reproductive assistance carries great moral authority, for reasons to be explored in part II. Nonetheless, Ayatollah Khamene'i's unprecedented permission of third-party donation, including sperm donation, egg donation, embryo donation, and surrogacy, has created new possibilities in Shia-dominant Lebanon and Iran. How Middle Eastern men accommodate or resist these novel interventions—and the moral justifications they draw on to do so—are also the subject of part II.

Throughout this volume, we follow Middle Eastern men on their quests for ICSI, the reproductive technology that allowed Hamza to become a father. We examine the trials and tribulations of what men call *tifl unbub* (literally, "baby of the tube," or test-tube baby) or, simply, "the operation." Increasingly, the quest for ICSI involves "reproductive tourism," whereby infertile men travel between IVF centers and between countries in search of ICSI success. Such reproductive travel, I argue, is better understood as "reproductive exile,"[3] for many infertile couples feel forced to leave home in order to access reliable assisted reproductive health services. Such movements are all too familiar for most Middle Eastern men. Men such as Hamza are a population in motion, with a high percentage of men moving across borders in the course of their lifetimes for reasons having to do with politics, economics, and, in some cases, reproductive disruptions that require cross-border reproductive care (CBRC).

DISRUPTING OUR SCHOLARSHIP AND ASSUMPTIONS

This is a book about disruptions, with the term "disruption" taking on two important meanings. First, the term "reproductive disruption"—which I have used in my earlier writing[4]—captures the sense of disjuncture, asynchrony, loss, injustice, and stigma that many infertile people feel when they discover that they are unable to conceive a child. Male infertility, like female infertility, definitely constitutes a reproductive disruption, and one that comes as a surprise to most men, who have no idea that they are infertile until diagnosed through semen analysis, usually after marriage.

Second, I intend for this book to disrupt many taken-for-granted assumptions about men's lives, and particularly Middle Eastern men's lives. Preconceived notions about the malevolence of Middle Eastern men certainly come to us through the media, both cinematic and informational. As one of my colleagues summed it up, after attending a research seminar on my work: "You just can't buy a positive picture of a Middle Eastern man these days." This vilification of Middle Eastern-qua-Muslim men through both popular and scholarly discourses is the subject of the next chapter, "Hegemonic Masculinity." Suffice it to say here that one of the main goals of this book is to disrupt stereotypes, or what we think we know about Middle Eastern men as patriarchs, polygynists, protestors, religious fanatics, and terrorists—men who represent the very epitome of brutality, rage, and misogyny. This book purports to be an antidote to that kind of thinking, my attempt to humanize men who have been categorically condemned by the media and many politicians as "guilty" after 9/11.[5]

Part of the failure to humanize Middle Eastern men lies in the hands of scholars. In the new millennium, there is a dire need to retool our scholarship on Middle Eastern men's lives. In this regard, two contemporary anthropological theorists have urged scholars to engage in such scholarly disruptions and thereby unseat facile essentializations. One of our most esteemed Middle Eastern anthropologists is Lila Abu-Lughod of Columbia University, the author of the award-winning *Veiled Sentiments: Honor and Piety in a Bedouin Society*.[6] In her 1991 seminal essay, "Writing Against Culture," Abu-Lughod took issue with the way in which anthropologists were using the "culture" concept; by representing cultures as seemingly coherent, timeless, and discrete, they ignored history and engaged in a project of profound "othering."[7] She urged anthropologists to write against culture by focusing instead on discourse and practice, global connections, or ethnographies of the particular. Turning her critical gaze on the anthropology of the Arab world, she also challenged the discipline's obsession with particular ethnographic"prestige zones"(e.g., Morocco under the influence of interpretive anthropologist Clifford Geertz) and with particular"zones of theory"that were taking on a talismanic quality within Middle Eastern anthropology at the time.[8] These zones of theory included tribalism and segmentary lineage theory; harem theory, or the presumed "private"space relegated to Middle Eastern women; and Islam, which she called the "theoretical metonym" for the Arab world. She lamented the relative poverty of anthropological theory on political economy and class, or the anthropology of emotions. In both of her provocative works, she beseeched the anthropological discipline to"reform"itself through attention to history and power.

More than two decades later, Middle Eastern anthropology has yet to break out completely from its theoretical and ethnographic shackles. Of the approximately 420 ethnographies written by anthropologists over the past sixty years—exactly half of which have been published in the new millennium—most focus on only six of the twenty-two Middle Eastern nations, including in order, Israel/Palestine, Egypt, Morocco, Iran, Turkey, and Yemen. Afghanistan, Algeria, Jordan, Lebanon, Sudan, Syria, and Saudi Arabia constitute a second tier of ethnographic attention, with at least ten books on each country, many of them quite old and outdated. Geopolitically crucial countries such as Syria and Iraq, the countries of origin of many of the men in my study, have been difficult to access and, hence, much less studied. The small, petro-rich kingdoms of the Arab Gulf, where many of the men in my study, including Hamza, have migrated, have received the least ethnographic attention.

Works on the original"zones of theory"—namely, tribalism, gender (qua veiled women), and Islam—continue to form a kind of holy triumvirate, composing one-quarter of the entire anthropological corpus. These are followed by numerous ethnographies of place—namely, villages, towns, urban quarters, minority ethnic enclaves, and migrant neighborhoods— which are heavily overrepresented among the remainder. Thankfully, many newer themes have emerged over the past decade and are being celebrated at the 2011 Middle East Studies Association Annual Meeting under the title "Anthropology of the Middle East: A New Millennium."[9] Some of these newer themes include studies of mass mediation and popular culture, Middle Eastern youth and education, law and human rights, language and literature, colonial politics and modern violence, memory and subjectivity, fine arts and architecture, diaspora and transnationalism, forced migration, and tourism. There is now even one ethnography on sexuality and sexual practice from contemporary Iran.[10] However, ethnographies of science, technology, and medicine—the theme of my own work in the Middle East over the past twenty-five years[11]—are relatively few and far between.[12] Middle Eastern anthropology is decidedly out of touch with the up-and-coming discipline of science and technology studies, which has produced a decade's worth of award-winning anthropological ethnographies.[13]

Furthermore, ethnographies of masculinity—or "men as men," to use Matthew Gutmann's well-turned phrase[14]—are, to my knowledge, nonexistent for the Middle Eastern region as a whole. This glaring lacuna is indexical of problems in the wider discipline of anthropology. Gutmann, a professor at Brown University, has lamented the erasure of men from contemporary gender scholarship in anthropology. Ethnographic accounts of masculinity are rare and tend to focus on the "manly" subjects, such as physical training, sport, education, wage earning, and militarism.[15] Although the literature on masculinity is beginning to grow in anthropology, the majority of it hails from Euro-America and Latin America, and much of this Americanist scholarship centers on masculinity construction among men who have sex with men, given the grim specter of the HIV/AIDS epidemic.[16]

Within such studies, Gutmann notes that masculinity is often described imprecisely. Four distinct notions of masculinity can be found in anthropological discourse: masculinity as anything men *think* and *do*; masculinity as anything men think and do to *be* men; masculinity as reflected by some men being inherently *more manly* than others; and masculinity as anything that woman are *not*, emphasizing the central importance of male-female relations.[17] In his award-winning ethnography, *Fixing Men: Sex, Birth Control, and AIDS in Mexico*, Gutmann unpacks ten common misconceptions about men's reproductive lives and sexuality, including, for example, that men do not—and will not—take responsibility for birth control.[18] His research from Oaxaca shows that some men are embracing vasectomy as a permanent form of male contraception. Their reasons for doing so are varied but include conjugal empathy and sacrifice, themes that are also prominent in Middle Eastern men's narratives.

Like Abu-Lughod's and Gutmann's, my own work on gender and reproduction in the Middle East has caused me to reflect on such silences and misconceptions. In what follows, I examine scholarly erasures and policy assumptions regarding men, before describing my own ethnographic foray into the world of Middle Eastern men's reproductive lives.

REEMBEDDING MEN IN REPRODUCTION

According to a widely held but largely untested assumption in feminist social science, population policy, and lay circles, men are disinterested and disengaged in matters of human reproduction. Because men do not give birth, their power and attention lies elsewhere in social life, with the responsibility for pregnancy, parturition, breastfeeding, and childcare remaining solely in the hands of women. Drawing upon the title of Simon de Beauvoir's great feminist treatise,[19] my colleagues and I have argued that men are relegated to be "the second sex" in the scholarship of reproduction, including in anthropology.[20]

Case in point: When I surveyed the state of the art in the year 2006, I found that more than 150 ethnographic volumes on reproduction and women's health had been written in the past twenty-five years, with nearly two-thirds of those volumes published since the new millennium.[21] Only four ethnographies on men—two on men's experiences of childbirth and fathering in the United States,[22] one on soldiers' reproductive and sexual troubles after the first Gulf War,[23] and Gutmann's book on men's reproduction and sexuality in Mexico[24]—have ever been published, to my knowledge. To date, there are no ethnographic monographs devoted to male infertility or men's use of assisted reproductive technologies, including donor sperm;[25] erectile dysfunction or other sexual health problems;[26] sexually transmitted infections (STIs) other than HIV/AIDS; men's usage of the vast repertoire of contraceptives; older men's experiences with prostate cancer and reproductive aging; men's attitudes toward prenatal genetic testing and fetal demise; men's feelings about partners' abortions; men's experiences of pregnancy loss and child death; and men's reproductive health in general. Certainly, other vital topics could be added to this list if it were widened to include smoking, cardiac disease, diabetes, and the like. Although several new journals are devoted to men's health (e.g., *International Journal of Men's Health, Journal of Men's Health and Gender*), the empirical literature is still scant compared to that devoted to women and reproduction. Although men influence women's reproductive lives and health in a variety of ways, how women influence men's reproductive lives is rarely explored. Instead, when men are included in reproductive health studies, the focus is generally on the consequences of their actions for women's reproductive lives and well-being.

But are men truly so disassociated from reproduction? This book challenges that assumption, bringing men back into the reproductive imaginary as reproductive progenitors, partners, decision makers, lovers, nurturers, and fathers. Men not only contribute their gametes to human procreation but are often heavily involved and invested in most aspects of the reproductive process, from coupling to impregnation to parenting. Furthermore, men have their own reproductive issues and concerns, which may be connected to but also separate from women's reproductive health and well-being. Thus, men need to be reconceived as reproductive in their own right, and men's reproductive rights need to be acknowledged along with women's.

This insight—that men have reproductive issues and rights—was first suggested on a policy level at a major 1994 conference in Cairo, Egypt. Called the International Conference on Population and Development (ICPD), a broad new approach to population policy, called the Reproductive Health Initiative, was conceived.[27] Men were included in the new rubric of "reproductive health for all," and infertility was recognized as an impediment to "family planning" in the truest sense of that term. The Reproductive Health Initiative promised to move population policy beyond the narrow focus on fertility control. ICPD was hailed by many, including Third World feminist organizations, as a great historical achievement.

Despite the broad definition of reproductive health put forward at the ICPD conference, the Reproductive Health Initiative still remains heavily focused on population reduction through family planning. Some critics argue that the term "reproductive health" has simply replaced the term "family planning" in population and international health discourses, with little substantive change at the level of actual programs.[28] Moreover, the questions can be asked: Has the ICPD Reproductive Health Initiative actually improved the reproductive lives of men? And are men and women suffering from infertility actually better off than they were in 1994? The answers to these questions remain unclear.

Treatment of infertility in order to conceive a desired child is now being conceptualized as a fundamental reproductive right. However, reproductive rights discourse continues to be based on Eurocentric, neoliberal bourgeois notions of reproductive "choice" that may not apply to or be operationalized in many non-Euro-American societies, or among poor minority communities within Euro-American settings, where reproductive rights may be severely constrained.[29] Reproductive health discourses are still predicated on Western-generated notions of the right to choose (be it contraception, abortion, infertility treatments, or parenthood itself). These discourses assume, at some rudimentary level, a body of autonomous individuals who are free to make choices and who can come together in a concerted way to vocalize their resistance as political agents.[30] Yet, in many non-Euro-American societies such as the Middle East, individual agency is often subsumed within larger collectivities such as the extended family; hence, there may be limited opportunities for individual action and expression. Moreover, strategies of everyday resistance and group mobilization (e.g., infertility support and lobbying groups) may be severely constrained by the political contexts within which individuals live their lives.

Globalization, the concomitant spread of biomedicine, and neoliberal values of reproductive "choice" and "freedom" in a now privatized reproductive "marketplace" suggest that individuals bear responsibility for their health and illness, with every person expected to care for himself or herself

In the name of striving for a better quality of life.[31] Within this perspective, a person with a condition such as infertility should actively seek treatment or find other strategies to overcome the childlessness. With regard to male infertility in particular, seeking a solution becomes a challenge and test of a man's capacity to fend for himself, his wife, his marriage, and the future of his family. For those men who fail in this regard, they may be blamed for not availing themselves of their choices in the reproductive marketplace. Yet men's reproductive choices may be severely constrained by both biology (a lack of sperm) or access (a lack of ICSI)—constraints that the ICPD initiative has done little to overcome.[32]

In short, the neoliberal reproductive rights discourse first promulgated at the utopian Cairo ICPD conference has yet to materialize for many people around the world, including many infertile Middle Eastern men. The discourse is oriented toward women, is still focused on population control and the provision of birth control, and fails to account for the many ways in which people lack true reproductive agency.

In my own work on Middle Eastern infertility, I have been struck by the failure of reproductive rights discourse to resonate with most audiences. Namely, is the right to bear children a human right? Many individuals would answer no to that question, especially in the context of poverty or overpopulation (e.g., Gaza, or Cairo with its 20 million inhabitants). The suffering of the infertile in places such as the Middle East evokes little sympathy. Instead, most Westerners, and even some Middle Eastern elites, argue that Middle Eastern fertility levels should be dramatically curtailed, and individuals' reproductive rights to bear a child questioned and constrained. That I have argued vociferously for the right to IVF, ICSI, and other reproductive technologies in resource-poor settings such as Egypt seems incredibly naïve—even *ill-conceived*—to many.[33] A recent conversation, which occurred "behind my back," is just one of hundreds of examples I could recount over the ensuing years since I began my research. A member of my own extended family, a high school teacher in Ohio, recently asked my parents what kind of research I *really* do, and why Yale University would want to hire me for it. When my then eighty-three-year-old mother attempted to explain the importance of overcoming infertility in the Middle East, my cousin retorted, quite aggressively: "Why would she want to help terrorists have babies? They'll just bring future terrorists into the world!"[34]

Although Middle Eastern men are conceived of as particularly ominous reproductive actors, the *negative* contributions of men in general have emerged from ICPD reproductive health discourses. Men either impregnate women (sometimes against their will) or cause women's poor reproductive health outcomes, through HIV/AIDS, other STI exposure, sexual violence, or physical abuse. In addition, they have been regarded as formidable barriers to women's decision making about fertility, contraceptive use, and health care utilization in general.[35]

Two recent attempts to reframe men's contributions more positively are noteworthy. In the first, both men and women are seen as having reproductive rights, but men are also seen as having "responsibilities" toward their families.[36] "Responsible men" share in family planning; remain faithful to their partners; seek health care for their partners during pregnancy, birth, and postpartum; and participate as fathers in family life and child care. To wit, "real men" are "responsible men," whose role is to protect and ensure the reproductive rights and well-being of others.

But what are the problems of this framework? First, responsible men rhetoric is blatantly patriarchal, if men are primarily conceived of as paternalistic protectors of women and children. Second, in this framework, women's and men's contributions to reproductive health are seen as inherently unequal, and their experiences of reproductive health as fundamentally different. Interventions following from this framework remain focused on the reproductive health problems *caused* by men, along with approaches designed to *empower* women. Third, the fact that the reproductive rights of men and women coexist in relationship to each other is fundamentally ignored; if men, too, have reproductive rights, then women should also have "responsibilities" in protecting men's reproductive rights and health. Fourth, if men are conceived of as primarily responsible for others, then their own reproductive health problems are ignored; this is particularly problematic for integrating men into reproductive health interventions and programs. Finally, a framework that invests men with responsibilities suggests that men are fundamentally "irresponsible." This assumption is profoundly problematic, even denigrating. Many men are already responsible when it comes to reproduction and have been acting so for centuries, according to historical research on reproduction and contraception.[37]

The second framework for including men in reproductive health heralds them as "partners" to women.[38] Men as partners is a "client-based" approach, which seeks to provide sustainable reproductive health care for men without compromising (and hopefully improving) services for women. Such a perspective recognizes men's important contributions to reproductive health, as well as men's own reproductive health care needs. It attempts to reconcile conflicting reproductive goals within the context of reproductive "partnerships," primarily among married couples. Such an approach focuses on men as husbands and members of a family, with a significant locus of responsibility for reproduction.

What are the problematic assumptions of this framework? First, given the explicit focus on the cooperation of men and women in reproductive decision making, this framework downplays the different reproductive and sexual strategies and goals that men and women may pursue separately, including outside of the marital union.[39] A related problem is the ideological assumption of heterosexual monogamy and fidelity within marriage, which has become a programmatic goal of the men-as-partners approach. Third, this perspective has been difficult to implement, as the definition of "partner" has been difficult to operationalize, even within the context of marriage. Does marriage make a man a partner, or does "partnership" bespeak more nuanced notions of love, companionship, friendship, and the like? Fourth, on a programmatic level, this approach does not clearly answer whether services for men should be integrated or separate from those for women; this is a contentious issue that depends heavily on existing services as well as the kinds of services provided. Finally, the partner perspective also makes several implicit assumptions about men and reproductive health—namely, that educating men about men's and women's reproductive health needs will make men more sensitive and responsive to these needs and that incorporating men into reproductive health programs will improve both men's and women's reproductive health outcomes. Such assumptions may not hold in all contexts.

Men in the Middle East may feel greatly responsible for reproduction and may strive to be the best possible partners to their wives. This is true even though few Middle Eastern men have been "targeted" in the kinds of programs just described. Their sense of responsibility and partnership comes from other sources, including conjugal love, which, as I argue, has been virtually overlooked in population and reproductive health discourses (as well as in Middle East anthropology). That men—even Middle Eastern men—actually *love* their wives and will do what they can to meet their wives' reproductive desires and needs seems to have been lost in the popular imagination and by the population studies establishment. Middle Eastern men as responsible reproductive partners, in love with wives whom they wish to please, is, perhaps, the abiding theme of this volume.

UNSEATING PATRIARCHY

Implicit in much of the ICPD discourse is that the reproductive and sexual needs of women are culturally subordinate to those of men. In many locales around the world, this may be true: namely, men may have implicit rights *over* women's reproduction and sexuality. Thus, the achievement of equity in reproductive health requires unseating patriarchy wherever it is detected. The concept of patriarchy, or men's systematic domination of key structural and ideological resources and positions, does not fully explain poor reproductive health outcomes for women. Yet a strong argument can be made that patriarchy affects women's reproductive health on both macrostructural and microstructural levels.[40] On the macrostructural level, women's reproductive health is affected by male policy makers, male health care administrators, and male service providers, who may perpetuate a dominant "male definition" of what is important and what is not without taking heed of women's perceptions and felt needs. On the microstructural level, research shows that men are more likely to have more sexual partners over their lives; to have multiple partners simultaneously; to pursue commercial sex; to have extramarital sexual relations; and to commit an act of violence against women, adolescents and children, and other men.[41] Men have the option to be absent at childbirth; tend to commit smaller percentages of their income to children and childcare; and contribute less time to direct childcare.[42] In short, men's relative superior power and privilege in most societies may have dire consequences on women's lives and reproductive well-being.

Men's relative power and privilege over women has been the dominant trope in the Middle Eastern gender studies literature—much of it written by Middle Eastern–born scholars—where the concept of "patriarchy" has served as a theoretical metonym. Scholars have unearthed the patriarchy in Islamic scriptural representations of women and in Islamic personal status laws.[43] They have analyzed childhood socialization practices that produce patriarchy in Middle Eastern family life.[44] They have critiqued a variety of Middle Eastern patriarchal practices ranging from veiling to female genital cutting to honor killing.[45] They have analyzed women's resistance to men's violence, including through women's storytelling, poetics, and memoirs of war.[46] And they have hailed the emergence of Middle Eastern feminist movements, both historically and amid growing male-dominated Islamism.[47]

Furthermore, nearly one hundred ethnographies have been written by anthropologists about Middle Eastern women. Very few of these ethnographies have examined women's and men's actual relationships within the context of marriage. This lacuna reflects the highly gender-divided world of Middle Eastern anthropology: namely, women study women, and men study men. Ethnographers and ethnographies of what might be called "gender interaction" or "marital ethnography" are largely absent, not only for the Middle East but within the discipline of anthropology as a whole.[48]

As a result of this lopsided view of gender through the eyes of women subjects and scholars, very little has been written about Middle Eastern men as men. A growing interest in Middle Eastern homoeroticism can be detected,[49] as well as the study of what might be called "military masculinity."[50] Four recent volumes examine primarily discursive traditions,. including writings on Arab men's (and women's) sexuality since the early nineteenth century,[51] Arab men's portrayals in fiction since 1967,[52] and Arab men's representations in Hollywood post-9/11.[53] The fourth volume, which is a compendium, is appropriately titled *Imagined Masculinities*, to signal how little is known about the realities of men's lives in the Middle Eastern region.[54] Calling the Middle East "one of the seats of patriarchy," the editors nonetheless challenge women's studies scholars to focus on masculinity as a "complementary endeavour" to their various "feminist projects."[55] The editors argue that Middle Eastern patriarchy "is both more complex . . . more implicated in the structure of social relations than has sometimes been admitted, and at the same time not as monolithic as has been suggested."[56] For example, in her chapter on representations of maleness in the Arab popular media, Ghoussoub argues for "men's tortured conception of their own 'masculinity': its meanings, demands and projections." She poses the rhetorical question, "Who said it was easy to be a man?"[57] Through chapters on male circumcision, military service, and men's images in the Middle Eastern media, movies, and memoirs, the underlying purpose of the volume is to recalibrate understandings of Middle Eastern men's lives, including their oppression by other men. The editors and authors strive to show that men's lives may not be easy, particularly in a region that is highly militarized and where young men are often conscripted. However, the theme of patriarchy prevails throughout the volume. The editors remind us that men are "positioned at the thresholds and have often attempted to police the mobility and conduct of their sisters, daughters, companions, wives, and comrades, sometimes—quite often in fact—with the complicity of their mothers and other senior women."[58]

My own intellectual genealogy as a Middle Eastern studies scholar and the founding editor of the *Journal of Middle East Women's Studies* (*JMEWS*) is tied up in this feminist project. For more than two decades, I have focused on Egypt, writing a series of three books that one scholar has dubbed my "Egyptian trilogy."[59] The second volume, *Infertility and Patriarchy: The Cultural Politics of Gender and Family Life in Egypt*, represents my most extended contribution to this feminist genre. In the book, I localize patriarchy within the Egyptian context, offering the following formulation:

> Patriarchy is characterized by relations of power and authority of males over females, which are (1) learned through gender socialization within the family, where males wield power through the socially defined institution of fatherhood; (2) manifested in both inter- and intragender interactions within the family and in other interpersonal milieus; (3) legitimized through deeply engrained, pervasive ideologies of inherent male superiority; and (4) institutionalized on many societal levels (legal, political, economic, educational, religious, and so on).[60]

The remainder of the book examines the ways in which patriarchy is "lived" by poor urban infertile Egyptian women in their relationships with husbands, in-laws, and community members. I argue that the severe stigmatization, threats of marital dissolution, and social ostracism faced by infertile women are rationalized and perpetuated by the dominant procreative ideology in Egypt, which attributes life-giving powers to men through spermatogenesis of fetuses and blames women for thwarting men's procreative powers. The book concludes with an analysis of the social and cultural factors perpetuating emphatic pronatalism in Egypt and the resultant "cult of motherhood" that is increasing in importance with the rise of Islamism in the country.

In later publications, including contributions to edited volumes on *Islamic Masculinities*[61] and *African Masculinities*,[62] I describe the ways in which fertile Egyptian women are scapegoated for their husbands' infertility and impotence. In "'The Worms Are Weak': Male Infertility and Patriarchal Paradoxes in Egypt," I demonstrate four ways in which Egyptian women carry the social and physical onus of male infertility.[63] First, they are blamed for the reproductive failure and expected to bear their husbands' secret in silence. Second, lacking the signs of pregnancy, their gendered identities are diminished, while their husbands' masculine identities remain relatively intact. Third, they are expected to endure a childless marriage, while their husbands may become increasingly frustrated, demoralized, and divorce prone. And, finally, they are expected to seek treatment for their husbands' infertility, a form of asymmetrical, gendered embodiment that leaves men physically unscathed. As I conclude, infertile Egyptian men experience various forms of privilege in their marriages, social relations, and treatment experiences, often to the detriment of the wives who love and support them.

Similarly, in "Sexuality, Masculinity, and Infertility in Egypt: Potent Troubles in the Marital and Medical Encounters," I show how hegemonic constructions of masculinity prohibit frank marital and medical discussions of male sexual dysfunction, producing acute dilemmas for women who are labeled infertile by virtue of their childlessness.[64] In a culture that rewards and locates masculinity in a man's ability to father children, male sexual dysfunction is rendered invisible—particularly within a "don't ask, don't tell" regime upheld by impotent husbands and the male gynecologists who proceed to treat these men's wives. Although male sexual dysfunction represents a "crisis moment" for hegemonic Egyptian masculinity, this masculine crisis is lived most acutely by women, who must absorb both the sexual shame and the reproductive blame in public.

These publications were based on research conducted entirely with poor Egyptian women. As I wrote in the introduction to *Infertility and Patriarchy*, "I came to know much more about Egyptian *husbands*, as seen through the eyes of Egyptian wives, than about Egyptian *men* in either a general sense or individually."[65] However, my portrayal of poor Egyptian husbands was not entirely unsympathetic, one-sided, and unfair. The most important chapter of my book, "Conjugal Connectivity," described the ways in which many poor Egyptian men support and protect their infertile wives within an otherwise hostile social milieu. These men's desires for "companionate" marriages—characterized by loving connectivity even in the face of female infertility—was perhaps the major insight of the study. Relatively few of the infertile women that I encountered were living lives of brutal oppression by domineering patriarchs. Rather, many of them described their good fortune in having adoring spouses and satisfying sex lives—contrary, they admitted, to what was expected for a childless marriage within their social environment.

Since then, I have gone on to reconsider the ways in which I once systematically excluded men from my earlier studies. I returned to Egypt in the late 1990s to study elite women's utilization of in vitro fertilization and was literally overwhelmed by husbands' response to my study, with nearly half of them coming forward to speak with me, usually about their own infertility problems. The majority of these couples (70%) were seeking assisted reproduction because of male infertility in a society where infertility affects more than 15 percent of all married couples, and at least 60–70 percent of the infertility problems hail from men's own reproductive tracts. It was then that I realized the toll on men's bodies and lives entailed by male infertility, and I attempted to portray this embodied suffering and emasculation in my third book, *Local Babies, Global Science: Gender, Religion, and In Vitro Fertilization in Egypt.*[66]

The New Arab Man is my own act of scholarly contrition—my frankly apologetic attempt to render visible the lives of Middle Eastern men whom I once regarded as imponderable and forbidden research subjects. In this book, I challenge many of my earlier claims and assumptions about Middle Eastern patriarchy and men's lives. I argue that Middle Eastern patriarchy today is being unseated by Middle Eastern men themselves, who are questioning traditional notions of manhood. This does not mean that patriarchy is nonexistent in the Middle East; certainly, it does persist in a variety of forms. However, we need to rethink whether patriarchy should remain the dominant theoretical trope. Better empiricism—actually studying men's lives and their relationships with women—might help to undo patriarchal assumptions in Middle Eastern gender studies. In short, as Middle Eastern feminist scholars, we could do a much better job of nuancing our patriarchal polemics, if we only took ethnographic realities into account.

In my own long-term, feminist research project, I had argued to myself and others that Middle Eastern men were off limits to me, as a female anthropologist studying the intimacies of reproduction, sexuality, and infertility. However, the Egyptian men who volunteered for my study in the late 1990s proved that I might need to rethink many of my methodological assumptions. One Middle Eastern–born colleague, Lahoucine Ouzgane, was also especially helpful in this regard. When I discussed with him my reluctance to move forward with a post-9/11 project on Middle Eastern male infertility, he surmised that I might possess superior access to this sensitive research subject by virtue of my positionality. First, if Middle Eastern men regard fertility as an important and somewhat competitive attribute of manhood, then it might be very difficult for them to discuss infertility with another man, he surmised. As a woman, I might be better positioned to enter this secret world of reproductive shame, providing at least some men the only opportunity for frank discussion. Second, a Western woman is assumed to be knowledgeable in the ways of sex and conception, so that sexually troubled Middle Eastern men might be able to discuss their problems and questions more freely. Third, as an educated *duktura* and professor of medical anthropology and public health, I might be considered a potentially knowledgeable and empathic confidante, sworn to secrecy by virtue of research ethics. Fourth, as a middle-aged woman "past my prime," I could represent a quasi-maternal and comforting presence, especially to younger men. Finally, as a temporary visitor to these men's social worlds, I might be seen as taking "men's secrets" far away, providing a fleeting moment in their tortured lives for honesty, candor, and catharsis.

NARRATING MEN'S REPRODUCTIVE LIFE HISTORIES

The New Arab Man is the outcome of my own ethnographic attempt to render men's lives visible. I have made the collection of Middle Eastern men's stories my major research project in the post-9/11, wars-in-Iraq-and-Afghanistan world in which we live. Hundreds of Middle Eastern men have come forward to tell me their "reproductive life histories." What is a reproductive life history? This is a term I have coined to merge the methodological genres of cultural anthropology and epidemiology, the two disciplines in which I have received advanced training.[67] The "reproductive history," as used in epidemiology, explores the important reproductive events in individuals' lives through a process of structured interviewing. Questions revolve around premarital and marital sexuality, contraception, conjugality, infertility, pregnancy, pregnancy loss, childbirth, and maternal and neonatal mortality. Reproductive epidemiology also focuses on so-called risk factors (e.g., smoking, sexually transmitted infections) that may lead to so-called disease outcomes (e.g., infertility, stillbirth). Carefully rendered reproductive histories can provide an incredible wealth of information on both epidemiological and demographic variables. Through systematic and detailed reproductive histories, reproductive disruptions of all kinds may emerge.

When combined with anthropological ethnography, reproductive histories take on additional meanings, transforming into full-fledged reproductive life histories. In anthropology, the "life history" is one of the most important ways in which ethnographers elicit chronological accounts of persons' lives, through processes of gentle questioning and probing.[68] Life histories are, in my view, the sine qua non of ethnography—that which takes our field to a different level of subjective inquiry. In medical anthropology, some of the most compelling and award-winning ethnographies adopt the life history genre.[69] Psychological anthropologists, too, have argued for the importance of "person-centered ethnography," which attempts to develop "experience-near ways of describing and analyzing human behavior, subjective experience, and psychological processes."[70]

Here, I have attempted to conjoin the two disparate genres— epidemiological reproductive history with anthropological life history—to elicit nuanced reproductive life histories from Middle Eastern men. The resulting person-centered, reproductive accounts take us to places well beyond reproduction, providing rich entrée into experiential worlds, local moralities, and embodied subjectivities. The exploration of Middle Eastern men's subjectivity is at the heart of this endeavor. I am inspired in this regard by my medical anthropologist colleagues at Harvard and Princeton, who have challenged us to "rethink subjectivity" in the modern era:

> In the many settings in which anthropologists now work, the vagaries of modern life are undoing and remaking people's lives in new and ominous ways. The subjects of our study struggle with the possibilities and dangers of economic globalization, the threat of endless violence and insecurity, and the new infrastructures and forms of political domination and resistance that lie in the shadows of grand claims of democratization and reform. Once the door to the study of subjectivity is open, anthropology and its practitioners must find new ways to engage particularities of affect, cognition, moral responsibility, and action.[71]

My own ethnography is a foray into these multiple domains: of politics, war, globalization, economic stresses, emotions, identities, religious subjectivities, and moral and practical responses to technological innovation. My research is based on reproductive life history interviews carried out with more than 330 Middle Eastern men in Egypt (1996), Lebanon (2003), United Arab Emirates (2007), and so-called "Arab Detroit," Michigan (2003-8), the capital of Arab America.[72] In these four places, I have interviewed men from fourteen different Middle Eastern countries. These include the Levantine countries of Lebanon, Syria, Palestine, and Jordan; the Arab Gulf countries of UAE, Bahrain, Oman, and Yemen; the North African countries of Egypt, Sudan, and Morocco; the war-torn country of Iraq; and the non-Arab Middle Eastern countries of Iran and Turkey. In addition, during my 2007 research project on "Globalization and Reproductive Tourism in the Arab World," I interviewed Muslim men from many different parts of South and Southeast Asia (e.g., India, Pakistan, Sri Lanka, Malaysia, Indonesia), as well as East Africa (e.g., Somalia, Djibouti, Tanzania), who were coming to the UAE to access ICSI.

As a result of this research over more than a decade, I have come to know, *inter alia*, Lebanese taxi drivers, Syrian university professors, refugees in Palestinian camps, wealthy Egyptian businessmen, Iraqi Shia clerics, Hizbullah police officers, Yemeni American auto workers, Lebanese Christian house painters, Emirati engineers, Armenian Lebanese jewelers, Syrian Bedouin shepherds, Druze *shaykhs*, Sudanese doctors, Syrian construction workers, Bahraini oil men, wealthy Lebanese in the African diaspora, and many poor and middle-class men, mostly from Lebanon, Syria, Palestine, and Iraq. The list goes on, but it is united by one fact: all of these men have shared their reproductive life histories with me.

In this book, I focus primarily on the Lebanese, Syrian, and Palestinian men who participated in my three-year study called "Middle Eastern Masculinities in the Age of New Reproductive Technologies," which began in Beirut, Lebanon, in January 2003. There, I met Hamza, as well as 220 mostly childless men who were visiting Lebanese IVF clinics. Throughout this book, I present basic statistical information about these 220 men—120 of them infertile, and 100 of them fertile—all of whom hailed from the Levant (Lebanon, Syria, Palestine). Usually, I present this information in the form of simple percentages, with many accompanying tables of information derived from their reproductive life stories. I also believe it is important to say a few words about these men, as well as the ways I "studied" them. I firmly believe that anthropologists should share their methodological tool kit with readers, with students, and with each other. Too often such details are submerged in footnotes or erased altogether from ethnographies. This, in my opinion, is an unfortunate omission, which reduces the credibility of anthropology to the wider world.

Who were these 220 men? Most were Lebanese citizens, born and raised in the country and survivors of the civil war. Seventy-five percent were currently residing in the country, and 16 percent were expatriates, who either were born outside the country or had fled to other countries during the war years. These expatriate Lebanese lived all over the world, but primarily in South America, West Africa, North America, Europe, and the Arab Gulf. Additionally, 6 percent of the men in the study were Syrians, both Muslim and Christian, who were traveling to Beirut with their wives (and sometimes an accompanying Syrian doctor) as reproductive tourists. They hoped to access assisted reproductive technologies in Lebanon, a country that they viewed as technologically superior and more open to the West than their politically and economically isolated home country. The remaining men in the study were Palestinians, almost all Sunni Muslims. Most were living in the country as refugees, their families having fled there in 1948 after the founding of the nation of Israel. Two of these men were living in refugee camps; a few had achieved middle-class status as professionals; and a handful of these men were living more successful but also more complicated lives in the Arab Gulf Palestinian diaspora.

The men in this study came from all social classes and religious backgrounds, but they were generally united by their experiences of the Lebanese civil war, many attributing their current infertility problems to this collective trauma. Like Hamza, the majority of the men in this study were Muslim (70%), about half Shia (35%), half Sunni (30%), and a small number of Druze (4%) and Alawi (1%), both minority Shia Muslim subsects. Interestingly, only two of these men were of mixed Muslim parentage, and nine men, all Muslim, refused to define a religious sect or declared themselves atheists or nonpracticing. (Issues of religious affiliation and dissent are taken up in chapter 8.) The remaining men in the study, nearly one-third (30%), were Christians from a variety of denominations, including Maronite Catholic (14%), Greek Orthodox (8%), Armenian Orthodox (2%), and Roman Catholic (2%). One man was a Lebanese Jew, and he was living outside the country.

As in my earlier Egyptian study, which was based in two of Cairo's major IVF clinics, I was fortunate to gain ethnographic access to two of the busiest and most successful IVF clinics in Lebanon, both located in central Beirut. One clinic was part of a large, private university-based teaching hospital and catered to a religiously mixed patient population of both Sunni and Shia Muslims, Christians of a variety of sects, Druze, and various immigrant and refugee populations. All of the IVF doctors were male and Maronite Catholics; all of the embryologists and nursing staff were Muslim women.

The other research setting was a private, stand-alone IVF clinic catering primarily to southern Lebanese Shia Muslim patients, but with occasional Christian and Sunni Muslim patients from both Lebanon and neighboring Syria. In this clinic, all of the IVF doctors were Muslim, half Sunni and half Shia, with the only practicing female IVF doctor (a Sunni Muslim) in the city. In Lebanon and in the Muslim Middle East more generally, the gender and religious affiliation of physicians can matter to patients, especially in the morally contentious world of assisted reproduction. For example, Sunni Muslim patients may prefer Sunni Muslim physicians who

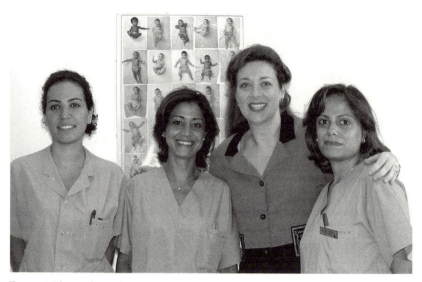

FIGURE 1. The anthropologist with Lebanese IVF clinic staff

are similarly opposed to gamete donation. Furthermore, the most pious Muslim couples are generally uncomfortable if male physicians conduct gynecological exams; thus, they may seek out a female infertility physician, as was the case in this clinic.

Between these two clinics, I conducted formal tape-recorded interviews with six IVF physicians, two embryologists, and one IVF clinic head nurse (figure 1). With the help of some of these clinic staff members, I was able to recruit 220 Lebanese, Syrian, and Palestinian men into my study. Because of my interest in merging ethnographic and epidemiological analysis, I designed the study in a classic "case-control" fashion, with 120 infertile cases and 100 fertile controls. I was able to assess men's fertility status not only on the basis of their interviews but also on the results of their semen analyses, which were provided to both me and the men in the study by the on-site IVF clinic laboratories, and which were based on the guidelines set out by the World Health Organization.[73] Infertile men in this study generally knew that they suffered from this condition, as a result of multiple semen analyses, sometimes carried out over many years. In a few cases, however, infertile men in this study had assumed that they were fertile and first learned about their infertility condition upon visits to the IVF clinics where I was conducting my research.

The fertile men in this study were all husbands of infertile women seeking IVF. Although some of these men "misclassified" themselves as infertile, their semen analyses carried out on the day of the interview proved to be normal. The inclusion of fertile men in this epidemiological case-control study served important ethnographic purposes; it allowed me to understand the experiences and perspectives of infertile men, as well as men who were not infertile but who were experiencing childless marriages. Their stories—usually of love and support for their infertile wives—were often deeply moving and are included in this volume. I met many of the wives of both fertile and infertile men in Lebanon, and in 20 percent of the interviews, wives were present, sometimes actively participating in the interview responses and discussions.[74]

As in my Egyptian study, more than half of my interviews were conducted in Arabic (57%) and about one-third in English (35%), with the remainder involving both languages (8%). Many of the men in the study had lived outside the Middle East and spoke excellent English (along with other languages in many cases). I conducted about half of the interviews alone, and half with a research assistant, especially in the initial stages of research when I was familiarizing myself with a distinct colloquial dialect of Arabic (Levantine versus Egyptian).

All of the men were recruited into my study, usually by a physician, nurse, or other clinic staff member, while in the midst of seeking or undertaking an IVF or ICSI cycle. I interviewed most men alone, in a private room secured for the purposes of interviewing. Because virtually all of the men in my study were literate, they read the informed consent form (required by both my home and Lebanese host universities)[75] with great intensity and interest, signing their names in Arabic and/or English. On the consent form, I asked for a separate signature allowing tape-recording of the interview, an option to which few men agreed.[76] Once men had signed and been given a study number, I gave each man a copy of the consent form, as well as my business card, to keep in their personal records. After being convinced of the confidential, anonymous nature of our conversations, many of the men in the study opened up with rich interviews that were often deeply personal and poignant. Interviews sometimes lasted two to three hours, with a friendly exchange of phone numbers or email addresses at the end.

A large amount of data was collected during the eight-month study period in Beirut. This included 220 completed eight-page reproductive history questionnaires, which I administered verbally to each man in the study; 1,200 pages of qualitative interview transcripts, generated from open-ended interviews with all of the men in the study and some of their wives or other family members; 550 pages of field notes, based on participant observation and informal interviews and conversations with clinic staff and patients in clinic waiting areas, as well as two pharmaceutical company representatives, several American egg donors and sperm recipients, and three Shia Muslim clerics; and more than 200 blood samples, which were frozen in the Beirut IVF laboratories and then hand-carried by me via airplane to the United States for the purposes of later toxic metal analysis.[77]

In addition, I gave four major presentations on my research while in Lebanon: one grand rounds in the Department of Obstetrics and Gynecology at the American University of Beirut hospital; one lecture in the AUB Faculty of Health Sciences (i.e., the public health school); one seminar at the Middle East Reproductive Health Working Group annual conference; and one keynote presentation at the European Society for Human Reproduction and Embryology, which took place that year in Madrid.

A few crucial points also bear mentioning here. First, the problem with formal methodological description is that it cannot capture the "feeling" of fieldwork—or, for me, what it was like to spend hundreds of hours in Middle Eastern IVF clinics, to meet strangers who became interlocutors and friends, and to become the privileged confidante of men's deepest secrets and sorrows. I have tried to describe my experiences as an ethnographer in the private spaces of Middle Eastern IVF clinics elsewhere,[78] and some of those ethnographic vignettes emerge in the pages that follow.

Second, there were many men who were asked to participate in my study but refused—sometimes directly to my face and quite coldly. This problem of outright refusal—or, in gentler terms, "nonresponse"[79]—is taken up in chapter 2, as it is a problem that has plagued male infertility research around the world. Having said that, many men were quite willing to talk with me, some of them volunteering after reading my study ad placed in clinic waiting areas. Why did men volunteer to talk? I believe that there are many reasons, some more important than others.

First, most of these men were seeking answers; they wanted to understand *why* they were infertile and were willing to talk with me about their etiological beliefs and suspicions. Second, there is inordinate down time for men in IVF clinics, where they must sit patiently in waiting areas while their wives undergo the gynecological procedures that are part of any IVF or ICSI cycle. Sometimes, I sat in the waiting areas with them, striking up individual and group conversations on a variety of topics. My presence in the waiting areas could sometimes lighten the tense and somber mood as men waited for hours—sometimes rubbing prayer beads or staring at their cell phones—for their wives to finish the operation. During these long waiting periods, many men agreed to participate formally in my study.

In addition, fluent English speakers often enjoyed the opportunity to use their English with me or, as one friendly Hizbullah member joked, "to have a dialogue with an American." Many of the fluent English speakers had spent time in the States, and reminded me, in their demeanor and remarks, of their "quasi Americanness." In fact, many of the Lebanese men in this study had relatives in Michigan, and were delighted to know that I was a professor (at that time) at the University of Michigan. As one man quipped, "Are you from Michigan? (Yes.) All my family is in Michigan! All of Lebanon is in Michigan!"

For most men, the opportunity to tell their full reproductive story—often for the first time to anyone—was therapeutic, cathartic, even confessional. Once in a private interview room, men's stories often came tumbling out, with seemingly taciturn men warming up, even becoming garrulous. Conversations with these mostly war-scarred men could become quite emotionally intense. Some men became teary-eyed while recounting the war dead and their own harrowing wartime experiences. In other cases, men who had lost precious ICSI babies through neonatal mortality or stillbirth described the beauty of their children, their names, their burials, and showed me, if they had them, their babies' photographs. As the mother of stillborn twin daughters, I shared my own deep sense of loss and expressed my condolences to these very sad, childless men.

Although the mood of this research was heavy—far from the lighthearted and sometimes bawdy humor that characterized my earlier Egyptian research with women—suffice it to say that there were many sweet and funny moments, as men gushed to me about their beautiful wives, or conveyed the exciting news of an ICSI pregnancy, or showed me their ultrasound pictures of growing fetuses. Some men who had completed interviews subsequently convinced other men in the waiting areas to talk to the "nice American *duktura*," even though "she comes from the land of George Bush!" A few men invited me to their homes (although this has always been rare in the secretive world of IVF and ICSI).[80] Many men thanked me profusely, expressed appreciation for research that was "helping our people and our country," and promised to stay in touch with me. Some of them did, emailing me to ask follow-up questions or sharing the joyous news of ICSI births.

After eight months in Lebanon, I returned to Michigan in August 2003 to begin the next phase of my male infertility research in Dearborn, home of North America's largest Arab American population. Working through an Arab-serving IVF clinic in the heart of the Dearborn ethnic enclave, I met fifty-five Arab immigrant men, most of them still lacking American citizenship rights. The majority were refugees, having sought political asylum from the Palestinian conflict, the Lebanese civil war, or the First Gulf War in Iraq. In addition, I met several Yemeni men who had come to the United States to escape grinding rural poverty but whose lives in impoverished Yemeni American enclaves remained difficult. I met forty of the wives of these men, most of them veiled, including with black facial veils if they were Yemeni. Nine of these women were interviewed alone, and thirty-one with their husbands.

In general, these Detroit Arab men and their wives were unassimilated and spoke Arabic as their primary language. As a group, they were poorly educated and marginally employed in the low-wage service and industrial sectors. Their existence on the margins of mainstream American society has been exacerbated in recent years by the slow death of Michigan's industrial economy and the rise of U.S. homeland security surveillance. Despite the support of a variety of mosque communities and Islamic social services, these men's economic and political situations in America continued to worsen with each passing year of my research, which began in 2003 and ended in 2008 with my move to Yale University.[81]

I must juxtapose this despair of postindustrial Detroit to the "glitter" of global Dubai, where millions of men like Hamza have gone to seek their fortunes. There, I spent the first half of 2007, conducting a study of globalization and reproductive tourism in a large, multinational IVF clinic on the border of Sharjah and Dubai.[82] I met Middle Eastern men from across the region, including Lebanon, Syria, Palestine, Morocco, Tunisia, Sudan, Iran, and Turkey. For the first time, I interviewed men from the Arab Gulf, mostly Emiratis dressed in their long white robes and headscarves, but also men from neighboring Bahrain and Oman. Taken altogether, more than 330 men in four field sites—Egypt, Lebanon, Arab Detroit, and UAE—have provided me with what might be the largest single "masculinities data set" of any scholar, past or present, working in the Middle East.

Finally, as noted in the prologue, I also traveled to Iran in March 2006 to deliver a keynote address at a University of Tehran–sponsored conference on "Embryo and Gamete Donation." Although I am a non-Muslim, American female anthropologist, I was invited by the Iranian Shia Muslim male conference organizers to represent the Sunni Muslim view on assisted conception, given my extensive research on this topic in Egypt. Iran is an especially important country in this high-tech world of assisted reproduction, hosting more than seventy clinics, one of which I visited. Muslim men's and women's attitudes toward the newest technological variants are being shaped by male Shia clerics, particularly in Iran, who are using *ijtihad*, or religious reasoning, to interpret and make sense of these new technologies.[83] Their *fatwas*, or religious decrees, outlining rules for assisted reproduction, third-party gamete donation, and adoption, have had an enormous impact on infertile Muslims' lives, shaping the contours of acceptable reproduction. For Muslim men in particular, these rulings on technologically assisted fatherhood have had significant effects on masculinities in ways that could never have been imagined when the technologies were introduced to the Muslim world nearly twenty-five years ago.

Emerging Technologies and Masculinities

As seen in the aforementioned description, my engagement with Middle Eastern infertility and assisted reproductive technologies—or ARTs, as they are now called by clinicians and scholars—has been one of long duration. I have been studying this same topic, in its various manifestations, since the introduction of IVF to Egypt in 1986. By following infertility and assisted reproduction in the Middle East over the past twenty-five years, I have been able to witness the introduction of new biotechnologies, the new social and cultural accommodations and innovations accompanying these technologies, and the important moral discourses and transformations resulting from this technological emergence. These various forms of emergence—of biotechnologies themselves, of accompanying social and cultural phenomena, and of moral deliberations—are at the very heart of this ethnography.

The world of assisted reproduction is characterized by constant discovery and innovation. Biomedical understandings of and solutions for infertility have emerged almost continuously since the birth on July 25, 1978, of England's Louise Brown, the world's first test-tube baby. Louise Brown is now thirty-three and the married mother of a young son, Cameron, who was conceived naturally and born on December 20, 2006. In 2010, Robert G. Edwards, a retired professor of physiology at the University of Cambridge, received the Nobel Prize in Physiology or Medicine for the invention of in vitro fertilization, which he developed in consort with British obstetrician Patrick Steptoe.

Since this British invention of IVF more than thirty years ago, the world has seen the rapid expansion of a host of assisted reproductive technologies, including: *in vitro fertilization* to overcome female infertility, especially blocked fallopian tubes; *intracytoplasmic sperm injection* to overcome male infertility; *third-party reproductive assistance* (with donor oocytes, sperm, embryos, and uteruses, as in *surrogacy*) to overcome absolute sterility; *multifetal pregnancy reduction* to selectively abort multiple-gestation IVF pregnancies; *ooplasm transfer* (OT), of cytoplasm from a younger to an older woman's oocytes, to improve egg quality in perimenopausal women; *cryopreservation* (freezing) and storage of unused sperm, embryos, oocytes, and now ovaries; *preimplantation genetic diagnosis* (PGD) to select "against" embryos with genetic defects and to select "for" embryos with specific and/or desired traits, including sex; *human embryonic stem cell* (hESC) research on unused embryos for the purposes of therapeutic intervention; and *human cloning*, or the possibility for asexual, autonomous reproduction, which has already occurred in other mammals (e.g., Dolly the sheep).[84] Most of these technologies are discussed throughout the course of this book and are more fully defined in the Glossary of Medical Terms, which contains a complete list of medical vocabulary found in this volume.

With the advent of these various technologies, men's lives and bodies have become increasingly medicalized. Male infertility provides a case in point. Once regarded as a source of male shame, imperfect manhood, or God's will—with most men told by their doctors that the source of the problem was "idiopathic," or unknown—male infertility has been reclassified as a biomedical disease category, with recognized causes, precise diagnostic techniques, and new technological fixes. In a twenty-first century marked by DNA microscopy, genetic karyotyping, four-dimensional ultrasonography, gamete micromanipulation, and preimplantation genetic diagnosis, male infertility has entered an era of profound biomedicalization—or the regulation of bodily processes themselves[85]—with men submitting their genitals to needles, knives, scopes, ultrasounds, and operating theaters in the hopes of conception.

Throughout this book, we examine Middle Eastern men's entrée into this high-tech world of biomedicine, where diagnoses of infertility are proffered and solutions recommended. Beginning with masturbation and ending at ICSI, we follow this arduous, embodied process and men's quests for conception. Part of the questing process involves the search for understanding. "Why did this happen to me?" Men have ample time to contemplate this question, sharing their insights with a curious anthropologist. In men's indigenous theories of causality, "weak" sperm are often tied to conditions beyond men's control, from God's will to family inheritance to relentless war and associated stress.

It is important to point out here that this medicalization of male infertility is relatively new. In the Middle East, the advent of laboratory-based semen analysis did not become widespread until the 1970s,[86] nor did it become fully reliable according to World Health Organization standards until much later.[87] Furthermore, until the early 1990s in the West, the only known solution to male infertility was donor insemination, the oldest of the reproductive technologies, but one still shrouded in secrecy and stigma.[88] The introduction of ICSI—pronounced "ick-see"—in Belgium in 1992 was a watershed event. A variant of IVF, ICSI solves the problem of male infertility in a way that IVF cannot. With standard IVF, spermatozoa are removed from a man's body through masturbation, and oocytes are surgically removed from a woman's ovaries following hormonal stimulation. Once these male and female gametes are retrieved, they are introduced to each other in a petri dish in an IVF laboratory, in the hopes of fertilization. However, weak sperm (i.e., low numbers, poor movement, misshapen) are poor fertilizers. Through "micromanipulation" of otherwise infertile sperm under a high-powered microscope, they can be injected directly into human oocytes, effectively aiding fertilization to occur

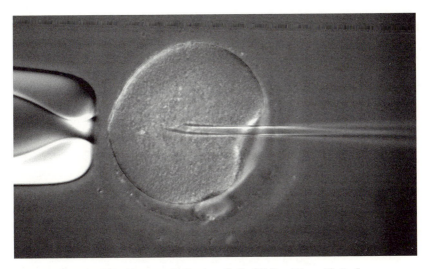

FIGURE 2. Intracytoplasmic sperm injection. Spike Walker/Stone/Getty Images

(figure 2). As long as one viable spermatozoon can be extracted from an infertile man's body, it can be "ICSI-injected" into an oocyte, leading to the potential creation of a human embryo. With ICSI, then, otherwise sterile men can father biogenetic offspring. This includes azoospermic men, who produce no sperm in their ejaculate and must therefore have their testicles painfully aspirated or biopsied in the search for sperm. In short, ICSI gives infertile men a greater chance of producing a "take-home baby."[89]

The coming of ICSI to the Middle East in 1994, where it was introduced in an IVF clinic in Cairo,[90] has led to a virtual "coming out" of male infertility across the region, as men acknowledge their infertility and seek the ICSI solution. The coming of this new "hope technology" has repaired diminished masculinity in men who were once silently suffering from their infertility. Furthermore, ICSI is being used in the Middle East and elsewhere as the assisted reproductive technology of choice, effectively replacing its predecessor IVF. Why? Basically, IVF leaves fertilization up to chance, whereas ICSI does not. Thus, ICSI provides a more guaranteed way of creating "the elusive embryo."[91] When patients' success rates increase, so do clinics' reputations. Thus, the world is beginning to witness the replacement of IVF by ICSI.[92] With ICSI, human fertilization is increasingly aided and abetted by human embryologists working in IVF laboratories around the world.

ICSI may be a breakthrough technology, but it is by no means a panacea. For one, the precisely timed collection of semen—what Lisa Jean Moore has called "man's most precious fluid"[93]—can produce deep anxiety

TABLE 1. Middle Eastern men in the diaspora: Fifty countries of stated residence

North America	South America	Europe	Middle East	Africa	Asia	Australia-Pacific
United States (19)	Brazil (4)	United Kingdom (10)	Lebanon (17)	Cote d'Ivoire (7)	Kazakhstan (1)	Australia (2)
Canada (6)	Panama (2)	France (9)	Saudi Arabia (11)	Sierra Leone (3)	Taiwan (1)	
	Venezuela (?)	Russia (7)	United Arab Emirates (10)	West Africa unspecified (3)		
		Switzerland (6)	Kuwait (7)	Liberia (2)		
		Netherlands (4)	Syria (6)	Nigeria (2)		
		West/East Germany (4)	Egypt (3)	Gambia (1)		
		Belgium (4)	Iraq (2)	Senegal (1)		
		Sweden (3)	Iran (2)	Gabon (1)		
		Greece (3)	Jordan (2)	Mauritania (1)		
		Cyprus (2)	Libya (2)	Zaire (1)		
		Armenia (1)	Yemen (2)	Zambia (1)		
		Ukraine (1)	Oman (1)	Ethiopia (1)		
		Romania (1)	Tunisia (1)			
		Luxem-bourg (1)	Turkey (1)			
		Unidenti-fied (1)	Gulf Un-identified (1)			

Note: Total number of countries in each region: North America, 2; South America, 3; Europe, 15; Middle East, 15; Africa, 12; Asia, 2; Australia-Pacific, 1.

and even impotence, but it is imperative for all ICSI procedures. Second, ICSI has not supplanted sperm donation entirely, because some men produce no spermatozoa whatsoever. Third, ICSI sometimes does not succeed, leading to endless rounds of fruitless repetition among some couples. Fourth, when it does succeed, ICSI may be perpetuating genetic defects into future generations. Male infertility seems to have a strong genetic ba-

TABLE 2 Men's stated reasons for periods spent abroad

Reason	Number of Men
Political exile/refugee	44
Education	31
Employment	27
Medical/reproductive tourism	55
Family unification	3
Father's work	3

sis, through mutations of the Y chromosome and other inherited disorders that may be passed by ICSI to male offspring. The ethics of passing genetic mutations to children has been a cause for concern.[94] Fifth, ICSI involves a grueling surgical procedure for women. And it is also highly dependent upon the complicated stimulation and extraction of healthy oocytes from women's bodies. Whereas the fecundity of older men can often be enhanced through ICSI, women's fertility is highly age sensitive, with oocyte quality declining at later stages of the reproductive life cycle.[95] In short, older women may "age out" of ICSI, causing highly gendered, life-course disruptions surrounding women's "biological clocks."[96] Finally, men may arrive at ICSI after years of other failed treatment options. ICSI is expensive, usually costing thousands of dollars, and is often deemed a last resort, especially for men without adequate financial resources.

Throughout this volume, we follow men's stories of heartbreak as well as their ICSI successes. Male users of these technologies are often well aware of the social messages encoded in their ICSI quests, and this knowledge shapes what might be called men's "medically assisted ways of being men."[97] In the end, individual men may wholeheartedly adopt, experimentally adapt, or altogether reject these technologies in their attempts to embody idealized norms of masculinity.

Furthermore, these technologies would not have reached the region were it not for Middle Eastern IVF doctors—schooled in places such as London, Sydney, Tokyo, and Los Angeles, and at institutions such as Harvard and Yale[98]—who have brought their learning back home, taking pride in the development of new Middle Eastern IVF clinics and practices. Through these entrepreneurial physicians, these technologies have arrived, one by one, in the Middle East, eventually spreading (although unevenly) across the entire region. Although rarely portrayed as a high-tech location, the Middle East is, in fact, awash in assisted reproductive technologies, with some Middle Eastern countries—especially Egypt, Saudi Arabia, Turkey, and Iran—claiming well over fifty IVF clinics each. Urban centers in these countries have become major hubs for medical innovation and tourism. Iran, for example, leads the way in gamete donation and surrogacy, as well as organ transplantation, sexual reassignment surgery, vasectomy, and a therapeutic stem cell industry.[99] In IVF clinics in Tehran, Arabic translators are employed to facilitate communication between Arab reproductive tourists and the Farsi-speaking physicians and clinical staff. These therapeutic border-crossings—what I have called "quests for conception" in my early work[100]—are part and parcel of regional transnationalism and mobility.

In fact, the Middle East is a region in constant motion. Middle Easterners are circulating from country to country for the purposes of medical treatment, education, employment, trade, and pilgrimage, as well as leaving the region, both temporarily and permanently, for purposes of resettlement. The degree of Middle Eastern mobility cannot be understated. In my study of 220 Middle Eastern men, exactly 100, or nearly half, had lived outside their countries for extended periods (table 1), either to escape the war, to pursue education or employment opportunities, or to be united with family elsewhere (table 2). One-quarter of these men—37 Lebanese living outside the country and 18 Syrians—had traveled to Beirut as reproductive tourists, attempting to access IVF and ICSI.

EMERGENT MASCULINITIES

In part I of this book, I argue that Middle Eastern men's own conceptions of masculinity are changing, not only as a result of these transnational experiences and global influences but also in response to emerging health technologies that are entering the region. Change is also coming from *within* Middle Eastern societies, as men reconceptualize their own lives, contrasting them to their fathers' generation. Men are quite cognizant of traditional stereotypes; they can articulate these and can explain how their own lives differ. In short, manhood is not static; new masculinities are emerging in the Middle East and require our consideration.

In this book, I examine Middle Eastern men's lives in relation to what I call "the four M's": masculinity, marriage, morality, and medical treatment seeking. I argue that Middle Eastern masculinity is in a state of flux, with shifting praxis in the realms of reproduction, sexuality, marriage, and family life. I examine the ways in which Middle Eastern men are rethinking what it means to be a man, especially in the context of infertile marriages.

The focus of this volume is on "emergence": that which is "new" is highlighted. As Raymond Williams reminds us in his seminal essay, "Dominant, Residual, and Emergent": "New meanings and values, new practices, new relationships and kinds of relationship are continually being created."[101] Drawing upon Williams's notion of the emergent, I argue that an "emergent masculinities" approach is needed to understand Middle Eastern manhood. In other words, manly selfhood is not a thing or a constant; rather, it is an act that is ever in progress. Men enact manhood in different ways from moment to moment, as they move through the different social contexts that form their daily lives. Individual masculinities also change in response to larger life changes; these may include health problems such as infertility, job change, marriage, or fatherhood. Importantly, men live out all these changes in bodies that are also ever changing; these changes include aging, becoming ill or well, or being altered through medical treatment, exercise, or neglect. By calling for an emergent masculinities approach, I call for attention to this ongoing, relational, and embodied process of change in the ways men enact masculinity. In short, I argue that any theory used to understand the *practice* of masculinity must account for the *emergence* of change, physically and socially, over time.

In the next chapter, I examine R. W. Connell's theory of "hegemonic masculinity,"[102] which has been widely adopted by most gender scholars and which I have used in my own work to understand societies' dominant forms of manhood.[103] I explore what "hegemonic masculinity, Middle Eastern style" might look like, on the basis of a reading of the existing literature. However, I argue that many, if not all, Middle Eastern men are striving for a much different notion of masculinity. By searching for evidence of hegemonic masculinity in the patriarchal Middle East, it is too easy to promote sterile reifications and facile judgments about men's lives, reinforcing harmful caricatures. Such caricatures have fed into notions of Middle Eastern "exceptionalism": namely, that the Middle East is exceptionally prone to violence, because the men there are exceptionally brutal, irrational, even psychopathic, and their predispositions are fueled by a hyperzealous, extremist religion.

I hope to challenge such stereotypes by telling stories of ordinary Middle Eastern men from a range of nations and backgrounds. Not all of the stories are happy ones: far from it. Nonetheless, they should serve to humanize the discourses of hegemonic masculinity, Middle Eastern style, which are constantly fed to us through the Western media. In this regard, I could not agree more with my medical anthropologist colleagues in Lebanon, who assert in their article, "Challenging the Stereotypes: Men, Withdrawal, and Reproductive Health in Lebanon":

> We think it is vital for more nuanced research on sexual relationships, particularly in areas of the world where powerful stereotypes— traditional families, women's low status, oppressive religion, early marriage, high fertility, male dominance, vulnerability to divorce,

need to produce sons—influence the questions we ask and the interpretations of what we see and hear. While acknowledging the complexity of people's sexual lives, our modest research suggests that it might be useful to credit women with some measure of agency, and men some measure of altruism and humanity.[104]

In this same spirit, part I, "Emergent Masculinities"calls for a theoretical and ethnographic reframing of the relationship between hegemony, patriarchy, masculinity, marriage, and reproduction. The variability, hybridity, and transformation of masculinity that I detect in the Middle East today defy easy categorization. Middle Eastern men are appropriating diverse styles of masculinity, drawing from both indigenous and global forms. In so doing, they are reconceiving manhood in ways that have yet to be properly described but deserve our empirical attention.

Islamic Masculinities

In part II,"Islamic Masculinities,"I examine what it means to be a moral man in the context of emerging, and sometimes ethically controversial, reproductive technologies. I ask what is at stake for ordinary Muslim men as they attempt to make health-related decisions in a way that is morally satisfying and consistent with local religious norms. What do Muslim ICSI seekers think about making a test-tube baby? When faced with the need for donor eggs or sperm to overcome infertility, what do ordinary Muslim men (and women) actually do? Is the search for human gametes one of the major motivating factors for reproductive tourism in the Middle East?

Given the ongoing emergence of reproductive biotechnologies in the region, these are all open questions. It is imperative to examine what Harvard medical anthropologist Arthur Kleinman has called"local moral worlds"or"the moral accounts, [which] are the commitments of social participants in a local world about what is at stake in everyday experience."[105] Through an"ethnography of experience,"Kleinman urges medical anthropologists to pay close attention to moral issues of spiritual pain and social suffering, which may accompany the arrival of new biotechnologies, such as ICSI, around the globe. Local moralities are perhaps best exposed when new health technologies confront deeply embedded religious and ethical traditions.[106] Such traditions may embrace new biotechnologies (e.g., lifesaving health technologies) but prohibit aspects of those technologies that do not meet with religious moralities (e.g., sperm donation). For individuals confronting the moral stances and ambiguities of their local religious traditions, they must attempt to make sense of such religious responses, while at the same time invoking their own moral subjectivities to find acceptable solutions to their often dire health needs and concerns.

Middle Eastern men, most of whom are practicing Muslims, must now make sense of a dizzying array of reproductive possibilities to overcome their childlessness. Quite importantly, Islamic institutions and individual clerics have provided considerable guidance in this regard, usually in the form of written *fatwa*s, or authoritative religious decrees. But how do individual Muslim men of varying degrees of piety respond to these discursive fields of authority? As Talal Asad has argued in "The Idea of an Anthropology of Islam," "A practice is Islamic because it is authorized by the discursive traditions of Islam, and is so taught to Muslims." However, as Asad reminds us, "the resistances they encounter (from Muslims and non-Muslims) are equally the concern of an anthropology of Islam."[107]

Religious resistances are incredibly important to any discussion of masculinity and assisted reproduction. On the one hand, three potential solutions to childlessness—third-party gamete donation, gestational surrogacy, and child adoption—are widely resisted, both religiously and socially, in Middle Eastern Muslim communities. On the other hand, not all Muslim men react similarly to these religious bans. There is emerging evidence of discordance and dissent across the region. Minority religious responses, on the part of both Shia Muslims and Christians, have been an important part of this equation.

In short, if we are to speak of an emerging "Islamic bioethics,"[108] then it is important to bear in mind that Muslims do not agree on some set of common global norms or "best practices." The assisted reproductive technologies and Muslims' attitudes toward them provide a compelling nexus for the study of what might be called "Islamic technoscience in practice," a topic about which very little is currently understood.

As noted by anthropologist Mazyar Lotfalian in his unique volume, *Islam, Technoscientific Identities, and the Culture of Curiosity*, there is a glaring lacuna in the study of science and technology in the Islamic world.[109] According to Lotfalian, there are "really only two strains of relevant work"—on the Islamic medieval sciences and on philosophical arguments for civilizational differences between Islamic and Western science and technology (i.e., Samuel P. Huntington's "clash of civilizations" thesis).[110] This dearth of relevant scholarship clearly applies to the cross-cultural study of reproductive technologies. For example, in the seminal volume on *Third Party Assisted Conception across Cultures: Social, Legal and Ethical Perspectives*, not a single Muslim society is represented among the thirteen country case studies.[111]

Yet, as these assisted reproductive technologies become further entrenched in the Muslim world, and as additional forms of biotechnology, including stem cells and perhaps cloning, become available, it will be crucial to interrogate new local moralities, as well as new manifestations of masculinity and conjugality that are likely to arise in response to these technological innovations. Thus, as anthropologist of science and technology David Hess rightly observes, "Anthropology brings to these discussions a reminder that the cultural construction of science is a global phenomenon, and that the ongoing dialogue of technoculture often takes its most interesting turns in areas of the world outside the developed West."[112]

Clearly, the time has come to examine the globalization of assisted reproductive technologies to diverse Islamic contexts, particularly given the rapid technological development and globalization of these biotechnologies. Currently, there are about a dozen researchers who are engaging in empirical studies of assisted reproduction in the Islamic world, including in such countries as Iran, Turkey, and Malaysia.[113] Their studies point to interesting variations in both the Islamic jurisprudence *and* the cultural responses to assisted reproduction, particularly between the two major branches of Islam, but even among co-sectarians from different countries (among Shia Muslims in Iran versus Lebanon).

In short, Islam, as a global religion, is not monolithic, timeless, and unchanging. As noted by Gelvin in his recent compelling history of *The Modern Middle East*,

> The doctrines and institutions associated with Islam or any other religion are not frozen in time. They exist within history, not outside history. And while there are continuities of religious doctrines and institutions, the meaning those doctrines and institutions hold for society, and the function they play in society, evolve through time.[114]

Furthermore, Lahoucine Ouzgane has importuned scholars to render "Muslim men visible as gendered subjects."[115] He has adopted the term "Islamic masculinities" as a way of thinking about Muslim men *as men* from a social constructionist perspective. The term "Islamic masculinities," according to Ouzgane,

> is premised on the belief that men are not born; they are made; they construct their masculinities within particular social and historical contexts. Thus, masculinities in Islamic contexts emerge as a set of distinctive practices defined by men's positionings within a variety of religious and social structures.[116]

Although the literature on Muslim women's lives has truly flourished over the past thirty years, this literature has treated "Muslim men as an unmarked category," according to Ouzgane.[117] He reminds us that Muslim men's lives are enacted in relationship to women; that the Muslim world is diverse and ever changing as a result of religious and political agendas,

Western imperialism, and the marked effects of globalization; and that, unfortunately, Muslim men's lives are now steeped in Eurocentric, anti-Arab, anti-Islamic bigotry. Thus, he calls for scholars to exercise caution, to provide accounts that militate against such essentialisms, and to make the consideration of local realities a priority. Only when masculinity studies are "grounded in historical, cultural, and geographical context" will the diversity of masculinities in the Muslim world become apparent.[118]

In short, not all Muslims, including Muslim men, are alike. Some are pious, while others are not. Some are scripturally oriented, while others value independent reasoning. Some follow particular clerics, while others consider their primary relationship to be with God. Some know that they are "rule breaking" but hope for God's mercy and forgiveness. Others simply do not care, having left the religion, or having identified themselves with secular humanism, communism, atheism, or science. This great diversity within the world's Muslims cannot be emphasized enough. As will be shown in the chapters that follow, Muslim men do not follow a single path. Their responses are mediated by a wide variety of ever-changing values and social forces, including the emergence of ICSI and other assisted reproductive technologies across the Middle East and many other parts of the Muslim world.

Indeed, the transformative effects of technology in Muslim men's lives cannot be overstated. The 2011 revolutions across the Middle East are a testament to the power of technology in reshaping the political landscape of an entire region. However, Facebook and Twitter are not the only transformative technologies in the Middle East today. Through their embrace of assisted reproductive technologies, Middle Eastern Muslim men are demonstrating their emerging masculinities, marital commitments, and moral subjectivities—and, in doing so, questioning many taken-for-granted assumptions about men *as men* in this critical region.

PART I

Emergent Masculinities

CHAPTER 1

Hegemonic Masculinity

HISHAM, THE SYRIAN ACCOUNTANT

On a scorching summer day in 2007, I met Hisham in a blessedly air-conditioned IVF clinic in the United Arab Emirates. Hisham's wife was having her eggs "harvested" under anesthesia, and so Hisham had time to kill and was more than happy to talk with an anthropologist. As I soon learned, Hisham hailed from the relatively poor country of Syria, where he was the oldest of six children. Like so many other young Syrian men, Hisham and his two brothers had all left the country, the brothers to the United States and Hisham to the Arab Gulf. Following an unpleasant stint in Saudi Arabia, Hisham moved to the Emirates. There, he accrued enough financial resources to marry, agreeing to an arranged marriage with a Syrian woman named Rana, who was ten years his junior.

In preparation for the wedding, Hisham decided to undergo premarital semen analysis to ascertain his fertility. Although the test was not required by law or by Rana's family, Hisham—like increasing numbers of Middle Eastern men—thought this the sensible thing to do, given the growing recognition in the region that men, too, may be infertile. Although Hisham was not deemed infertile per se, his sperm count was considered "borderline." Consulting a fellow Syrian urologist at an Emirati hospital, Hisham was convinced by the physician that he could improve his fertility by undergoing a varicocelectomy, an invasive genital surgery designed to remove varicose veins from the testicles. Eager to please his new young wife, Hisham underwent the varicocelectomy shortly after marriage. This is a decision that Hisham now deeply regrets. Not only was the surgery unsuccessful, but it was actually iatrogenic, causing irreparable physical and emotional harm. Hisham's sperm count plummeted after the operation and has never returned to normal. As a result, his only hope of producing a child is through ICSI.

When I met Hisham, he and Rana were trying their second cycle of ICSI, carried out in secrecy from both of their families. Hisham told me that he was not at all embarrassed about his fertility problem. Rather, he explained that feelings of empathy would lead the relatives to worry and intervene with long-distance phone calls. It was simply less stressful for both him and Rana to tell their families about the ICSI once they had obtained a successful result.

As educated, middle-class professionals with a science background, Hisham and Rana realized that ICSI could not guarantee a successful pregnancy. Their first ICSI attempt at a Lebanese-run clinic was "a very bad experience," both interpersonally and physically for Rana. Hisham and Rana were far happier with the quality of care at this second clinic on the border of high-tech Dubai. But in Dubai, the cost of an ICSI cycle was much higher—nearly $5,000 as opposed to only $2,000 in Lebanon— which had required Hisham to use his credit card and take out a bank loan. "I'm now in a lot of debt trying to make a baby," Hisham explained. "Plus, I'm afraid for her. I don't know if there are bad effects from the hormones. She started feeling dizzy and vomiting. She was feeling very weak, feeling always sleepy. I don't want to see her suffer this way."

Hisham is thinking of returning to Syria if the current cycle of ICSI is not successful. According to Hisham, ICSI is now widely available in the cities of Damascus, Aleppo, and Homs, but for only one-third the cost of an ICSI cycle in the UAE. Furthermore, in Syria, he can rely on his family and in-laws to take care of his beloved wife, Rana, who he feels has "suffered" for him. Hisham is full of love, respect, and empathy for his wife, which he expressed throughout his interview.

> *Insha'Allah* [God willing], she'll get a baby. She's suffering, actually, and I'm feeling pretty awful about it. She is trained as a chemist, but she works long days as a secretary with a horrible commute to Dubai. I wish if she gets a baby, she can quit her job and maybe I can bring her mother, one or two months, then my mother, just to take care of her. Like they can help her so that she can just sit, because she's very, very active, and I'm afraid for her.

According to Hisham, he often volunteers to cook and do housework, because they both work twelve-hour days, six days a week. But his wife is adamant about carrying out what she perceives to be her domestic duties. "It's really exhausting for her," he said, "with lots of tension, pressure. And for nothing! We don't have children, so it seems like all of this work is not worth it."

Never once did Hisham mention his own masculinity throughout the course of a two-hour, wide-ranging interview. He does not consider male infertility to be a problem of manhood; rather, it is a problem of sperm counts, with a now widely accepted medical solution of ICSI. The only blame Hisham assigns is to the Syrian urologist who "tricked" him into undertaking a dangerous surgery.

Furthermore, Hisham is not the only infertile man in his social world. One of his close Syrian friends, Eyad, is also infertile, and they share their trials and tribulations openly. Eyad led Hisham to the Emirati IVF clinic, where he is also pursuing ICSI with his wife. If necessary, both Eyad and Hisham will take their wives back to Syria to undergo future ICSI cycles.

However, Hisham remains hopeful that he and Rana will achieve a successful ICSI pregnancy in the Emirates. No matter what happens, Hisham and Rana remain committed to each other, and to God's plan for their lives. "Even if there is no success, this is God's will," Hisham concluded. "We did our best, and we'll say *mash Allah* [what God wills]."

THEORIZING MASCULINITY

How do we begin to analyze Hisham's masculinity with few if any clues from Hisham himself? Hisham was one of many infertile men in my study who appeared unconcerned about the masculinity effects of male infertility. Hisham, like Hamza, was a long-term migrant, having lived in the UAE for eleven years. Both men suffered from male infertility, leading them on ICSI quests undertaken with their beloved wives. In Hisham's case, however, he had experienced the embodied suffering of a futile varicocelectomy, and he was now very concerned about how hormones and egg harvesting might affect Rana's current and future health. Embodiment—of invasive surgeries and artificial hormonal medications—was what Hisham lamented most vociferously in his interview.

Hisham's story is a fine exemplar of emergent masculinities—the term that I have coined as a key conceptual trope to understand new forms of masculinity in interaction with new forms of medical technology.[1] My concept of emergent masculinities has been inspired by my own ethnographic findings, as well as the conceptual work of two social theorists, R. W. Connell and Raymond Williams, both of them influenced by the Marxist scholar Antonio Gramsci. R. W. Connell has been the world's most influential authority on masculinity. (Connell was "he" when formulating and reformulating hegemonic masculinity theory, but is now Raewyn. I use "he" to refer to his earlier work.) In Connell's case, he has applied Gramsci's notion of hegemony to a theory of masculinity.[2] In Williams's case, he has examined processes of historical and cultural change, which he calls "emergence."[3]

In my view, any ethnographic study of masculinity must begin with Connell's theory of hegemonic masculinity. It has been incredibly influential in masculinity research since the 1980s, and it has greatly influenced my own early work on Egyptian masculinity and sexuality.[4] In this chapter, I apply the notion of hegemonic masculinity to discourses about Middle Eastern men, as brought to us through both scholarly and popular media. I then explore the theory's utility—or lack thereof—for understanding someone like Hisham as a masculine subject and for analyzing masculinity in the Middle Eastern region as a whole.

HEGEMONIC MASCULINITY

As the only social constructionist analytic developed specifically for studying masculinity, hegemonic masculinity has been widely used since its 1985 introduction.[5] Drawing explicitly from feminist theory and Marxist sociology, Connell sought to reconcile the lived reality of inequality among men with the fact of men's group dominance over women. This new theory sought to examine hierarchical inequality among men, relate analysis of masculinity to feminist insights on the social construction of gender, and resist the dichotomy of structure versus the individual plaguing contemporary studies of gender and class.[6] To achieve these goals, Connell used Gramsci's concept of hegemony, a social mechanism through which various groups develop the "will to conform" with a leading group's way of being, thereby facilitating class-based domination.[7] He argued that by using hegemony to understand masculinity, scholars could reveal the historical production of various masculinities, the way power functioned to mediate the production of these masculinities, their hierarchical relationships, and the dialectical relationships between social structures and practiced masculinities.[8]

Connell defined hegemonic masculinity as the strategy for being a man that legitimizes patriarchy in current, local practices of gender. In this formulation, masculinity is shaped by, but not necessarily an incarnation of, cultural ideals of manliness.[9] Specifically, he argued that most men are not fully able to practice hegemonic masculinity, because it requires access to particular social resources. Hegemonic masculinity thus creates inequality among men, making some men dominant over others, and subordinate men complicit with its practice as they aspire to act out elements of this idealized way of being manly.[10] Crucially, the theory of hegemonic masculinity is about *relationships*—among men, between men and women, and between men and their ideas of other men. Connell argues that masculinity must be understood in terms of relationality and that the relationships *within* gender (i.e., between men) are based on the relationships *between* genders (i.e., between men and women), relationships that are hierarchical. However, the notion of hierarchy and competition *within* masculinity is, for Connell, of cardinal importance. He argues, "We must also recognize the *relations* between different kinds of masculinity: relations of alliance, dominance, and subordination. These relationships are constructed through practices that exclude and include, that intimidate, exploit, and so on. There is a gender politics within masculinity."[11]

Because there are different ways of being a man, masculinities are differently valued. In the Weberian sense, hegemonic masculinity is a normative "ideal type," which, while varying cross-culturally, exhibits general patterns. Hegemonic masculinity often concentrates ideal masculine attributes, including wealth and command of other resources, attractiveness, virility (i.e., sexual potency), physical strength, heterosexuality, and emotional detachment. These ideal qualities are often associated with the ruling class—men who control and dominate other men. Hegemonic masculinity is thus associated with masculine power, but a form of power that exists more through persuasion and consent than through the exercise of force.[12]

Connell is equally concerned, if not more so, with what he describes as "subordinated" (a.k.a. "marginalized,"""alternative," or "subaltern") masculinity, which embodies some of the opposites of these ideal hegemonic attributes. Connell points in particular to gay, working-class, and nonwhite men, contrasting their experiences to those of the white, heteronormative, ruling class in Euro-America. Because hegemonic masculinity is unattainable for so many ordinary men, it may lead to distress for those unable to achieve normative expectations. Moreover, subordinated men may be conflicted about their desire to achieve hegemonic masculine ideals, which they may perceive, critique, and protest as oppressive. Indeed, Connell defined "protest masculinity" as "a pattern of masculinity constructed in local working-class settings, sometimes among ethnically marginalized men, which embodies the claim to power typical of regional hegemonic masculinities in Western countries, but which lacks the economic resources and institutional authority that underpins the regional and global patterns."[13]

Clearly, masculinity cannot be isolated from its institutional context, including the state, the workplace or labor market, and the family. Because masculinity is an aspect of institutions, it is tied to three distinct but related domains—namely, exercise of power, division of labor, and objects of desire. Men's exercise of power in many societies ranges from the institutionalized connection of masculinity with political authority and the use of military force to the legitimization of sexual and other forms of intimate violence, leading some men to violate, while others are violated. Class-based divisions of labor affect men's differential access to work and income, leading some men to be marginalized in the labor market. Finally, gender informs systems of desire, influencing the kinds of bodies that are deemed desirable and the conditions under which they are desired. According to Connell, "masculinities as cultural forms cannot be abstracted from *sexuality*, which is an essential dimension of the social creation of gender."[14]

Although Connell is most concerned about demonstrating relationalities *between* forms of masculinity, his conceptualization of hegemonic or subordinate types has led to an unfortunate dualism, which masculinity theorists have subsequently problematized. In one of the most sophisticated evaluations, Demetrakis Demetriou argues that Connell has followed Gramsci too closely. Gramsci viewed hegemony as culminating in the formation of a historic bloc, achieved through leadership of a fundamental class; similarly, Connell sees masculine power as "a closed, coherent, and unified totality that embraces no otherness, no contradiction."[15] According to Demetriou, the contributions of the subordinate class to the formation of hegemonic masculinity must be taken into consideration: even subaltern men resist total subordination and emasculation. For Demetriou, the formation of hegemonic masculinity involves a "dialectic of appropriation/marginalization," or a reciprocal process of masculinity construction *between* hegemonic and subordinate groups of men. Connell, however, following Gramsci, assumes that hegemonic masculinity resides *within* a hegemonic class of men; thus, he leaves no room in his formulation for masculine *hybridity*, or the ways in which both dominant and subaltern men may appropriate diverse elements from various masculinities through complex forms of negotiation.[16]

From a somewhat different angle, Mike Donaldson examines the outcome of theoretical overdetermination in the new masculinity studies, in which the dominance of hegemonic masculinity as a key theoretical trope has led to its unfortunate reification. In his essay "What Is Hegemonic Masculinity?" Donaldson portrays hegemonic masculinity as a kind of conceptual cul-de-sac.

> A culturally idealized form, it is both a personal and collective project, and is the common sense about breadwinning and manhood. It is exclusive, anxiety-provoking, internally and hierarchically differentiated, brutal, and violent. It is pseudo-natural, tough, contradictory, crisis-prone, rich, and socially sustained. While centrally connected with the institutions of male dominance, not all men practice it, though most benefit from it. Although cross-class, it often excludes working-class and black men. It is a lived experience, and an economic and cultural force, and dependent on social arrangements. It is constructed through difficult negotiation over a life-time. Fragile it may be, but it constructs the most dangerous things we live with. Resilient, it incorporates its own critiques, but it is, nonetheless, "unraveling." What can men do with it?[17]

Donaldson's final question, although posed in playful jest, is still highly relevant: How does hegemonic masculinity translate, if at all, into the realm of quotidian practice? How would we begin to study the enactment of, or resistance to, hegemonic masculinity in men's lives? As a qualitative sociologist, Connell was fascinated by the potential of ethnography—or what he has called "ethnographic realism,"[18] discovered primarily through the kind of life history research described in the preceding chapter—to account for hegemonic masculinity within a global and historical framework, thereby moving beyond psychological and sociobiological portrayals of masculinity, which he found to be inherently ethnocentric. According to Connell, ethnographic accounts of masculinity "might lead to a comparative sociology of masculinity capable of challenging many of our culture's received notions."[19]

However, the difficulty of operationalizing hegemonic masculinity becomes apparent when the concept is applied to ethnographic data. While the theory is designed to account for masculine relationality, as well as fluid and shifting power between men, its ethnographic applications often seem to reify specific masculinities as static manly types, which hold particular positions within a set social hierarchy. Namely, the pigeonholing of ethnographic participants as examples of "hegemonic" or "subordinated" males casts them as static subjects and serves to solidify the types themselves. This obscures the lived reality of different forms of masculinity as *ever-changing social strategies* enacted through practice. Actual men's performances of gender are constantly in flux and may change radically as their social and physical circumstances change.[20]

As a result, applications of hegemonic masculinity theory may have the unintended consequence of reducing masculinity to a typology, instead of elucidating masculinity as a dynamic social practice. This essentialization of hegemonic masculinity precludes the study of change, internal tension, and disjuncture in individual men's enactments of manliness. For example, the ethnographic portions of Connell's own work use individual men's life histories to represent different types of masculinity, as if men's lives culminate in a particular sort of masculinity rather than moving through many variants.[21] This sort of application undoes the goal of the theory; it casts men as either normal or deviant in relationship to some fixed masculine ideal, thereby hampering study of various masculinities' interrelationships and historical contingencies. When applied, then, the theory of hegemonic masculinity frequently obscures the very relationality, fluidity, and dynamism that it was developed to explain.

Further, because hegemonic masculinity theory is based in a Marxist sociology more focused on structures and power than embodiment, applications of hegemonic masculinity often fail to account for the way men's bodies and physical ways of being are constituted by gender practices. As poststructuralist gender theory demonstrates, the physicality of masculinity is integral to practices and understandings of what it is to be a man. While the theory of hegemonic masculinity can be useful for comparing different men's relative social positions at a specific point in historical time, it cannot account for individuals' changing embodiments of masculinity

over the individual life course. The social, physical, structural, and technological changes that occur throughout a man's life force him to enact masculinity in ever-changing ways. Thus, a theory is needed that can account
not only for hierarchical relationships among men and between men and
women but for the relationships between the different masculinities that a
man may embody and perform over his lifetime. In short, scholars not only
must attend to differences and power-laden relationships between men
who act out recognizably different types of masculinity but also must examine and explain the nuanced ways of "being a man" through embodied
practices that change over the life course.[22]

Reformulating Hegemonic Masculinity Theory

Having listened carefully to these criticisms over the years, Connell himself argues, "If the concept proves still useful, it must be reformulated in
contemporary terms."[23] In his view, five major challenges to the theory
must be taken into account. First, the concept of multiple masculinities—
"hegemonic" and "subordinated"—has tended to produce a static, dualis-
tic typology, instead of portraying a diverse field of masculinities in practice
within particular social settings. Second, inconsistencies and ambiguities in usage of the concept have stripped hegemonic masculinity of its
intended historicity and applicability to the lives of real men. Masculinities
not only differ across generation, social class, and cultural setting but also
are subject to change over time. Third, the concept of hegemonic masculinity has been reified and associated with an "assemblage of toxic traits."[24]
Hegemonic masculinity is no longer seen as a "dominant" type but rather as
a negative trait complex, associated exclusively with men who are unemo-
tional, nonnurturing, dispassionate, aggressive, violent, and even criminal.
Fourth, hegemonic masculinity is based on an unsatisfactory theory of the
masculine subject, leading to the loss of visibility and agency for individual
men. Men may adopt hegemonic masculinity when it is desirable, but they
may also distance themselves from it, resisting hegemonic masculinity at
strategic moments over the life course. Finally, hegemonic masculinity is
portrayed as a self-contained, self-reproducing system in a functionalist
model of gender relations. In such a portrayal, the historicity of gender is
ignored, such that patriarchy is left unchallenged.

Having enumerated these main criticisms, Connell points to four areas
in which the concept of hegemonic masculinity requires reformulation:
the nature of gender hierarchy, the geography of masculine configurations,
the process of social embodiment, and the dynamics of masculinities. With
regard to gender hierarchy, Connell notes that the concept of hegemonic masculinity was originally formulated in tandem with the concept of

"hegemonic femininity," which was soon renamed "emphasized femininity" and which acknowledged the asymmetrical relations of masculinities and femininities in a patriarchal gender order.[25] However, because of the problem of "separate spheres" research—that is, feminist scholarship by women and men's studies scholarship by men—the relationship between men and women soon dropped out of focus in hegemonic masculinity discussions. This omission requires correction, according to Connell, and will serve ultimately to reduce the isolation of men's studies and to emphasize the relevance of male-female gender dynamics to a variety of social problems. As Connell and his colleague James W. Messerschmidt state,

> Focusing only on the activities of men occludes the practices of women in the construction of gender among men. As is well shown by life-history research, women are central in many of the processes constructing masculinities—as mothers; as schoolmates; as girlfriends, sexual partners, and wives; as workers in the gender division of labor; and so forth. The concept of emphasized femininity focused on compliance to patriarchy, and this is still highly relevant in contemporary mass culture. Yet gender hierarchies are also affected by new configurations of women's identity and practice, especially among younger women—which are increasingly acknowledged by younger men. We consider that research on hegemonic masculinity now needs to give much closer attention to the practices of women and to the historical interplay of femininities and masculinities.[26]

Second, with regard to the geography of masculinities, Connell acknowledges that change in locally specific constructions of hegemonic masculinity has been an important theme of the emerging masculinities research, along with the significance of transnationalism and global institutions for local gender orders. Connell argues that a new tripartite framework is needed for analyzing empirically existing hegemonic masculinities: *local*, constructed in face-to-face interactions in families, communities and organizations, and typically discovered through ethnographic and life history research; *regional*, constructed at the level of the culture or nation-state, and typically found through demographic, political, or various kinds of discursive research; and *global*, constructed in transnational arenas (e.g., long-distance migration, multinational businesses, global media), and evident in the emerging research on masculinities and globalization.[27] Although Connell stresses the importance of global influences on local gender orders, he seems most interested in "regional masculinities," which provide a "symbolic model" and "cultural framework" for society-wide formulations of masculine reality.

Third, Connell argues for more work on social embodiment, or particular ways of representing and theorizing men's bodies in research on hegemonic masculinity. Connell admits that bodies "are involved more actively, more intimately, and more intricately in social processes than theory has usually allowed."[28] Yet, Connell is least specific in suggesting how embodiment and hegemony might be productively studied together. He points to work on transgender practice and transsexuality but says little about other embodied social phenomena, including men's health, illness, aging, medical treatment, or the use of medical technologies (e.g., sexual and reproductive health technologies).

Finally, Connell urges attention to change, or what he calls "the dynamics of masculinities," which were not articulated clearly enough in the original formulation of hegemonic masculinity. These dynamics include change over the male life course, as determined through life history research; change over time, particularly as the generation of male children become men; and change brought about by social contestations, such as women's and gay protest movements, which open the possibility for democratizing gender relations over time. According to Connell, "Both at a local and a broad societal level, the situations in which masculinities were formed change over time. These changes call forth new strategies in gender relations (e.g., companionate marriage) and result in redefinitions of socially admired masculinity (e.g., the domestic partner rather than the Victorian patriarch)."[29]

Connell concludes by advocating for the "renovation" of hegemonic masculinity, following these reformulations. The term should be retained, he argues, but opened up to "new usages."[30] In short, hegemonic masculinity is a "traveling" concept, which acquires new meanings when applied to new problems and settings.

Hegemonic Masculinity—Middle Eastern Style

Most of the empirical research on hegemonic masculinity has been carried out in the West and Australia, the latter representing the site of Connell's earliest work on the role of men in Australian labor politics.[31] But what do we know about masculinities in other regions of the world, including the Middle East? How are ideas of masculinity conceptualized, embraced, experienced, challenged, and sometimes resisted? Is it fair to speak of a Middle Eastern form of hegemonic masculinity? If so, what are its elements?

Here, I attempt to formulate a notion of "hegemonic masculinity, Middle Eastern–style," based on my long-term engagement in Middle East studies, as well as my reading of four different types of sources: the selective representations of the Western mass media, ethnographic portrayals by mostly male anthropologists, Middle Eastern feminist writings, and what we might call the "self-stereotypy" or *residual indigenous Oriental-ism* of Middle Eastern men and women themselves.[32] Together, these four sources have coproduced a version of Middle Eastern hegemonic masculinity as follows.

In the Middle East, the hegemonically masculine man is said to be a *family patriarch*. He is socialized into patriarchy during boyhood, where he learns to dominate his sisters and even his mother, although he is still subordinated by the senior males of the family. Eventually, he achieves patriarchal control over his own family when he reaches adulthood, marries, and produces offspring, especially sons, who are necessary for the perpetuation of his lineage. Because he is a patriarch, he may exert his power and authority over the women, junior males, and children in his family through coercion and even force. This is especially true if *family honor* is threatened. Women who shame themselves through perceived licentious behavior simultaneously shame their families. The family patriarch (or his surrogates) must respond swiftly and definitively to defend the family honor, even through *honor killing* of the offending female family member. As a hegemonic male, he is supported in his exercise of power and violence by other male relatives.

These hegemonic males live in close proximity. This is because family life in the Middle East is said to be strictly *patrilineal* and *patrilocal*, meaning that kinship is defined through men and men alone, and these men form extended family residences together with their wives and children. Within these patrilocal compounds, women who have married in are subordinated by men of the patrilineage, as well as by men's mothers and sisters. This is because women *buy into patriarchy*. To receive the support of men in their natal families, they turn against in-marrying women in a cruel form of intragender patriarchal rivalry.

Women who marry into the patriarchal, patrilineal, patrilocal extended family are in an extremely vulnerable position. If they challenge their husband's authority, they are at risk of an *Islamic form of divorce* in which a man need only utter his intentions without recourse to formal legal proceedings. Hegemonic masculinity allows men to exercise these divorce rights liberally and freely. Marriage is not characterized by love, because it is *arranged* by families, often for the purposes of familial and tribal alliance. Without conjugal intimacy, men's primary emotional commitments remain with their own mothers.

In this context of fragile marital bonds, hegemonically masculine men enjoy their rights to *polygyny*. Muslim men may marry up to four wives simultaneously, as long as they promise to treat them equally. Equal treatment demands *hypervirility*: The polygynous man not only enjoys sexual variety but must be sexually potent to quell rivalries between competing co-wives. Furthermore, the Islamic mandate to reproduce an Islamic "multitude" encourages *pronatalism* within polygynous marriage, with some men producing their own small tribes of children from multiple spouses. *Tribalism* itself requires large families, not only for the purposes of nomadic pastoral labor but also for tribal raiding and defense. Hence, men's tendencies toward *violence* and *militarism* are perpetuated, indeed encouraged, through tribal structures, as well as through Islamic *jihad*, or the mandate to defend the religion when it is threatened by outside forces.

The role of *Islam* in reinforcing hegemonic masculinity is crucial. Islam organizes daily life through prayer and ritual; it dictates men's attitudes toward women, including through gender segregation and prohibitions on intimate contact with unrelated women; it channels men's economic relations through tithing and restrictions on credit; and it supports religious extremism, even *fanaticism*, including violent hatred of non-Muslims. Muslim men follow all-male clerics who shape the contours of Muslim manhood through their preaching and their written discourse, particularly *fatwas*, or religious proclamations outlining which attitudes and practices are *halal* (permitted) or *haram* (prohibited). In the *umma* (community of the faithful), seeking one's own fortunes through *bazaar* culture is a noble form of masculine livelihood. Muslim men are encouraged to seek wealth, for Islam does not condone voluntary penury, as shown in the example of the Prophet Muhammad, who was a successful merchant.

Within this context of Middle Eastern hegemonic masculinity, men vie with each other for economic and social success. The hegemonic male is *homosocially competitive*. He accumulates greater wealth than other men. He fathers more children, especially sons, through his marriages to multiple women. He is perforce a *heterosexual*, as homosexuality is one of the gravest forms of *zina*, or illicit sexuality in Islam. He demonstrates his piety more fervently than other men through his attendance at the mosque, his physical appearance (e.g., untrimmed beard and calloused forehead from praying), and his willingness to take up arms in the name of Islam. He is socially powerful through his patriarchal control over other men, including those in his family, his business, and his communal *jihad*. In short, in his performance of hegemonic masculinity, he is a force to be reckoned with—a *rajul* (man) who is not only respected but also feared.

ORIENTALISMS: NEW AND INDIGENOUS

This long description of Middle Eastern hegemonic masculinity represents my best effort to concatenate a list of masculine traits as they are presented to us in various Western sources. Clearly, such a composite sketch of Middle Eastern hegemonic masculinity is extremely essentializing and deeply vilifying—a "toxic trait list," to use Connell's own term. Contemporary masculinity in the Middle East is rarely captured in such stereotypic portrayals, even if elements of this hegemonic masculine caricature may, at times and in certain places, be "true" to the lives of some men. Rather, masculinities in the Middle East, as elsewhere, are plural, diverse, locally situated, historically contingent, socially constructed, and performed in ways that require careful empirical inspection. Yet, empiricism concerning Middle Eastern manhood has been the exception rather than the rule. In the West at least, we have allowed our perceptions of Middle Eastern men's lives to be overwhelmed by recent media portrayals of Taliban, al-Qaeda, Hamas, and Hizbullah religious zealots, suicide bombers, ruthless dictators, and petro-rich Gulf moguls. Such contemporary representations of Middle Eastern men as medieval theocrats, violent barbarians, oil despots, and patriarchal oppressors are part of a much longer history of Orientalism, through which the West has viewed the East with simultaneous prurience, repugnance, and outright fear (figures 3–5).[33]

Post-9/11 representations of Middle Eastern masculinity bespeak a *new Orientalism* replete in American popular culture. It can be found in the political fear-mongering of presidential candidates such as John McCain, who argued that "Islamic terrorism" (i.e., perpetrated mostly by men) is the single worst threat facing American society. In the election battle between McCain and Barack Obama, McCain supporter Gayle Quinnell claimed

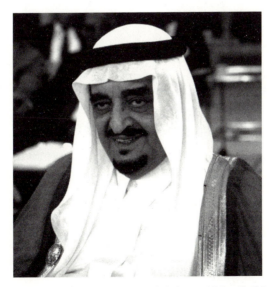

FIGURE 3. Media image of King Fahd bin Abdul Aziz Al Saud of Saudi Arabia, before his death on August 1, 2005. Thomas Hartwell/Time & Life Images/Getty Images

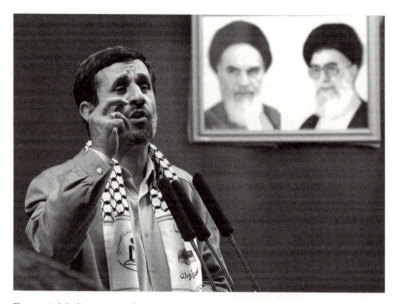

FIGURE 4. Media image of Mahmoud Ahmadinejad, president of the Islamic Republic of Iran. Atta Kenare/AFP/Getty Images

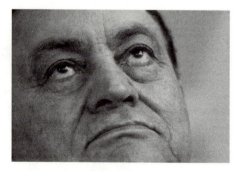

FIGURE 5. Media image of Hosni Mubarak, president of Egypt before his resignation on February 11, 2011. Andreas Rentz/Getty Images News/Getty Images

on camera at a GOP rally that she was scared of Obama because he is "an Arab." McCain's response: "No. No, ma'am. He's a decent family man with whom I happen to have some disagreements." In John McCain's world—and evidently in the thinking of many Americans—"Arab" and "decent family man" are mutually exclusive categories. That Arab men should be vilified in this way reflects the new post-September 11 landscape of America, where "Arab" and "Muslim" are, indeed, deemed "indecent." The 2010

Islamophobic frenzy over the building of a mosque and Islamic community center near Ground Zero, the site of the former World Trade Center, has renewed hate-mongering diatribes against Arab and Muslim men. For many right-wing American Tea Party advocates, Obama's own middle name, Hussein, as well as his Kenyan Muslim paternal origins, disqualify him from a legitimate claim to the presidency of the United States. The conspiracy theories about Obama as a "Muslim terrorist plant" can only be called insanely malevolent.

In Obama's case, he shares a third discredited status because he is black. Both Arabs-qua-Muslims ("Arab/Muslims" for short) and black Americans are vilified by many white Americans, who regard Arab/Muslim and black men in particular as dangerous, untrustworthy, and inherently violent (as well as fanatical, if they are Muslims). The very possibility that Arab/Muslim and black men might be trustworthy, loving, law-abiding citizens—who may want to conceive and nurture children as responsible father figures— seems to have eluded both the media and popular imagination, leaving deeply entrenched caricatures that are difficult to overcome.[34] These caricatures of Arab/Muslim and black men include notions of hypersexuality and hyperfertility (e.g., Newt Gingrich's descriptions of Obama's father as a "Luo tribal philanderer"). Arab/Muslim men are seen as polygamous fathers of children from multiple wives, harkening back to Western Orientalist fantasies of the harem.[35] Similarly, black men are often portrayed as informal polygamists, spawning offspring with multiple, unmarried sexual partners (as well as spreading HIV/AIDS to them).[36]

The dangerous hypervirility of Arab men is the dominant theme of the post-9/11, Harlequin "Desert Romance" series, in which Middle Eastern Bedouin men—typically hegemonic male "sheikhs"—abduct (usually blonde) Western women to remote desert harems, only to unleash, via their hypervirility, these women's unbridled passions there. The books' covers and titles—exemplified in table 3—bespeak the themes of violence, captivity, and terror, even if the Western heroine, lacking any other form of agency, learns to love and desire her abuser. In short, "romance equals rape" in this pop-culture series destined for middle-aged American women, with Arab men cast as hegemonic, villainous, sexual predators.

In a less benign form, this new Orientalism is seen in the movie *Sex and the City 2*, which was released in American theaters in summer 2010. Described by one Film Salon reviewer as "an Orientalist's wet dream,"[37] the four American female protagonists—Carrie, Samantha, Miranda, and Charlotte—embark on an expense-paid trip to Abu Dhabi, idealized as "the new Middle East" by the wealthy Emirati "sheikh" who hosts them. These four "material girls" are enthralled by the lavishness of the sheikh's private jet, the white limousines waiting for them at the Abu Dhabi airport, the $22,000-night penthouse suite in the sheikh's desert hotel, and

TABLE 3. Selected titles from the Harlequin "Desert Romance" series

In the Enemy's Embrace

Taken by the Sheikh

By the Sheikh's Command

The Sheikh's Unsuitable Bride

Bedded by the Desert King

The Desert Prince's Mistress

King of the Desert, Captive Bride

The Desert Sheikh's Captive Wife

The Sheikh's Unwilling Wife

The Desert King's Virgin Bride

the four turbaned Indian manservants assigned to cater to the American women's whims and desires. However, outside this Shangri La, Carrie and her friends encounter the "real" Middle East, which includes silent women in burqas and grim, oppressive men who cannot handle Samantha's open displays of sexuality. These range from strapless dresses and kisses on the beach, to the performance of fellatio on a water pipe and a handbag literally bursting with condoms. Because of Samantha's Western-style sexual "liberation," the four women are kicked out of the hotel, and then chased by an angry mob of bearded Arab men dressed in traditional Emirati robes and headscarves. The women are "saved" by "oppressed" Arab women in their black facial veils and abbayas. Once the "burqas" are removed, the women are shown to be wearing designer fashions hidden from "their" men. As the Film Salon reviewer concludes, quite aptly, "The movie uses only two broad colors to paint the Middle East: one depicting an opulent Eden for our blissfully ignorant protagonists to selfishly use as a temporary escape, and the other showing an oppressive dungeon populated by intolerant men [who] cannot comprehend cleavage or bare shoulders."[38]

Such Orientalizing, fearsome portrayals make no room for ordinary Middle Eastern men such as Hisham or Hamza, who defy such easy categorization as tyrannical misogynists, desert lotharios, or Muslim zealots. What are we to make of their masculinity? Is hegemonic masculinity, Middle Eastern–style, always patriarchal, hypervirile, brutal, and religiously fanatical? Are Hisham and Hamza simply "subordinated" men, unable to achieve hegemonic masculine ideals? Or are their lives actually much more representative of masculinity as it is emerging in the contemporary Middle East today?

To begin to answer these questions, I would like to make a number of preliminary points, based on my ethnographic fieldwork. First, the "new

Middle East"—to use the term put forward, then vigorously retracted in *Sex and the City 2*—is filled with men like Hisham and Hamza, who do not conform to any particular "type," and certainly not to the aforementioned caricatures. Second, men such as Hisham and Hamza are aware of such vilifying stereotypes of Middle Eastern men, in part through their exposure to English-language Western media. (Recall Hamza's vehement protestations: "But I am not a terrorist!") Yet, it is very important to point out that not all of these damning portrayals emanate from the West. A third important point is that Middle Easterners themselves make frequent reference to indigenous notions of "the Oriental man" or "the Eastern mentality," in a common form of self-stereotypy. It is partly these *indigenous stereotypes* of Middle Eastern manhood—or what I would like to call "residual indigenous Orientalism"—that men such as Hisham and Hamza are rejecting, a point that deserves further attention.

In the Middle East, the Arabic term *rujula* is used to describe "manhood" or "masculinity." When the term *rujula* is articulated in conversation (or *rujuli* in the Lebanese dialect), it tends to be associated with certain hegemonic attributes, including tribalism, the fathering of many sons, and the oppression of women. However, these notions of *rujula* are increasingly critiqued by Middle Eastern men as "backward," "old-fashioned," and "traditional." In interviews, men often took great pains to signal their "modernity," "education," and "culture," critiquing the past as oppressive to *both* men and women. Their comments on what they considered to be an "Oriental" or "Eastern-style" *rujula* were often quite funny and biting. As one man remarked,

> If you see on TV, or a video clip—I mean if you see on *Arabic* TV or a video clip—when a man puts on the *jallabiya* [i.e., the traditional male robe], what do you see? The horse and the sword! But that mentality, it's an old, old mentality. Seriously! Nobody has his sword anymore!

A second man quipped, "Arab manliness and all that sort of crap! Yeah, it's definitely still there. But for me, I take a wiser and bigger view of life."

Another man, speaking about the masculine side effects of male infertility, explained to me,

> You see, it's *rujuli*, the Oriental mentality. Most of them [infertile men], they don't talk at all [about it]. They don't even go to have tests to see [if they are infertile]. So, if they don't have children, it's the wife who can't have [them]. I think even the educated—no, maybe less with educated people—but they equate having children with being a man. So, when they go to have tests and see that it's male infertility, of course, they will feel affected. But I have an understanding wife.

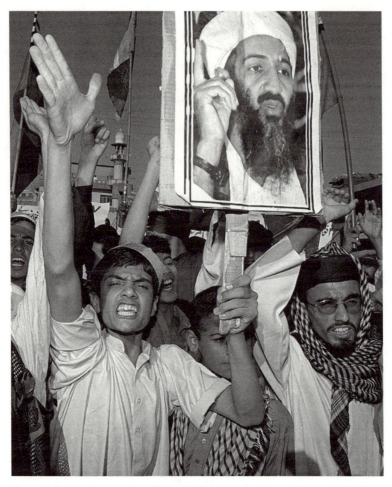

FIGURE 6. Media image of a rally by Al-Qaeda supporters. Shakeel Adeel/
AFP/Getty Images

All of my masculinity is here, within the couple. If a couple has good
relations, this will not affect them. It's a medical problem. Even in the
family, we were not raised in this Oriental way. It's not like, "He's a
boy, he's the boss. She's a girl, she has to obey." We were all raised
the same in my family.

As these quotes suggest, many men do not see their lives as resembling
the caricature of hegemonic masculinity, Middle Eastern–style, which has
been described in this chapter. The difficulty of fitting so many men into

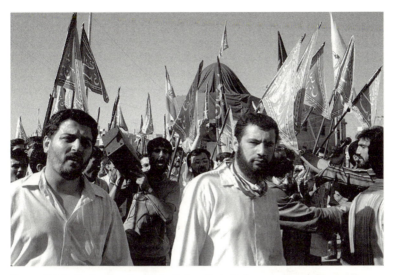

FIGURE 7. Media image of a Hizbullah rally in Lebanon. Kaveh Kazemi/ Hulton Archive/Getty Images

a single hegemonic mold suggests that hegemonic masculinity requires rethinking. In my own work, I have become less and less comfortable with the concept of hegemonic masculinity as the best way of characterizing Middle Eastern manhood. As we have seen, the term now carries with it many negative connotations, or a "toxic trait list," which, in the context of the Middle East, condemns all men as oppressive patriarchs, polygamists, religious fanatics, and terrorists. In Connell's own reassessment of the concept, he points to al Qaeda as the only Middle Eastern example, calling it a global "protest masculinity" and comparing it to white supremacist movements in the United States (figure 6).[39] These kinds of examples from the Middle East, be they Sunni or Shia "protest masculinities" (figure 7), are simply not "true" to the lives of most men.

Indeed, if there is a "protest masculinity" to be found in the Middle East today, it is in the lives of those ordinary men who, in January 2011, took to the streets in Tunisia, Egypt, and beyond to protest the dictatorial regimes, police brutality, corruption, poverty, and unemployment in their home countries. As young men, they called for many things, including democracy, freedom of expression, freedom from repression and fear, the right to vote, the right to work at a decent wage, and the right to afford marriage and family life within their home countries. It is these ordinary, "nonterrorist" men who are by far the statistical majority in the region, but whose individual stories of hope and fear, suffering and triumph are rarely told.

FROM HEGEMONIC TO EMERGENT MASCULINITIES

After more than twenty years of work in the region, I maintain that hegemonic masculinity theory must be rethought for the Middle East, and perhaps for men's lives everywhere around the globe. When I first began my work on male infertility and sexuality in Egypt in the late 1980s, I found the concept of hegemonic masculinity—which was quite new at the time—to be very useful in framing my analysis. Specifically, I used hegemonic masculinity as a way to describe male privilege and female blame when poor urban Egyptian couples confronted the embodied problems of male infertility and sexual impotence. Although I found elements of hegemonic masculinity in my informants' life experiences, I was also struck by the fact that many poor urban infertile Egyptian men were *not* engaging in wife blame or acting in an otherwise hegemonically recognizable fashion. Most poor Egyptian women prided themselves on having "good husbands," thanking God for their luck in marriage. Calling this empirical phenomenon "conjugal connectivity," I argued that Egyptian men—even poor "subordinated" men—were treating their wives as loving partners. Women who were infertile emphasized that such good treatment was not to be expected: namely, residual, indigenous Orientalist views of men suggested that they invariably divorce infertile wives. However, as I could show through my ethnography, this was not the norm. Rather, most men stayed in their infertile marriages, arguing that love prevailed over having children. In the late 1980s, this was my first evidence that men were changing in the Middle East and, in so doing, changing society with them.[40]

As the years have passed, I have met hundreds more "good husbands" from numerous Middle Eastern countries and social backgrounds. In this book, we will meet a wide variety of Middle Eastern men, seeing how they relate to their wives, their family members and friends, religious authorities, and physicians. We will witness their contemplations over emerging forms of medical technology, observing how they embody some and reject others. In order to understand their masculine practices, we must focus on two issues: emergence and embodiment.

"Emergence" is a concept that has been developed by Marxist scholar Raymond Williams, who, like Connell, is interested in cultural processes of hegemony.[41] In classic Marxist theory, hegemony is associated with the dominant class in society, which rules primarily through coercion and consent rather than through the use of force. In his essay, "Dominant, Residual, and Emergent," Williams asks how a dominant group maintains a cultural system and how this system might change over time. Through what he calls "epochal analysis," he contrasts "feudal culture" and "socialist culture" to the "bourgeois culture" found in capitalist systems. However, even dominant bourgeois culture is subject to change. As he explains, "*no dominant social order and therefore no dominant culture ever in reality includes or exhausts all human practice, human energy, and human intention.*"[42] Instead, "new meanings and values, new practices, new relationships and kinds of relationship are continually being created."[43] Williams calls this "emergence," to signify that which is novel rather than strictly alternative or oppositional to the dominant culture. These emergent elements may eventually be incorporated into the dominant culture, causing the social order itself to change over time.

Williams's focus on the emergent, rather than on the dominant or hegemonic, has helped me to think about new forms of masculinity. There is abundant ethnographic evidence from around the world that masculinity is changing, transforming patterns of gender in the process. For example, anthropologist Mark Padilla has shown how male workers in the Dominican Republic's booming tourism industry are experimenting with their conjugality and sexuality, emphasizing the "regional" and "situational" masculinities of Dominican men as they move through distinct social contexts over time.[44] In Mexico, anthropologists Gloria Gonzalez-Lopez, Matthew Gutmann, Jennifer Hirsch, and Emily Wentzell have shown that younger generations of Mexican men are questioning their fathers' *machismo*, which was characterized by harmful heavy drinking, risky promiscuity, and family violence.[45] Similarly, emerging ethnography from Japan shows that young middle-class men are rejecting the corporate, heavy-drinking "salary-man model" of masculinity, attempting instead to forge new forms of domestic partnership with Japanese women, whether they be wives or girlfriends.[46] Even men in the United States are changing. In an article entitled "Beyond the Bad Boys: A Quiet Revolution in Male Behavior," author Julia Baird defies the conventional wisdom that "men are bastards, men don't change, men always put their own desires before their families" (e.g., as in the examples of Tiger Woods, John Edwards, Arnold Schwarzenegger, or Jessie James).[47] Instead, she cites emerging evidence that men are spending more time with their children (double the amount found in 1977); men have dramatically increased their share of housework, especially among the working class; men are now feeling more torn over balancing work and family than their wives are; and taking care of a child is now part of what it means to be a father, even if "stay-at-home dads" are still in the minority. As Baird concludes,

> In the midst of the tabloid hysteria about bad boys and dirty dads, it's important to remember that some things are going right. It is such a simple and important change that we have almost missed it: more and more men are starting to care for their children. The consequences of this are enormous.[48]

The concept of "emergence" speaks to these processes of social change, as men navigate and adapt to their changing social worlds. In my view, the term "emergent masculinities"—intentionally plural—embraces social history and new forms of manhood in a way that "hegemonic masculinity" does not. Whereas hegemony emphasizes the dominant and ideal, emergence highlights the novel and transformative. When applied to manhood, emergent masculinities encapsulate change over the male life course as men age; change over the generations as male youth grow to adulthood; and changes in social history that involve men in transformative social processes (e.g., male labor migration, the rise of companionate marriage, the introduction of computers and the Internet into homes and workplaces). In addition, emergent masculinities highlight new forms of masculine practice that accompany these social trends. These would include, for example, men's desire to date their partners before marriage, men's acceptance of condoms and vasectomy as forms of male birth control, men's desires to live in nuclear family residences with their wives and children, and men's encouragement of daughters' education. All of these masculine practices are, in fact, emerging in the Middle East, but are rarely noticed by scholars or media pundits.

The "emergent" is omnipresent in the Middle East. The region now hosts, *inter alia*, the world's tallest building and other architectural marvels; a global satellite television culture headlined by the homegrown product, Al Jazeera; Internet cafés frequented by youth; a mass cell phone culture even among domestic servants and day laborers; multistory shopping malls selling European designer labels, as well as local Islamic fashions; rates of university matriculation among women now outstripping those of men; entrance of large numbers of women into the government bureaucracy and retail service sector; mass migration of men to the Arab Gulf and to virtually every other continent; concomitant delays in marriage, as young men and women establish themselves in new careers, new nuclear residences, and new lives different from their parents; and emerging social movements, including recent protest movements against dictatorial regimes, which have been largely initiated by younger-generation men and which have spread like wildfire across the region. In short, a veritable revolution in men's and women's social worlds—and their interactions with each other—is abundantly observable across the Middle Eastern region and requires scholarly attention.

Thus, an emergent masculinities approach that takes new forms of masculine practice seriously as an object of empirical investigation serves us better than resort to a worn-out notion of Middle Eastern hegemonic masculinity, the pitfalls of which have been highlighted in this chapter. It is time, I would argue, for new thinking about manhood in the Middle East. This, of course, requires ethnographic documentation of gender *in practice*—of men acting *as* men, in relation to women and to other men—rather than as mere representatives of nation-states, religious sects, political parties, tribal groupings, and the like. The Middle East is, in fact, an excellent site for rethinking masculinity, as men themselves recast their own lives in relation to globally diffused, but toxic Orientalist stereotypes. In short, the Middle East is ready for an emergent masculinities approach to be applied.

Furthermore, emergent masculinities must enjoin the notion of embodiment, a concept that is widely used within medical anthropology and the other social sciences.[49] The embodiment of emergent masculinities implies the physical, in this case, changing notions and practices of the male body itself. Men's bodies are often thought of as embodying their masculinity, and notions of masculine embodiment are locally and historically situated. For example, the physicality of bulging biceps and "six-pack abs" may signal youthful masculinity in the contemporary West, whereas handle-bar mustaches were a sign of masculinity in a former era. Furthermore, a man's pot belly or double chin may be a sign of poor fitness in one society, but a marker of masculine prosperity and well-being in another. In addition, men's bodies change over time, as they engage in physical labor or exercise, gain or lose weight, become ill, or grow old, with attendant losses of sight, hearing, physical vigor, and sometimes mental lucidity. How men react to these physical changes—and how they judge their health over the life course—are important aspects of embodiment that deserve to be studied.

What men do with their bodies is of equal concern: Do they play soccer? Do they dance? Do they overeat? Do they drink alcohol? Do they smoke? Do they sit in front of a computer all day at work? Do they masturbate? Do they have sex with or without condoms? Do they go to the doctor when feeling ill? These kinds of questions are often framed in terms of "risk" or "risky behavior," an epidemiological concept. However, the answers to these questions are also tied to embodied masculinities. For example, in the Middle East, many men smoke because this is what men are socialized to do *as men*; smoking is equated with masculinity, whether or not it is perceived as dangerous (and it often is not). Furthermore, as will be shown in chapter 5, men in the Middle East are conflicted about masturbation, because of religious injunctions about appropriate versus inappropriate sexuality. Studying these bodily enactments of manhood, whether culturally valorized or not, is a crucial subject for a new anthropology of masculinity.

Finally, emergent masculinities intersect with emergent health technologies. These technologies include pharmaceuticals, such as vitamins, testosterone, performance-enhancing drugs, antidepressants, insulin, antihypertensives, antiretrovirals, erectile dysfunction treatments, and many other forms of life-prolonging or life-enhancing medication. However, men's engagement with medical technology spans other dimensions as well. Ultrasounds are no longer confined to pregnancy; they are used to examine men's testicles. Men undergo a variety of physically demanding diagnostic tests and therapeutic technologies, including MRIs, fine-needle biopsies, and x-ray-guided angioplasty. Men's increasing willingness to embody these medical technologies and practices is another aspect of emergent masculinities that certainly deserves our attention.

In the Middle East, men are self-consciously acting out emergent masculinities in relationship to their changing bodies and to new technologies that mediate these changes. In the world of assisted reproduction, men's engagement with medical technology can be quite agonizing, when their sexual organs are scrutinized and opened up in various ways, or quite liberating, when their ICSI twins and triplets are born. The stories presented throughout this book show men engaging creatively with these new medical possibilities, forging new ways to be men and become fathers in the process.

In conclusion, I argue that masculinity theory must become dynamic enough to account for these emergent and embodied changes in Middle Eastern manhood. Previous work on hegemonic masculinity has established the nature of masculinity as hierarchical, relational, and located in specific cultural contexts. I believe that it is crucial to develop new theoretical approaches that, when applied to ethnographic cases of real men's lives, do not reify them into particular "types" of men but instead account for their nuanced and constantly evolving responses to their changing social worlds and physical bodies. Men's experiences of infertility and new assisted reproductive technologies such as ICSI represent a quintessential example of emergent masculinities that are deeply embodied.

As an anthropologist, I am committed to ethnography as the best way to explore men's changing social worlds, their evolving understandings of manhood, and their embodied experiences. In addition to Hamza and Hisham, we will meet many Middle Eastern men in this book, who are enacting emergent masculinities within changing local worlds of marriage, morality, and medicine. I urge others to engage in similar studies of "lived" masculinities on the local level. By doing so, we can establish the empirical base upon which to further develop an emergent masculinities approach and to bring masculinity theory up to date in the new millennium.

CHAPTER 2

Infertile Subjectivities

"I Am the Problem," Said Ziad

While writing up notes in an IVF clinic waiting room one day, I found myself seated across from two men who were chatting amiably with each other. This was surprising, given that most men are quiet and tense—sometimes holding prayer beads—while waiting for their wives to emerge from the operating theater. Soon, one of the men left, leaving me alone with the other man, whose appearance was not typical for Lebanon. He had long, dark hair, slicked back with shiny pomade into a ponytail. He also wore a gray striped suit with a black shirt and no tie, giving him the appearance of either a fashion model or a mogul—it was hard to tell. The man began reading my study advertisement placed on the waiting room table, soon entering my phone number into his mobile. Detecting his interest in the study, I introduced myself to him, asking if he wanted to participate. He agreed without hesitation, and we found a quiet spot in a nearby ultrasound room. As soon as we were seated, he blurted out, "I'm Ziad, and *I am the problem*. I would have called you if you hadn't found me, because I assume I am the only one in Lebanon with this problem." With little further prompting, he began to tell his story, which began with the Lebanese civil war.

The only son of a Lebanese Greek Orthodox family, Ziad joined a Christian militia at the tender age of thirteen. "I will never forget the fear and the stench of the B7 missiles I carried," he told me, after asking for repeated assurances that the interview was confidential. Ziad's militia involvement interfered with his education, and like many young men of his generation, he barely finished high school. Smart, handsome, and self-taught, Ziad found a job in the men's fashion industry when the war ended. Beginning as a salesman, he soon became a buyer, traveling monthly to Europe on purchasing expeditions. There, he was exposed for the first time to the wide world of Western sexuality. Ziad admitted that he engaged in numerous one-night stands, with at least three hundred women. Although he used condoms on occasion, he often did not. Thus, he lived in fear of accidentally impregnating a woman during one of his casual trysts. This was especially worrisome in his home country of Lebanon, where premarital sexuality and out-of-wedlock pregnancies are socially taboo. Nonetheless, Ziad estimates that at least fifty different Lebanese women agreed to sleep with him during his twenties. He was treated for sexually transmitted infections at least ten times, noting "I took a lot of medicine in my life."

By his late twenties, Ziad was a successful businessman, owning two high-end men's clothing stores in the booming postwar city center of Beirut. He had also fallen in love with a beautiful, university-educated, Lebanese Christian woman named Jinan, who was his "type" and who agreed to marry him. When Jinan did not become pregnant after two years of marriage, Ziad decided to undergo semen analysis at one of the hospitals in downtown Beirut. On his first semen test, no sperm were found. Ziad explained,

> Really, I was shocked when I learned about my problem for the first time! I learned about it in Trad Hospital, and I left and walked all the way to Verdun [several miles away], without even taking my car. I was thirty years old, and I asked myself, "How could I never have known about this problem?" I never imagined I would encounter this. All the times I worried about getting someone pregnant, and this was in vain!
>
> I repeated the test seven or eight times in Lebanon that first year, and there were always zero sperms. In Lebanon, they told me, "No hope for you!" This was in 2000, the first time that I knew about my problem. So, I went to see many doctors. But, you know, in the Middle East, we're very business oriented. Everything is "for business." Every time I would go to a new doctor, they would say, "You need an operation!" "You need this." "You need that." "You need, need, need!" They told me that I have a big, big problem. They cut my life, really.

Demoralized by his azoospermia problem and the confusing medical care in Lebanon, Ziad decided to visit a Lebanese doctor in Brussels, Belgium. There, the doctor ordered a specialized semen test, and a very small number of sperm (seventy to eighty) were detected in Ziad's ejaculate. As Ziad explained, "This doctor told me, 'We don't need more than ten sperms to do in vitro. So it's no problem; you're not zero.' " Still, Ziad felt emasculated.

> It *really* influenced my sense of manhood for a year, that first year in 2000. I encountered moments in my life when I asked questions about my identity. "Am I really a man?" All the people in my business are gay, homosexuals. And I got afraid of this topic. At first, they used to joke with me about being gay, and I used to accept their jokes, given that I worked in this business. I used to accept these jokes easily.

But after I found out I had this problem, I used to get upset. I found the joking to be very aggressive. You think too much, you ask a lot, "Why me?" But now, I've managed to get over this bad feeling about myself. I asked doctors many questions, without giving the doctor any background about my problem so as not to influence him. Even though I didn't get a university degree, I asked many questions, and I've done research [on male infertility] all over the world.

Ziad is now convinced that his male infertility problem is strictly medical, not a problem of manhood. He notes that he was born with an undersized right testicle, and his left testicle has a small varicocele, or cluster of varicose veins. Most doctors have also explained that male infertility can be caused by a genetic problem that runs in the family. But because Ziad is the only son (with three sisters), he cannot prove a familial connection. He notes, however, that his mother's brother has no children. Discounting any genetic connection, Ziad's mother is convinced that the infertility stems from childhood mumps, which nearly killed Ziad at age seven. She told Ziad that she prayed to many saints to keep him alive. "I lived," Ziad quipped, "but not without medical problems!"

Today, Ziad has high cholesterol, which he attributes to ten kilograms of extra weight (well hidden through fashion). He also suffers from a chronic problem of severe migraine headaches, for which he takes multiple medications. Ziad commented,

The migraines and the cholesterol are affecting my sex drive. After intercourse, I feel very tense, and then I get swollen eyes and the aura of a migraine. Then one to two hours later, I get the migraine. So sex makes me feel tension, not relaxation! I feel hysterical because of the migraine. I need to relax and sleep [to overcome it], but I have no time because of my work. I like to work, but then I have no time to relax and to enjoy sex. And I'm worried about having a migraine after sex.

Ziad claims that he desires his wife sexually and is faithful to her, but that their sex life is now infrequent because of the migraines, his hectic work schedule, and the stresses of infertility treatment. Currently, Ziad and Jinan are undertaking their sixth ICSI cycle, including one failed cycle undertaken in Belgium. Only the fifth ICSI cycle led to a confirmed pregnancy, but it was ectopic (in the fallopian tube), requiring emergency treatment. When I asked Ziad if he was worried about undertaking ICSI again, he replied,

Worries, sure! Everyone worries, not about the ICSI itself, but about how many embryos will develop, the possibility of death of some embryos. The whole procedure is stressful. Every time we go through this, she's very hyper and stressed. I feel the tension is more for her, even though I'm the only guy in my family, and so I'm supposed to care about having children.

Ziad paused, then added,

Me, I only want kids "fifty-fifty." I'm mostly doing this for my wife, for her mother, for my mother. I could easily adopt a child, but I can't really mention it in front of my wife. She wants to feel pregnant, and this is only natural for a woman. She's smart, so she doesn't pressure me. But the people in Lebanon, they pressure us—especially they pressure her. They don't pressure me because I set limits. They ask me, "When will you have children?" And I say, "*Insha'Allah* [god willing], *insha'Allah, insha'Allah.*"

Here in Lebanon, people live *for* other people, not for themselves. They live *for* other people. So the parents, the neighbors, other people can be gratified that you have a child. Other people are more concerned about having children than the couple themselves!

I'm just preoccupied about this for my wife, my parents, and my wife's parents. I feel sorry for my wife and our parents. Had I known I had this problem before age thirty, I would never have married, because I feel bad for my wife.

For the sake of Jinan, Ziad tries to remain hopeful. He trusts his current Lebanese physician, whom he describes as "very natural, very humanistic." He was also encouraged by Jinan's pregnancy on the last ICSI attempt. If he had his wish, Ziad would like to be the father of three children, two boys and one girl. "Definitely two boys so that one wouldn't turn out to be an only son like his father. And definitely more than one child, because in Lebanon, they think an only child is really pampered." According to Ziad, if the sixth ICSI attempt fails, he has no choice but to try again.

MALE INFERTILITY

Ziad's story is illustrative on many levels. He suffers from a very serious case of male infertility, and this problem was first detected after marriage. Because male infertility is not a visible medical condition, most men have no idea that they are infertile until they attempt to impregnate their wives. Second, Ziad assumes that his infertility problem is unique. He knows no other infertile men and so does not realize the high prevalence of this condition across the Middle Eastern region. Third, Ziad has never been able to answer the "Why me?" question. Without sophisticated DNA analysis, the causes of most cases of male infertility remain strictly speculative. Fourth, Ziad has questioned his own masculinity, including the nature of his sexual orientation and the meaning of his previous sexual encounters. This conflation of male infertility with problems of virility (i.e., sexual potency) is common. Fifth, Ziad has bought into the medicalization thesis. Over time, he has accepted both a medical cause and a medical solution for his infertility problem, thereby disentangling his masculinity from what he has now come to view as a health condition. Sixth, Ziad is pursuing ICSI mostly "for her"; that is, he cares more about his wife's feelings and desires for children than about his own procreation. Seventh, even though Ziad is the only son in his natal family and is expected to continue his patriline, he admits ambivalence about fatherhood. Happy in his successful career and his marriage to a beautiful, intelligent woman, he argues that having children is more about pleasing other people—especially the prospective grandparents—than about fulfilling the desires of the man or the couple. Finally, Ziad thinks of himself as part of a couple; he does not need children to make his marriage, or his masculine identity, complete.

Ziad's story is interesting in that it conveys a full range of masculine responses to male infertility, including shifts in subjectivity over the course of a man's lifetime. In this chapter, we explore the infertile subjectivities of other Middle Eastern men. Male infertility does not lead to an inevitable crisis of masculinity. Rather, men in the Middle East live with their infertility in a variety of ways, ways that have changed since the emergence of ICSI.

To understand men's infertile subjectivities, a few initial points about infertility as a biomedical problem bear mentioning. A standard biomedical definition of infertility is the inability to conceive after twelve months of regular, unprotected intercourse.[1] By this definition then, infertility affects more than 15 percent of all reproductive-aged couples worldwide.[2] So-called male factors contribute to *more than half* of all these cases.[3] Yet this high percentage is rarely acknowledged, because women tend to bear responsibility—even if misattributed—for failures of reproduction.[4] Because male infertility is often idiopathic, or of unknown cause, it is recalcitrant to prevention, and among the most difficult forms of infertility to treat.[5] Male infertility can be solved by ICSI, but it is not a condition that can be cured per se. In other words, male infertility is a *chronic* reproductive health condition for millions of men worldwide.[6]

There are four major categories of sperm defects, any one of which leads to a diagnosis of male infertility: *oligozoospermia* (low sperm count), *asthenozoospermia* (poor sperm motility), *teratozoospermia* (defects of sperm morphology), and *azoospermia* (total absence of sperm in the ejaculate). Azoospermia may be either *nonobstructive* (due to lack of sperm production) or *obstructive* (*due to* blockages in sperm transport). These four types of male infertility account for about 40 percent of all infertility cases in the Western countries. However, in the Middle East, 60–90 percent of all cases presenting to IVF centers involve a diagnosis of male infertility, according to physician estimates.[7] Moreover, nonobstructive azoospermia is highly prevalent in the Middle East, as are cases of severe oligoasthenozoospermia (i.e., very low sperm count and poor motility). Because of advances in the field of genetics, it is now realized that a significant percentage of these kinds of severe cases are due to genetic abnormalities,[8] a point that was made by Ziad's physicians. That male infertility "runs in the family" is a theme to which we return in chapter 4.

In short, male infertility is especially common in the Middle East and quite common elsewhere, but this is not popularly known. Male infertility has been called a "neglected" reproductive health problem, and one that remains deeply hidden, including in the West.[9] Studies in the United States have shown male infertility to be among the most stigmatizing of all male health conditions.[10] The depth of this stigmatization may be even deeper in non-Western settings, casting a permanent shadow on a man's community standing.[11]

Such stigmatization is clearly related to issues of sexuality. Male infertility is popularly, although usually mistakenly, conflated with impotence (i.e., erectile dysfunction), as both disrupt a man's ability to impregnate a woman and to prove one's virility, paternity, and manhood.[12] This "fertility-virility linkage" means that men who are infertile are assumed to be impotent, even though most are not.[13] In the Middle Eastern context, they may also be assumed to be homosexual, as suggested by Ziad's own self-doubt in this regard.

On an even more basic level, male infertility casts doubt on a man's gender identity. Quite tellingly, the first definition of "male" in *The New Shorter Oxford English Dictionary* (1993) is as follows: "pertaining to, or designating the sex which can beget offspring; in organisms which undergo sexual reproduction, designating, pertaining to, or producing gametes (as spermatozoa) that can fertilize female gametes (ova)."[14] If biological "maleness" is, in fact, constituted by begetting offspring through the production of spermatozoa, then male infertility, or the inability to produce fertile spermatozoa, may come as a striking blow to men's gender identities, with far-reaching implications for the construction of masculinity.

The relatively small but growing body of social scientific literature on male infertility in the West suggests that male infertility can have these kinds of effects on men's gender identities. For example, in an article provocatively titled "The End of the Line: Infertile Men's Experiences of Being Unable to Produce a Child," Russell Webb and Judith Daniluk report their findings from an interview-based study of infertile American men, where the theme of male inadequacy was paramount.[15] According to the authors, "The participants used words and phrases like *failure, useless, a dud, inadequate, not a real man, garbage, loser,* and *defective* in reference to their self-perceptions as infertile men—men who were unable to 'give their wife a child.'"[16] Some men, furthermore, attempted to compensate for their feelings of inadequacy by acting like "super jocks," having affairs with other women, or throwing themselves into their work. In another American study, men reported that their male physicians attempted to "smooth troubled waters" by referring to their infertility as "shooting blanks"— masculinist, even militaristic language, which left men feeling estranged from their infertile bodies.[17] Both male infertility and its treatment have been reported in the West as resulting for some men in impaired sexual functioning and dissatisfaction, marital communication and adjustment problems, interpersonal relationship difficulties, and emotional and psychological distress.[18] In one of the few recent qualitative studies of infertile American men who eventually discontinued ICSI, researchers found that infertility threatened men's masculinity, in part because husbands were teased for being infertile, while their wives were pitied.[19] Men sometimes responded by casting blame on their wives, arguing that this was justified, because "it's different for men" to be infertile than for women.

It is very much an empirical question whether the effects of male infertility on men's sense of masculinity are culturally invariant; the topic has been even less researched in non-Western sites.[20] The few comparative studies tend to come from Israel, more Western than Middle Eastern in some ways. There, a handful of scholars have examined the impact of infertility treatment and especially donor insemination on masculinity.[21] In one Israeli study, infertile men were found to experience a profound sense of embarrassment and anomie in clinical treatment settings.[22] Poor semen analysis results were usually taken by men as indications of personal failure. Furthermore, infertile men felt as if they were expected to compete with another man, the sperm donor, who could easily substitute for them as a biological progenitor. Thus, the authors suggested that infertility may have a "diffuse, total impact" on men, who may become a "target of ridicule" if their infertility becomes known to family and friends.[23] In another Israeli study, a "conceptual link . . . between dysfunctional sperm, failed masculinity and impotence in sexual intercourse" was found among men presenting with their wives to Israeli IVF clinics.[24]

The most recent review of published scholarship on the sociopsychological impact of male infertility shows mixed results.[25] On the one hand, most recent studies confirm that infertility is more distressing for women than it is for men. Women invest more in having children, are more likely to initiate and continue treatment, experience higher levels of stigma, are likely to admit changes in mood and feelings of jealousy, and are aware that their "biological clocks are ticking away."[26] Women experience infertility as a "direct blow to their self-identity," whereas men experience infertility indirectly through the effect that it has on their wives.[27] However, this may be a predominantly Euro-American finding. According to the authors of the review, "It may be justifiable to think in terms of two worlds of infertility."[28] For example, studies of infertile men from Iran, Zimbabwe, and South Africa report higher scores for depression and anxiety than among men in the West,[29] leading the authors to conclude: "The infertility literature can also serve to remind us that it is not only women who reproduce, who undergo medicalisation and who experience stigma, and that men need to be a part of research on gender and health."[30]

My own early work on infertility in Egypt supports this conclusion: few men were willing to tell anyone, including their closest family members, that they were affected by male infertility.[31] Male infertility was described variously as an "embarrassing," "sensitive," and "private" subject for the Egyptian male, who would necessarily feel *ana mish ragil*—"I am not a man"—if others were to know that he was the cause of a given infertility problem. Because of the association between male infertility and manhood, men's wives were generally expected to participate in a two-person cult of silence regarding the male infertility, which usually meant that women shouldered the blame for the infertility in public. When women were questioned (as is often the case in Egypt) about the source of the childlessness, most told others that there was "nothing wrong" with either partner, and that the matter was "up to God." Sometimes women suggested to their acquaintances that they themselves were seeking treatment for the infertility. Women often explained that they "covered" for their husbands out of love and loyalty. However, some women also said that they feared the potential familial and marital consequences of exposing their husbands' secret.[32]

My Egyptian studies—and the available demographic evidence from the Middle East—suggest the existence of what I would call a "masculine reproductive imperative." Namely, men living in Middle Eastern communities are expected to have children, as reflected in the relatively high marriage and fertility rates across the region.[33] Men are presumed to acquire social power within the "classic" Middle Eastern family structure—that is, patriarchal, patrilineal, patrilocal—through the reproduction of offspring, especially sons, who will perpetuate this social structure into the future.[34] "Intimate selving" in Middle Eastern families also involves expectations of "patriarchal connectivity,"[35] whereby men assume patriarchal power in the family not only with advancing age and authority but through the explicit production of offspring, whom they nurture but also dominate and control. Thus, in this region of the world, men who do not become family patriarchs through physical and, ultimately, social reproduction may be deemed weak and ineffective,[36] and may be encouraged to divorce or take additional wives in order to continue the patrilineage and to prove their masculine virility.[37]

This masculine reproductive imperative is said to engender homosocial competition between Middle Eastern men in the realms of virility and fertility, which, as noted earlier, are typically conflated.[38] According to Lahoucine Ouzgane, a scholar of contemporary Arabic literature, virility emerges as the "essence of Arab masculinity" in the novels of some of the region's most eminent writers, with men in these stories both distinguishing themselves, and being distinguished from other men, through the fathering of children, and especially sons.[39] If this is, in fact, the case, as much of the literature from this region suggests, then the experience of male infertility for a Middle Eastern man can only be *imagined* as extremely threatening and emasculating,[40] particularly in a region of the world where men work hard to sustain their public images as "powerful, virile" patriarchs.[41]

The word *imagined* is significant. As noted earlier, one of the only scholarly books on Middle Eastern masculinity is titled *Imagined Masculinities* to signal how little is actually known about male identity and culture in the modern Middle East.[42] Male infertility is part of what I would call a *Middle Eastern masculine "black box"*: literally nothing is known about male infertility and masculinity, except for what I have discovered through my own research over the past two decades.

What have I found? The most important discovery is that male infertility is not necessarily a crisis of masculinity. Although some men feel that their manhood is diminished by male infertility, others deny any such association. Some men want to talk at length about their reproductive problems, whereas others do not. Some men are devastated by the thought of never having children, whereas others do not care if they ever become fathers. This range of infertile subjectivities is not expected but suggests that masculinities are emerging in a variety of forms in the Middle East today. Some men like Ziad are beginning to question the masculine reproductive imperative itself, reassessing whether fatherhood is always the route to a happy life.

Nonresponse

Ziad was perhaps not typical in his questioning of fatherhood. And he was also unusually willing to participate in my study and to talk about his reproductive and sexual problems quite openly and eloquently. Many other men were not. Requests to participate in my male infertility study in Lebanon yielded responses ranging from direct refusal to occasional voluntarism. If the willingness of Ziad represented one end of the participatory spectrum, then the refusal of many other men represented the other extreme. Most men were somewhere in between, willing to participate but with some reticence.

What do refusals and reticence mean in a study of Middle Eastern male infertility? Are they an indicator of the profound emasculation of male infertility in this region of the world? Perhaps, but not necessarily so. There may be many reasons for what Mike Lloyd has called "non-response in studies of men and infertility."[43]

Lloyd is one of the few ethnographers to study the lived experiences of male infertility directly. In his own study conducted in Wellington, New Zealand, Lloyd hoped to interview thirty infertile men, "but even this relatively small number proved difficult to attain."[44] Using multiple clinical and nonclinical networks, Lloyd was eventually able to conduct nineteen interviews over ten months' time, keeping track of refusals along the way. He claimed a nonresponse rate of 48 percent—"that is, for every man who agreed to talk to me, there was one man that refused."[45] These many refusals led Lloyd, a sociologist, to examine nonresponse in other qualitative studies of male infertility. Of the eight social scientific studies of male infertility, all of which were undertaken in Western countries, nonresponse was a recurring theme. Lloyd surmised that "researchers have often experienced great difficulty in gaining male respondents in studies of infertility."[46] Furthermore, in the absence of documentary evidence about why men refuse, researchers have applied their own commonsense cultural understandings, usually pointing to the "sensitivity," "secrecy," and "stigma" of male infertility. Lloyd concludes that infertile men's nonresponse is "condemned to be meaningful": namely, men may have simple reasons for not participating in male infertility studies (e.g., too busy at work), but, instead, researchers attribute psychosocial causes to men's reluctance (e.g., male humiliation). As a result, the "truth of infertility" in men's lives is poorly understood.[47]

Although I have been studying infertility in the Middle East for many years, I had never encountered this issue of nonresponse until I began working with men. Never once did a woman refuse to participate in my earlier studies of female infertility in Egypt. From the poorest slum dwellers to the wealthiest Egyptian movie stars, most women were eager to talk to me about their reproductive, sexual, and marital lives.[48] Thus, when I began my study of male infertility in Lebanon in 2003, I was somewhat surprised by men's reluctance. On any given day, one, two, or even more men declined to meet with me, even after careful description of the benefits of the study and its guarantees of confidentiality. On the basis of men's statements at the time, the reasons for refusal seemed multiple and varied. Generally, they fell into five major categories: pragmatics, politics, gender socialization, heightened emotions, and emasculation.

On the pragmatic level, men often felt very rushed in IVF clinic settings, where they were expected to meet with doctors, provide semen samples, make payments, and provide physical and emotional succor to wives, usually in the midst of their own busy workdays. Some men also had long drives homes, including across national borders. "Not enough time" was the most common reason for men's refusal and probably reflected men's honest, pragmatic assessments about the lack of time to conduct a thorough interview. On the other hand, on days when men spent hours in clinic waiting areas while their wives completed ICSI operations, refusals based on purported time constraints appeared disingenuous.

Politics also intervened in my study in Lebanon. I began my research there in January 2003, only two months before the United States invaded Iraq. During this period of heightened political tension, my Americanness was noted, with some men openly expressing their displeasure with the United States and its policies in the Middle East. In one clinic, which catered to many members of Hizbullah, I was clearly not welcome during March and April 2003, when virtually every Lebanese and Syrian man who was asked refused to participate in my study. Quite ironically, once George W. Bush announced "mission accomplished" in early April 2003, the bad feelings toward the United States ebbed somewhat, and my interviews at that clinic resumed in May.[49] However, my field notes from that clinic are filled with perpetual discomfort. One member of the mostly Shia Muslim clinical staff told me, "All Arabs are upset at America." Another stated bluntly, "You can't force people to talk." Pious Shia men at that clinic, some of whom were presumably allied with Hizbullah, were often reluctant to meet with me because of my nationality and my gender.[50] For example, one man refused quite apprehensively by stating, "If I talk to her, I'll end up in prison!" In short, the politics of research during wartime—particularly when it was my country that was going to war in a nearby Arab nation—clearly led to many refusals. I often found myself apologizing for my Americanness, introducing myself as being "from Michigan" rather than "from *Amrika*." Having said that, some men made generous attempts to put me at ease as an American researcher. For example, one man who agreed to talk to me stated, "Politics is politics. This has nothing to do with your study."

Many of these infertile men's wives were more supportive of my study, wanting their husbands to talk to me. Women's relative willingness versus men's relative reluctance to respond is clearly a reflection of gender socialization. As I was told by one of the IVF physicians, who had experienced similar refusals in a study of infertile men's genetic karyotypes, "Men here are shy even with their doctors. They let their wives do all of the infertility work and initiate everything." To some degree this is understandable; IVF clinics are, by definition, ob/gyn sites. They tend to be placed in ob/gyn or maternity units in Middle Eastern hospitals, where men feel out of place and uncomfortable in this female-dominated sphere.[51] Women in these spaces tend to talk with one another, offering comfort and condolences, whereas men do not. As one IVF doctor put it, "Women are socialized to talk about their problems, and men are not, even with their friends." The difference between husbands and wives in some of my couple interviews in Lebanon was quite striking. Lebanese women tended to be animated and forthcoming, whereas their husbands were often taciturn, even morose. When I asked one Lebanese male IVF physician why Lebanese men were like this—especially compared to the garrulous and friendly infertile men I met in Egypt—his answer was, "I could never be friends with an Egyptian. They talk too much! Everyone knows this about Egyptians."

Putting these kinds of national character assessments aside, the poor psychological state of many Lebanese men was something that I noted and was another major reason for refusals. Many men declined participation in my study by saying, "I'm not in a good mood," or "I don't feel like talking." The terms *nafsiya*, "psychology," and *asabi*, "nervous," were used repeatedly. In a few cases, men nearly pleaded not to have to participate in the interview, indicating a high level of distress over the subject. I told clinic staff members never to pressure men and to accept their refusals without any form of coercion. Men's heightened emotions were legitimate, I argued, given the stresses of "timed" ejaculation in clinic bathrooms, watching wives wince in pain during ICSI operations, or hearing bad news about semen test results or the "cancellation" of an ICSI cycle when embryos failed to develop. Men with financial problems experienced additional stresses at the time of payment.

For some men, talking about one's life and reproductive problems could also be highly emotional. Especially in Lebanon, but also for the Iraqi and Palestinian refugee men in my study, reproductive life histories were filled with memories of war. The psychologically exhausting fifteen-year Lebanese civil war, which was followed by at least seven years of postwar economic crisis, seemed to have generated high levels of poor mental health in Lebanon. Many men in my study openly admitted to feelings of stress, depression, and anxiety, for which some were taking medications. Even more of these men attributed their current infertility problems to *al harb*, "the war," which they believe had made them infertile.[52] In general, the Lebanese men in my study did not seem happy, an impression that was seconded by some of the physicians I also interviewed. Lebanese men rarely laughed, were somewhat reserved during interviews, and generally looked much older than their reported ages (presumably from a "weathering" effect attributable to the war, too much sun, and heavy smoking). Although I enjoyed my interviews with many men in this study, particularly after some of them started opening up as the interviews progressed, I found Lebanese men to be much less forthcoming and animated than Egyptians, the latter of whom are known within the region for their loquaciousness and good humor. Perhaps this tendency toward reserve made it more difficult for Lebanese men to admit deeply personal and potentially humiliating feelings of masculine inadequacy, leading to refusals.

Finally, some men invoked their rights to privacy, stating that "this is something confidential." As I had learned in my previous study of IVF in Egypt, both male infertility and ICSI were deemed "top secret," to be held in confidence between a couple and their physician.[53] When I encountered these same secrecy concerns years later in Lebanon, most of the IVF physicians and clinic staff members chalked this up to masculinity issues—or the "sensitivity" that Middle Eastern men feel about revealing their reproductive problems to anyone, including a Western researcher. Additionally, in Lebanon, some men were using donor sperm or oocytes, which may be forbidden in their religions.

I suspect that male infertility is, on some level for some Middle Eastern men, deeply humiliating—something to be hidden rather than revealed. In fact, when I first arrived at a Lebanese IVF clinic and explained my study to the staff members, a nurse predicted bluntly that my study would "never succeed" because of the stigma and secrecy surrounding this topic. She described how couples with infertile husbands tried to "hide from each other" in the recovery rooms and would sometimes stay there for hours if they saw an acquaintance who might expose their secret to the outside world. Although her prediction about my study's inherent failure did not come to pass, her point was well taken. At least some men in Lebanese IVF clinics probably refused to speak to me out of feelings of stigma and emasculation. Those who *did* agree to participate were probably the ones who felt least diminished by their infertility, or who had overcome feelings of emasculation, as in Ziad's case. One such man, who ended up speaking to me at great length about both his war traumas and his male infertility problems, sat in the waiting room with me one day and commented under his breath, "The shame men feel here; you can see it when you look in their faces and eyes, and no one speaks to each other. The doctors make it worse by coming and whispering to the patients. It reinforces the shame and secrecy."

Indeed, looking back on my research—including the hundreds of hours spent seated in uncomfortable waiting areas with quiet, morose, infertile men—I feel quite lucky and grateful. Somehow, more than three hundred men agreed to speak with me, a fact that I now find quite remarkable. In my own attempt to speak truth to their infertile subjectivities, what follows is my assessment of how male infertility affects Middle Eastern masculinity, and how men's infertile subjectivities are changing over time.

"Weak" Sperm and Emasculation

Clues to the emasculating effects of male infertility take many forms in the Middle East. The first clue comes from the high rates of nonresponse. The second clue comes when some infertile men, including a few in my study, present themselves at IVF clinics as being fertile "controls" rather than infertile "cases"—what epidemiologists term "misclassification." Their misclassification may be unwitting, as they may lack solid evidence of a male infertility problem. On the other hand, misclassification may be evidence of men's emasculation and what IVF physicians call men's "denial" of their infertility problems. Over the years, I have heard numerous stories of infertile Middle Eastern men refusing to go to doctors, preferring to "prove" their fertility through marriage to a second wife. However, with the widespread advent of semen analysis across the Middle Eastern region over the past three to four decades, resort to polygyny is no longer common in the current generation of reproductive-aged men. Nonetheless, it is said that some men still refuse to go for semen analysis or bribe laboratory technicians for falsely inflated reports. Although I cannot verify whether these patterns of male resistance are widespread, I did find instances where men in my study with severe sperm abnormalities attempted to downplay the seriousness of their infertility. Furthermore, I met some men, both fertile and infertile, who attempted to distance themselves from male infertility problems altogether, by insisting that "nothing was wrong" with either partner, despite clear medical evidence to the contrary.

As noted earlier, male infertility is not a problem that can be seen on a man's body, for the reproductive impairment is usually hidden deep in the testicles (or the brain's hormone-producing pituitary gland). Like Ziad, most men first learn of their infertility upon postmarital semen analysis. Only then does male infertility become a problem for masculinity, marriage, and the formation of family life. Or, as Ziad put it, "Had I known I had this problem before age thirty, I would never have married, because I feel bad for my wife." Another Lebanese-born man, who had spent most of his life in Latin America, described the effects of male infertility in this way,

> This is a hidden problem, but it is a huge issue for masculinity, especially if you're both Arab and Latino! It can affect your sexuality, leading to impotence, and it can affect your marriage. You start to wonder

if your partner views you as less than a man, because you can't give her a child. So it can damage your self-esteem and your relationship.

As suggested by this excerpt, emasculation stems from the fertility-virility linkage, a linkage that is made clear in the language used to describe both male infertility and impotence in Arabic. In what I would call "biomedical Arabic," infertility (both male and female) is referred to as *'aqam*, a term sometimes used interchangeably to denote erectile dysfunction. This fertility-virility linkage is even more apparent in popular spoken Arabic. Almost invariably, both male infertility and erectile dysfunction are referred to as *da'f*, or "weakness," with both sperm and erections being referred to as *da'if*, or "weak." Sometimes, men who are diagnosed as infertile are confused, because they have never experienced any sexual difficulties, and they conflate the two problems in their own minds. Doctors themselves use the language of weakness when describing both of these problems to their male patients. In fact, the language of weakness suffuses the Middle Eastern infertility realm. In IVF clinics, both physicians and patients speak of "weak sperm," "weak ejaculation," "weak erections," "weak periods," "weak ovaries," "weak ovulation," and "weak embryos." Not surprisingly, this language of weakness bleeds into personhood, with both infertile men and women sometimes describing themselves as *ana da'if*, or "I am weak." Men sometimes admit to feeling "weak" or "useless." They also worry that they may pass on their weakness to their male offspring.

This language of masculine weakness was less apparent in my 2003 Lebanese study than it was in Egypt in the 1980s and 1990s. This is largely because of detailed laboratory semen analysis methods, which are carried out in all IVF clinics, as well as in andrology laboratories across the region. While male infertility is defined outside IVF clinic walls by the perceived inability of a man to impregnate his wife, this definition changes radically once an infertile man sets foot in an IVF clinic, where a differentiated notion of male infertility comes into play. The concept of "severity" is applied in clinical settings, in order to locate the male patient along a graded infertility spectrum. Through the microscope in the IVF laboratory, experts examine sperm retrieved from semen—semen that is usually masturbated into a plastic cup or sometimes surgically removed directly from the testicles. The sperm are separated from semen through various spinning and washing techniques, then graded and quantified on the basis of numerous fertility-related factors, including count, movement, and shape. Quantitatively, a fertile man should have more than 20 million spermatozoa per milliliter of ejaculate (although the number has recently been reduced to 15 million by the World Health Organization); more than 50 percent of those spermatozoa should be motile, or moving (although 40 percent was previously accepted as a cutoff point); and more than 30 percent of spermatozoa should have normal morphology, or shape.[54] Thus, the diagnosis of male infertility reads as an equation: < 15 million/mL, $< 50\%$ motility, $< 30\%$ normal = male infertility. Those men with numbers much lower than this are deemed to have more severe cases. The degree of severity then determines the type of treatment that will be proposed. Intrauterine insemination (IUI), involving the injection of the husband's own sperm into his wife's uterus, is generally recommended for less severe cases of male infertility. But, when IUI fails, or when a man's sperm count, motility, or morphology is particularly poor, a man and his wife will likely be moved directly to ICSI.

Most men in my study had undergone semen analysis several times—even hundreds of times in some long-term cases. Because of this repeated ritual of semen analysis, many men had become quasi experts on their cases, including their numbers of sperm and the percentage of sperm motility, or movement. Most men in my study had an approximate idea about the numbers: namely, a fertile man should have "more than 20 million sperm and 40 percent active," per the WHO definition at the time. This is why men such as Ziad—who are diagnosed with zero sperm in their ejaculate—are often truly shocked and demoralized. Having no sperm is far different from having, say, 19 million. Nonetheless, azoospermia and very, very low sperm counts are quite common among infertile men in the Middle East. These cases are defined by the clinical adjective *severe*, as in "severe oligozoospermia" (e.g., < 100 or $< 1,000$ sperm found in the ejaculate) or "severe asthenozoospermia" (e.g., $< 10\%$ active). Sometimes men have both of these sperm defects together, a condition called "oligo-asthenozoospermia."

Men in the Middle East rarely use these Latin-based medical terms to describe their sperm defects. Rather, they use Arabic terms for sperm and motility, adding the adjective *da'if* as a qualifier. In Egypt, Iraq, and the Arab Gulf, sperm are generally known as *hayawanat al-minawi*, literally "spermatic animals." Lower-class Egyptian men use the term *didan*, or "worms," to describe sperm.[55] In the Levant region, including Lebanon, Syria, Jordan, and Palestine, men refer to their sperm as *bizri*, or "seeds," an agricultural metaphor of procreation that has been reported throughout the region.[56] Not surprisingly, in some parts of Palestine, IVF is known as "planting" (as in "planting seed").[57] In Iraq, the variation "implanting" is used. In my study in Lebanon, *tifl unbub* (baby of a tube, or test-tube baby) was used, similar to *tifl al-anabib* (baby of the tubes, or test-tube babies) in Egypt. In addition to these important terms, men are concerned about their sperm's *haraka*, literally "movement" or motility. Whether a man has any sperm—and whether enough of them are actively moving—determines whether ICSI can be undertaken.

Most infertile men become "sperm savvy" over time. In my study in Lebanon, many men could describe their sperm counts—and often motility and morphology percentages as well—with some degree of specificity and accuracy. When I asked about men's *tahlil bizri* (analysis of sperm), men had typical responses such as: "The first time after marriage, it was half a million, 500,000. But I took medicine and it increased to 5 million." Or "six months ago, it was 65 million, but only 20 percent motility." Or "I've had sperm tests more than ten times. The most recent was about 70 million, but the movement was only 8 percent."

Some men had a great deal to say about their semen analyses. Two examples of detailed "sperm talk" are representative of these kinds of discussions. As one man told me,

> I've had *a lot* of sperm tests, in both Syria and Lebanon. Maybe 100! It was 25 million the first time, then 28 million after the ampicillin, then 10 million, then 12 million, then 8 million sometimes, then 20 million, then 4 million, the minimum, one time only. The last time, it was 25 million, here at the hospital. But 75 percent are dead after one hour. Only 10 percent are active, and 5 percent are abnormal.

A second man, a Palestinian high school biology teacher, also had much to say about his "numbers,"

> Every year, I make two or three tests. But when I made a sperm test one year after marriage, the first time, it was 45 million, 30 percent active, 20 percent normal. The doctor said, "No problem." But there *is* a problem. And he didn't even mention that there is a problem. He didn't inform me accurately about the result. Every time, the activity is less than 40 percent, sometimes only 5 percent, or normally 5 to 10 percent. Now I know that this is a problem. My knowledge now tells me that 60 million, 60 percent active, and 60 percent normal [morphology]—these should be the numbers, and my numbers are always lower. Here, the last one [sperm test], one month ago, my count was 45 million, activity was 20 percent, and normal was 20 percent.

Despite this rhetoric of numbers and percentages, it is important to emphasize that "weakness" dominates men's vocabulary. Male infertility is still most commonly glossed as "weakness," and men like Ziad may begin to doubt their masculinity, even if they feel they are not to blame for the condition. In my interviews, men would occasionally relay how the discovery of male infertility had caused surprise, demoralization, and self-doubt. A few examples:

ELIAS: I was very devastated in the beginning—as a *man*. I don't think it's like this everywhere, but here in Lebanon, here you should have a baby straight away. So it took me some time until I realized that it's not the sperm that makes you a man.

MARWAN: Neither my parents or her parents know anything about my problem, because they might say, "Oh, he's not a man!" But, personally, I think this has nothing to do with manhood. My sperm cannot define my manhood in any way. To be honest with all people and to treat them as well as you treat yourself—this is manhood.

MAHMOUD: Even before marriage I wanted kids. I love children. So my masculinity was affected. Ah, yes! In all of the Arab world, if a man has a child, and especially if it's a boy, this "makes a man a man." If someone has four or five boys, this guy is strong! And if he only has girls, it's a big problem. Even now, everyone says this. But I believe it is what God gives. Sometimes I feel bad about myself, but then I remember God. If it [infertility] were not mentioned in the Qur'an, I would feel very bad. But it is, and when I remember this, then I feel good. I will have a child only when God wishes.

SAMIR: Sometimes I do, I do ask this question, "Why me? Why am I not like other men?" But I'm a believer in God. And I'm trying. I tried so many medications, so many treatments. And it's depressing, yes. Since 1993, when I started to see doctors, this is a long time. I feel guilt toward my wife. She wants to have a baby. Before, I didn't, I wasn't as much like her, I wasn't wanting a child so much. But now I'm starting to think about this. I love kids, yes. I love them. And, for the future, they will take care of my wife and me, later in life.

Mansour, an infertile, American-trained Lebanese Muslim physician, who was attempting with his wife to make a third ICSI baby (perhaps a son after the birth of two daughters), described the relationship between masculinity and male infertility this way,

Manhood. It's really an important factor in society. I know this as a pediatrician. The first thing people ask for at the first baby visit is to check the [male] baby's reproductive organs. They're worried from the first moment of life if [the child has] normal reproductive organs. If they will have a normal sexual life. It's about his future manhood. It's a strong feeling. And it's a deficiency if you can't have children. I do think people feel this. I would assume they do, because it's a secret kind of thing, male infertility. In my own case, who knows about this [his male infertility problem, involving abnormal sperm morphology]? My wife doesn't want *anyone* to know. So we come here [to the IVF clinic] in secrecy.

As is clear from all of these men's statements, male infertility is considered by society to be a threat to manhood. Thus, most infertile men are reluctant to reveal their condition in public.[58] Male infertility is still shrouded in secrecy, as suggested by many men's nonresponse to my study, as well as by the responses of men who agreed to be interviewed. Men often wanted multiple assurances that the information was confidential and anonymous and would not be tape-recorded (and potentially "leaked"). They also described to me how I was among the first to know about their infertility problems. These desires for secrecy were explained to me by Amin, a Christian engineer, in the following way,

> I think that, for Lebanese men, this problem [male infertility] affects their manhood. Maybe sometimes, I say something related to my problem, and people say, "Oof! How can you say that?" They want to maintain secrecy about personal things. They are shy; they don't like to tell their problems to other people. I know someone who had a problem like me [male infertility], but he never said so. If forced, he would say it was a problem with his wife. He told me, because he knows I don't have children and he was asking me about a doctor at the hospital, and I told him he should see my doctor also. So he was *obliged* to tell me he had male infertility. I told him, "I need to know your problem to tell you which doctor to go to!" But, in general, personal problems stay in the family.

Having said this, secrecy is not universal. In my study, men exhibited a wide variety of communication patterns, ranging from complete concealment to full disclosure. A significant number of men had consulted friends and relatives in order to obtain treatment advice and the names of good infertility specialists. In some families, close relatives took an even more active role by escorting the couple to the clinic, donating money for treatment, or caring for the wife after an ICSI cycle was completed. Other men preferred to avoid such intimate sharing of their cases and limited their communication with family members. They explained to parents and siblings that they were "receiving treatment" but did not divulge the timeline or technical details.

In short, men in the Middle East invest considerable energy in deciding whether, and to what extent, to share information about their male infertility and its treatment within their social circles. Within the wider social milieu, male infertility becomes a problem of impression management—namely, whether one should attempt to "pass for normal," thereby implicitly placing the blame for childlessness on an otherwise fertile wife. The fact that so few men are open about their infertility problems means that women are often blamed for the childlessness and sometimes face relentless social pressure because of this. Women being blamed for the childlessness of male infertility was certainly one of the major findings of my earlier studies in Egypt.[59]

However, in the past decade, some infertile men are speaking truth to this injustice, viewing it as inherently unfair and wrong. In fact, many infertile men in my study were like Ziad, who "claimed" his infertility at the outset of the interview in order to clear his wife of any responsibility. When I asked infertile men about their wives' fertility, a common response was *ma fii shi abadan*, or "there is nothing *at all*" wrong with her. Along similar lines, infertile men would sometimes respond *walla marra*, or "not *once*" when I asked them if they had ever impregnated a woman. The fact that Middle Eastern men are claiming their infertility, while expressing concern for their wives' "courtesy stigmatization,"[60] was an emerging theme of my interviews. Amin, the engineer quoted earlier, had the most to say on this subject,

> The first time I had my results, I didn't expect to have a problem like this, and I didn't expect that it couldn't have a solution. It was really hard for me, not because I have the problem, but because the solution is not clear. If I have a problem, I want to solve it. Just tell me the solution! But I've passed this way of thinking. I could have been born with this problem. It's not my fault, and it's not the fault of Yusra [his wife]. So, we just took it easy. It wasn't a big shock, because somehow, I was prepared. I suggested to Yusra that maybe this problem is from me. I don't know, but I didn't take it as a problem of manhood. For me, it's, it's not the "proof" [of manhood]. And thank God I'm being like this. Because women get more pressure, and especially here, because they don't think this problem is from the man. They think *she* is the problem. This is bad. Even my parents didn't understand. "Oh, no! Not possible." But I said, "If you want proof, I can show you." They didn't want to believe that their son had a problem. Instead, the whole family focused on her. When we got married and we went to the hotel, two days afterward, she met my aunt, who asked her, "Oh?" [are you pregnant?] Not like this, in only two days!

Other men talked about similar undue pressure placed on their own wives, and on Middle Eastern women more generally.

MOUSTAFA: Of course there's pressure. My mother and my brothers want me to have children—more than I'm wanting, in fact. An Arab person, if he's married and he doesn't have children, it's like he's not married. And the pressure is *a lot* on the woman. It's like if she didn't have children, she'll die, because motherhood to a woman means a lot to her. So 10 percent of the pressure is on the man, and 90 percent on the woman.

ISSA: I will tell you, people think that *she* has something "missing" when the man, he can't make a child. The women, they're degraded by society. And this is completely wrong.

These men's sense that a grave gender injustice was being committed was something new to me. Although I had analyzed this gender inequity in my earlier work in Egypt, my analytical frame was based on women's sad stories of being blamed for their husbands' infertility.[61] In my research in Lebanon, I was truly surprised to find men making feminist critiques of this inequity on their own. Men's desires to remove the *daght*, or "pressure" on their wives—based on what they saw as the inherent unfairness of a fertile woman being blamed for male infertility—was a recurring theme of my interviews in the new millennium. For example, a Palestinian man living in Dubai, who had traveled to Beirut for ICSI, had a great deal to say about this injustice,

> When I was married, I went to a doctor, and he was all secretive. I told him, "Why must it be secret? I'm not shy about it. It's a sickness, and I'm looking for treatment." I wouldn't do like other men [do]. They say it's a problem with their wives. I wouldn't do this. I say it's from me, and I have to go for treatment. But in the Middle East, for a man to go to a doctor [for infertility], they feel like he's not a man anymore, and they always blame the woman. My wife, she *would* tell other people, "No, it is not from him, it's from me," so that I don't feel hurt. But then she found out there's nothing wrong with her, so why should she do this? Men's exams are much less [invasive] than women's, so men should pursue it. But Palestinian, Jordanian men, they think it affects their manhood. But I and my wife are the same. A man is like a woman, there's no difference. She can get sick, and I can get sick. It's just a disease. So I tell people it's from me. But, on the contrary, other [men] will say [to me], "I'm a man because I have children. If you don't have a child, you're not a man."

NORMALIZATION

As suggested by this and other men's statements, new trends are emerging: some men desire to spare their wives from social pillory by public acknowledgment of their own male infertility. Some men are beginning to chastise physicians for shrouding male infertility in secrecy. Some men are disassociating male infertility from masculinity by turning to religious theodicies (i.e., "God made me this way"). Other men are destigmatizing male infertility by treating it as a medical condition (i.e., "it's a disease like any other"). All of these trends speak to emerging normalization: what was once perceived as a masculine character defect has been turned into a God-given disease category. For the religiously inclined, God sends diseases so that humans may seek solutions to their own suffering.[62] For men with more secular orientations, male infertility is being treated as a *marad*, or a "disease," which has helped to desocialize it, removing it from the realm of gender.

Increasing medicalization—or the growing acknowledgment of male infertility as a medical condition with a high-tech solution through ICSI—has led to major changes in the Middle East over the past decade and a half. The conspiracy of silence surrounding male infertility is beginning to fade, as men point to the increasing openness about male infertility within their social circles. Many men now admit to having infertile relatives and friends, who share information with each other, even helping out with the costs of treatment. Furthermore, the widespread advertisement of ICSI services across the Middle Eastern region has led to general acknowledgment within Middle Eastern society that men can be infertile, and that men's infertility can be overcome through a medical solution.

In short, widespread medicalization of male infertility in the new millennial Middle East is leading to greater social acceptance and decreasing stigma. Once inside IVF clinics, Middle Eastern men seem to begin accepting the fact that male infertility is a medical problem, "like any other medical condition." As George, a Lebanese Christian oil executive, explained to me, there are two views of male infertility, an "insider's" point of view and an "outsider's" perspective,

> In Lebanon, yes, male infertility does affect manhood. Men don't want to admit they can't have children. They're not men any more. But this is not the view of people inside treatment. People who are "in" know it *is* a medical problem. So we don't feel this problem of manhood or womanhood. In our company [where he works], four to five people have IVF babies. One guy was married for fifteen years, and he went to Singapore [for IVF]. Then another one went there. So, in my company, people talk about it. I tell everybody about it. I don't mind. Because it's easier to tell everyone what you're doing. Even at work, it's easier to tell them, so that they just stop asking. My boss said, "You've been married for more than two years and you didn't get your wife pregnant yet?" I said, "I'm trying, but I couldn't get my wife pregnant yet." Two days ago, I told him I'm coming for IVF. But this is *very* uncharacteristic of Lebanese people. People think like, "Manhood. He can't have children." So a lot of people blame the woman, even when it's male infertility. This is because people are secretive. They don't know the problem is male infertility, and so they say [it's from] the woman.

This insider's view—that male infertility has "nothing to do with manhood"—was the most common refrain in my interviews with men.

TABLE 4. Middle Eastern men's statements about male infertility and manhood

Country	Religion	Comment
Lebanese	Druze	Personally, I don't think my sense of manhood has been affected. My psychology is fine, because I'm seeing that infertility is very common, and more and more people are doing ICSI.
Lebanese	Shia Muslim	It hasn't affected my psychology or my manhood, because I believe male infertility has nothing to do with this. It is God's will. I accept whatever God wants.
Lebanese	Shia Muslim	I think when you are not having children, it's from some disease. It's a medical, organic problem. It has no connection with manhood.
Syrian	Sunni Muslim	No, never! Some people are born like that, and I have to accept my case.
Lebanese	Sunni Muslim	Male infertility, in the older generation, they blamed it on the woman. But this is dying out. Our generation, we know about male infertility, and we go to doctors.
Lebanese, living in the UAE	Sunni Muslim	I don't feel shy, actually, about this. I just feel this is a medical problem. This is something normal. I haven't done anything wrong, so why should I feel shy?
Lebanese	Shia Muslim	What makes a man a man is his ability to persevere and find a solution.
Lebanese	Shia Muslim	A man's reasoning abilities take precedence over physical problems. Manhood is about mind over body.
Lebanese, living in Tunisia	Shia Muslim	Never! No connection at all. Masculinity here is reflected more through sexual intercourse, to be able to live with your partner, and whether you have a good sexual relationship, regardless if you have children. As long as you can have sex!
Lebanese	Shia Muslim	Providing for the family is the most important thing in being a man. Because you have no choice to eat!
Lebanese, living in Nigeria	Shia Muslim	(Laughing) Manhood! I knew exactly what I could do [sexually], and that's no problem for me!
Lebanese	Sunni Muslim	Manhood. Never! I don't feel embarrassed in front of other people. I don't think manhood is related to the ability to have children. It's about how I treat my wife. I insure that she's completely satisfied and I provide everything for her. We have a very close relationship. I'm living my life as a man in all venues of my life.
Syrian	Sunni Muslim	It's not having children that defines manhood. It's his mentality, his personality, his understanding. There are some men who consider themselves men through their sexual relations, but not me. The way a man treats his wife doesn't even really define his manhood. I treat my wife on an equal basis, as a friend.

TABLE 4. Middle Eastern men's statements about male infertility and manhood *(continued)*

Country	Religion	Comment
Syrian	Alawi Muslim	Manhood. I don't think male infertility affects it, because this reflects narrow-mindedness. In my environment, there is no such mentality, or maybe I personally don't mingle with people who think like that. As long as a man is educated and open-minded, he would never be affected by this.
Lebanese	Shia Muslim	There is no relation to manhood, unlike for a woman. A woman feels she needs a child. For a woman, because she will feel when she holds the child that she is a mother. But for a man, no. When he holds a baby, he will look like a father, but not a man. In Lebanon, what makes a man a man is his reasoning, his mind.
Lebanese	Shia Muslim	What proves a man is a man is the way he thinks.
Lebanese	Maronite Catholic	Nah! Even if I don't have kids, I'm okay. It's not about manhood. I'd like to have kids because I'm making money, and so as many as I can afford, I don't mind.
Lebanese, living in Senegal	Shia Muslim	Maybe in the past it used to be a problem of manhood. At first, it used to be something which is not good about a man. In the old days, they would say, "He's not a man." It used to affect his manhood. But not anymore. Now male infertility is normal.
Lebanese	Shia Muslim	Male infertility? I believe that everything comes from God, for a reason, and this is unchangeable. A person who has faith in God is not affected by such things. So me? No! My psychology is not affected. As long as my relation with God is strong, everything will come as it should.
Lebanese	Sunni Muslim	I am not happy about this [azoospermia]. But I am a believer in God, so this is not a disaster for me. I believe in God. I believe in science. God creates science, and this is life, our life, to live it very well. Not to put a hole in our head! So I'm not blaming myself or my manhood.
Lebanese	Shia Muslim	My manhood is not affected at all. A man is a man by his reason, *not* by his appearance. Because if a man is defined by his physical potential, then nothing differentiates a man from animals.
Syrian Bedouin	Sunni Muslim	My psychology has *never* been affected! Sometimes I think of it [male infertility], but it doesn't affect my psychology, or my manhood. Because I think of it like this: I have sperm and medicine is advancing, so I think at some point, I may have the chance to have kids. At some point, God will give me a child.
Lebanese	Sunni Muslim	[Azoospermia] has no effects on my masculinity. Sure, it's not, "Oh great! I'm so happy!" But it has nothing to do with manhood. This does not affect me, like "I'm less than a man." Sure, you'll feel that something is wrong with you, but not your sense of self. It is upsetting, but what can I do about it?

TABLE 4. Middle Eastern men's statements about male infertility and manhood *(continued)*

Country	Religion	Comment
Palestinian	Sunni Muslim	I don't feel that way at all. Maybe I should!
Lebanese	Shia Muslim	Manhood? Maybe some people think that manhood is just bringing children. But this is traditional thinking, not modern and scientific. There is a proverb in Arabic, "If you can find medicine, your happiness will be secured."
Syrian	Sunni Muslim	Male infertility has no relation to manhood. Having children is from God. Manhood is your ability to provide for your kids, your living, your income. Manhood is providing for children, not making them.
Lebanese	Sunni Muslim	Manhood, no, it has nothing to do with it! Male infertility, it's from God. You could be very fit, lifting weights, doing boxing, and yet have no kids. So this is just a medical problem. Manhood is the understanding between a husband and a wife. Women have their rights, just like men. Manhood is being fair to women.
Lebanese, living in USA	Sunni Muslim	It's not a big deal. It's not under my control, because it's a physical problem. It won't make me less male or more male.
Lebanese, living in USA	Shia Muslim	The Arabic nature is to ask, "Why is this happening?" But God chose me to be like this. It's a test of my patience and faith.

Although I expected to hear consistent reports of infertility-related emasculation, I found instead significant levels of disassociation. Men were denying to me that they had ever experienced male infertility as an assault on their masculinity. Rather, I was told by numerous men that manhood is measured in different ways—and not only by the fertility of one's sperm. Table 4 provides a diverse sampling of some of these quite powerful comments about manhood and what it means. These Middle Eastern men are clearly voicing emergent masculinities that are independent of their fertility.

Having said this, some additional information must be considered when assessing these emergent masculinities. First, Lebanon generally has higher educational and literacy rates than most other Middle Eastern countries. Thus, many Lebanese men in my study were highly educated—with at least a high school diploma and many with advanced degrees—and virtually all were literate. Many of these men had educated, working wives, and thus presented to IVF clinics as "career couples." Presumably higher levels of education and satisfaction with professional careers may have offset the potential effects of emasculation and contributed to men's acceptance of a "medical model" of male infertility. In addition, Lebanon has never fully recovered economically from two wars, the most recent in the summer of

2006. For some men, then, manhood is more about the ability to persevere and to provide for loved ones under harsh conditions than about proving one's fertility per se.

Men in particular feel the stress of societal expectations to support both nuclear and extended family members, especially aging parents. Thus, male infertility may seem like a relatively trivial concern, especially given a current economic climate that is seen by most Lebanese as not conducive to raising a family.

MANHOOD BEYOND FATHERHOOD

As seen in Ziad's case, some men feel that having children is more "for the family" than for themselves. As we will see in chapter 4, men's families often invest heavily in their sons' ICSI quests, hoping to produce offspring for patrilineal continuity. For example, Ziad, who was an only son, lamented the fact that he was seeking ICSI more to satisfy the demands of his in-laws and parents than out of his own innate desire to have children or become a father. Becoming a father—and hence a family patriarch— was not necessarily a personal life goal. Another man explained it this way, "I don't have a problem with not having kids, but the problem is the family. I truly don't have a problem if I never have children, but *they, the family*— they want children!"

In my study in Lebanon, I found 14 out of 220 men, or 6 percent, who admitted to "not caring" about having children. Most told me that they were pursuing ICSI with their wives mostly out of a sense of familial obligation, not because of their own inherent desires to become fathers. Some of these men were infertile themselves; others were married to infertile women. Most expressed happiness in their marriages and felt that they lived well as childless couples. They were adamant that fatherhood was not necessary to "complete" their lives, their marriages, or their masculinities. Simply put, they did not associate manhood with fatherhood, and they distinguished between their families' wishes for children and their own needs as happily married men. One of these men said,

> On the first day I found out I had this problem, I got really upset by the situation. But then I decided I must overcome it. My own sense of manhood comes from my ability to persevere and to "go for it" through treatment. But if we don't ever have kids, it's not a big problem. Family members here do ask, "Why no kids?" But, now, people are accepting that you can wait after marriage [to have children], and we easily say to them, "No, we don't want kids now."

Another Lebanese man, married to an infertile woman, stated even more forcefully,

I'm willing to keep trying [IVF], but, to me, it doesn't matter one way or another. [Really?] *Really!* To her, it does, but to me, it doesn't. I guess, my nature, I'm a happy person. I really love kids, don't get me wrong. But whatever God, the creator, gives me, I'm fine with. And I'm honestly not that religious. So, it doesn't matter to me. I let her know. I try to tell her that it really doesn't matter to me.

Although the neighboring country of Syria is sometimes deemed more "traditional" and less "progressive" than Lebanon, I found this attitude of "not caring" among Syrian men as well. One of them told me, "The problem of the baby, I don't care a lot. If it comes, *ahlan wasahlan!* [Welcome!] I love children, but it is not an obligation." Another Syrian man, in a long-term marriage to an infertile woman, insisted, "Children are for the purpose of continuity in life, but they are not a basic thing in life. I can live without them. I'm really not caring."

I would argue that these statements exemplify an emerging trend in Middle Eastern family life—namely, the "childless-by-default," happily married, infertile couple. These couples have usually tried to conceive but have not succeeded. The infertility experience has solidified their commitments to one another and led to the acceptance of life together without children. This form of "childlessness-by-default" is not exactly the same thing as "child-free living"—a term that has emerged in Euro-American discourse to describe voluntary childlessness.[63] It is often argued that voluntary childlessness is only viable in the Western countries;[64] apparently, non-Westerners are unable to live without children. However, this assumption is both Eurocentric and outdated. According to my ethnographic findings, childlessness-by-default—a different form of "child-free living"—*is* becoming a viable option in the Middle Eastern region. There, married couples who are unable to produce a child are often deciding that they are happy to be together. Men in these marriages are usually grateful for their conjugal connectivity with "good wives." And because their subjectivities surrounding manhood are changing (as shown in table 4), fatherhood itself has become less socially mandatory.

In short, a notion of "manhood beyond fatherhood" is emerging. This trend is extremely important but is rarely acknowledged in the various commentaries or scholarship about the region. Middle Eastern men themselves, however, are speaking eloquently about this subject. For example, Michel, a Lebanese Christian man from a small mountain village, whose infertile wife had undergone eight exhausting cycles of IVF, asserted,

I love my wife, and she loves me. I'm the only married son in my family, so my wife feels pressure to do treatment, but I don't. It's just the name. I have the problem from my mother and father to keep the family name going. But, for me, I don't care! Because life is the most important thing, to live comfortably and to live happily. For me, I believe the man needs his wife and the wife, she needs the husband. We're in need of each other. Even if we had children, maybe in the end, we'd still be alone if the children left our village. So a happy marriage is the most important thing. I know that I am the 2 [percent] from 100 percent. Ninety-eight percent [of men] are not like me. [Why?] Because they have "blocked brains" in Lebanon!

Michel is not as rare a masculine subject as he believes. Many childless men in the Middle East are professing their abiding love for their wives and are seeking IVF and ICSI with them. Many men claim that happy marriages are more precious to them than fathering children. This finding is not new to me; even in the late 1980s, I found poor Egyptian men who were utterly devoted to their infertile wives. Furthermore, wives of infertile Egyptian men had some of the happiest marriages, which were marked by tenderness, intimacy, and companionship.[65] Those findings were based on my interviews with women. However, in the new millennium, it is the Middle Eastern men in my studies who have spoken powerfully about the importance of love and marriage over fatherhood.

CONCLUSION

In the end, it is fair to say that male infertility provokes a variety of masculine responses in the Middle East. It may be true that many men still feel deeply emasculated by male infertility, engaging in a "blame game" that implicates their fertile wives and damages their marriages. However, this pattern is changing. With the emergence of semen analysis in the twentieth century, followed by the emergence of ICSI at the turn of the new millennium, a normalization process has been set in motion. In the Middle East today, male infertility is increasingly construed as a medical condition with a high-tech solution. Thus, emergent masculinities speak to new realities, including the questioning of the secrecy and shame surrounding male infertility; the critiquing of patriarchal gender inequities that blame women for childlessness; the resistance to patrilineal family obligations requiring the production of offspring; the acceptance of happy "childless-by-default" living; and the valorization of conjugal love over paternity. Emergent masculinities are incorporating all of these new masculine subjectivities. As a result, male infertility no longer impugns Middle Eastern manhood in the way it once did a generation ago.

CHAPTER 3

Love Stories

HATEM'S SECRET EGG QUEST

I met Hatem and Huda just as they were getting ready to leave the hospital in Beirut. But when I explained my research to them, Hatem seemed especially eager to join the study. Hatem and Huda were not Lebanese, having traveled from rural Syria to undergo a cycle of IVF in Lebanon's capital city. Like most of the Syrian reproductive tourists whom I met in my study, Hatem was convinced that Lebanese IVF clinics were superior to the fledgling clinics in neighboring Syria, a Middle Eastern nation-state that has long been isolated from, and even sanctioned by, the West. Hatem had been bringing his wife to Beirut for IVF since 1997. He had another reason for bringing Huda to Lebanon: there, they could access donor eggs, which were unavailable in the Sunni-dominant country of Syria, where third-party gamete donation is strictly prohibited.

Double first cousins (through both the paternal and maternal sides) and married for seventeen years, Hatem and Huda clearly loved each other, despite the perplexing dilemma of her premature ovarian failure. Although Huda was only thirty-six at the time of our interview, she had entered menopause in her twenties. She required hormonal stimulation followed by IVF in order to achieve a pregnancy. After five unsuccessful IVF attempts, the physicians in Beirut recommended egg donation as the most likely successful option. As Sunni Muslims, Hatem and Huda knew that egg donation was forbidden in the religion. Yet, as Hatem explained, they rationalized their use of donor eggs in a previous IVF cycle in the following way,

> As long as the donor agrees, then this would reduce the *haram* [forbiddenness] based on our religion. Because she, the donor, is in need of money, she gave nine to ten eggs, and the doctor divided the eggs between that couple and us. We took five, and that couple, who were recently married, took five. And I personally entered into the lab to make sure that *my* sperm were being used. It's okay because it's *my* sperm.

After IVF with donor eggs, Huda became pregnant with twins, a male and a female. At six months and seventeen days of pregnancy, however, she began to miscarry, and Hatem rushed her to a hospital in Syria. As Hatem recounts,

> They opened her stomach [by cesarean], and there were twins, who still lived for forty-eight hours. They had lung deficiency because they were little and not fully developed. The girl died twelve hours before the boy.

After this traumatic experience, Huda could no longer accept the idea of egg donation. According to Hatem, who spoke for Huda as she sat quietly in the room,

> She was tortured [during the pregnancy]. She stayed four months vomiting whatever she ate, and she lost weight—from eighty-eight to fifty-five kilograms. And she was under a lot of stress because of our social environment in Syria. In our [farming] community, they stare at babies and see if they resemble the mother and father. We are not living in a city of 4–5 million. We are in a closed community of 15,000 people. And so, the first time, when we had twins, they did a blood test [because blood was needed] and everyone was surprised. Their blood group was AB, and it didn't match ours. Now everyone will *really* examine the personal traits of this [donor] baby if we do it again. They will look at us suspiciously. Not the doctors; they keep everything confidential. But people in the community who might come to visit and look at us curiously.

For his part, Hatem is willing to accept donor eggs again and has already made inquiries about finding a willing Shia Muslim egg donor in Syria. On the day of our interview, we also spoke about the possibility of finding a willing donor within the Beirut IVF clinic. Hatem saw no other way to achieve parenthood, given that he loves his wife and refuses to divorce her. Even though Hatem is an affluent farmer from a large family of twenty children (by one father and three co-wives), he has resisted all forms of social pressure to divorce or marry polygynously. His commitment, he says, is based on his deep love for Huda. As he told me,

> Had I not loved her, I wouldn't have waited for seventeen years. I would have married another. By religious law, I can remarry, but I don't want to. She told me I should marry another woman, and she even offered or suggested that she would get me engaged, because we're already old. We've reached middle age without kids. We're living in a large family with six of my brothers, and they all have children. That's why she's feeling very depressed and very angry that she's alone without children, although she's always surrounded by children. But, of course, she keeps these feelings to herself.

He continued,

> The love between us—I love her *a lot*. I was the one who considered going for IVF, for her sake. But we must keep it secret, because if my parents knew about us having an IVF child, the child would be marginalized and living a lonely life. So we keep everything secret, and we just mention to our families that she's receiving treatment.

As in so many IVF and ICSI stories, Huda and Hatem were ultimately unsuccessful in their seventh attempted IVF cycle. Huda's own eggs failed to mature under hormonal stimulation, and no egg donors were currently available at the clinic. Thus, Hatem and Huda returned home quietly to Syria, with little remaining hope of achieving parenthood, but with the love that had kept them together for nearly twenty years.[1]

Notes on Love in the Middle East

Although Hatem's love for his infertile wife Huda may seem exceptional, I would argue that it is not. Husbands' loving commitments toward their wives are a major part of Middle Eastern conjugality and an important feature of emergent masculinities in the region. Even seemingly traditional men such as Hatem—a farmer from a "closed" rural Syrian community—defy masculine stereotypes. Although conventional wisdom suggests that Middle Eastern men routinely divorce their infertile wives, Hatem's case provides evidence to the contrary. His story—and hundreds of others that I have collected over the past twenty years—suggest that enduring conjugal commitments are a key feature of emergent masculinities in the Middle East, even in the face of intractable infertility. Men such as Hatem love their infertile wives, just as wives love their infertile husbands. In many if not most cases of infertility, conjugal love prevails. According to my studies, this is as true among lower-class Middle Eastern couples—both urban and rural—as it is among cosmopolitan elites.[2] For example, Hatem hails from a relatively remote farming community, where he is surrounded by fertile family members, who urge him to remarry in order to have children. However, he defies such cultural expectations, and instead does everything in his power to help his wife Huda overcome her infertility. This includes covert and costly travel to Beirut for repeated IVF cycles, as well as secret quests for donor eggs, which are prohibited in Sunni Muslim countries. Hatem's love for his wife prevails over religious orthodoxy and is a love that he proclaims ardently and freely—to Huda and to the American anthropologist. In short, for Hatem, Huda is his *habiba*, his loved one, and nothing can tear them apart.

If, as I argue, Hatem and Huda's marital love story is quite typical, then it is important to begin by attempting to describe what love is and means in the Muslim Middle East. Understanding love is also anthropologically timely, in light of the increasing theorization and empirical investigation of this concept in the new millennium.[3] Recent anthropological inquiries have taken up the topic of love, focusing primarily on so-called romantic (or passionate) love and its biological, cognitive, and social parameters. One of the major goals of this growing body of literature has been to disprove an early scholarly notion—one found within the discipline of anthropology itself—that romantic love cannot be found in non-Euro-American contexts. Many early studies promoted an ethnocentric claim that romantic love "is a European contribution to world culture."[4] However, in their groundbreaking cross-cultural study of romantic love in 166 societies, William Jankowiak and Edward Fischer discovered that romantic love was a "near-universal" feature of the societies they studied, with romantic love being defined for the purposes of their investigation as "an intense attraction that involves the idealization of the other, within an erotic context, with the expectation of enduring for some time into the future."[5] They contrasted this definition of romantic love with "the companionship phase of love (sometimes referred to as attachment) which is characterized by the growth of a more peaceful, comfortable, and fulfilling relationship; it is a strong and enduring affection built upon long term association."[6]

Such dualities are common in the scholarly literature on love. As noted by Victor de Munck in his study of "Love and Marriage in a Sri Lankan Muslim Community,"[7] anthropological studies in South Asia have tended to divide marriage into two types: "arranged" versus "love" marriages. The increasing frequency and acceptability of love marriages in otherwise arranged-marriage societies throughout the region has generally been attributed to processes of social change, including industrialization, modernization, urbanization, and Westernization, all of which are seen as correlated with the decreasing importance of the joint or extended family as a corporate unit and the consequent growth of nuclear families and individual autonomy. However, as de Munck discovered in his own study in a Muslim community in Sri Lanka, "love can be accommodated to an arranged marriage model," with many arranged marriages being, in fact, "romantically motivated."[8]

The division of conjugality into oppositional types—"romantic" versus "companionate" and "arranged" versus "love"—is inherently problematic, as many marriages around the world may combine all of these features simultaneously. In the Middle East, for example, the widely held expectation is that romantic love and sexual desire will develop over time *within* arranged marriages, such that arranged marriages *become* love marriages over time. Furthermore, as in de Munck's South Asian example, many so-called arranged marriages in the Middle Eastern region begin with desire, longing, and sexual attraction, or, to use de Munck's term, "romantic motivation." Similarly, the romantic versus companionate marriage duality is inherently problematic, in that many long-term "companionate" marriages in the Middle East are characterized by ongoing "romance" and satisfying sexual lives. The assumption that romantic love somehow fades over time into a friendly but asexual, platonic "companionship" needs to be questioned for marriages in the Middle East, as elsewhere.[9]

Furthermore, what Jankowiak and Fischer call "the validity of an affectionless past"—namely, that love is a fairly recent European invention with no historical tradition outside of the West—is patently untrue. As shown by anthropologists working in non-Western societies around the world, "long traditions of romantic love"[10] may be found and even valorized in many societies through fables, songs, poetry, and other forms of popular culture.[11] In her seminal study, *Notes on Love in a Tamil Family*, anthropologist Margaret Trawick shows how love saturates Tamil society in South India.[12] Speaking of her informants' lives, Trawick writes, "They had been exposed to many formal teachings expounding upon and extolling love, and they were surrounded, filled, and made into human beings by a culture that said in a thousand ways that love was the highest good."[13] As these studies suggest, the challenge for anthropology, then, is to interrogate the very real possibility that love exists in "unlikely places"—including the supposedly violent and loveless Middle East.

In *The Map of Love*, Egyptian novelist Ahdaf Soueif writes,

> "Hubb" is love, "ishq" is love that entwines two people together, "shaghaf" is love that nests in the chambers of the heart, "hayam" is love that wanders the earth, "teeh" is love in which you lose yourself, "walah" is love that carries sorrow within it, "sababah" is love that exudes from your pores, "hawa" is love that shares its name with "air," and with "falling," "gharm" is love that is willing to pay the price.[14]

Among these nine forms of love, *hubb* is the base, and it is among the most highly extolled virtues in Middle Eastern society, expounded upon in many formal spiritual teachings and literally omnipresent in everyday popular culture. The Middle Eastern region is replete with love stories in music, literature, and poetry, both now and in the past. The most popular Arabic songs and movies depict *hubb* as involving longing, attraction, desire—often unrequited—thus leading to even more pronounced longing, attraction, and desire, as well as heartbreak and suffering. It is fair to say that Middle Eastern culture is imbued with *hubb*.

Even more important from an anthropological perspective, love permeates the actual affective relations between spouses, parents and children, and other close kith and kin. Across the Arabic-speaking Middle East, husbands and wives, parents and children, close kin, and close friends refer to each other by terms derived from *hubb*. Among the most uttered phrases in everyday life are *habibi* (male) and *habibti* (female), literally translated as "my love" or "my loved one," but also glossed semiotically as "my dear," "my dear friend," or simply "my friend." The fact that one of the most common terms of reference in the Arabic-speaking world is derived directly from the word *hubb* reflects the importance of love and its salience for connecting people into deeply enmeshed relations of emotion, affection, and care.

Furthermore, *hubb* is a major part of the spiritual realm in the Muslim world. The ascetic and mystical tradition known as Sufism has been implicitly present in Islam ever since its inception, eventually becoming explicit during the first Islamic centuries (the seventh and eighth centuries C.E.).[15] Sufi mystics have devoted their spiritual quests to God's limitless grace, mercy, and divine majesty. As noted by Sufi scholar Alexander Knysh, this emphasis on the "love of God" finds justification in the Qur'anic verse, "He [God] loves them, and they love Him" (5:54/57). Knysh explains, "Inspired by this and similar verses and traditions, the early mystics began to celebrate their longing for the Divine beloved in poems and utterances of exceptional beauty and verve. It was this exalted love and longing which, in their eyes, justified the austerities to which they subjected themselves in order to demonstrate their faithfulness to the heavenly Beloved."[16] Love of an inherently loving God continues to be extolled as one of the most important elements of Islam, not only in its mystical form. The Qur'an and other Islamic scriptures describe God as loving, compassionate, and merciful, particularly toward those Muslim believers who are faithful and loving to God in return.

Having said this, it is important to note that human love—including conjugal love and affection—receives no particular ideological valorization in the Islamic scriptures. The right to sexual fulfillment and marital fidelity are explicitly mandated in Islam,[17] but marital love itself is not idealized. Instead, some Middle Eastern feminist scholars have argued that Islam militates *against* strong, loving marriages by way of Islamic personal status laws that lead to the "fragility of marital bonds."[18] One of the strongest statements of this position can be found in feminist sociologist Mounira Charrad's award-winning volume, *States and Women's Rights: The Making of Postcolonial Tunisia, Algeria, and Morocco.*[19] According to Charrad, "Far from fostering the development of long-lasting, strong emotional ties between husband and wife, the law underplays the formation and continuity of independent and stable conjugal units. This shows in particular in the procedure to terminate marriage, the legality of polygamy, and the absence of community property between husband and wife."[20] With regard to infertility, Charrad notes that the legality of polygamy allows a man to marry a second wife in the hope of having heirs, particularly sons. However, she also notes that despite Western stereotypes of widespread marital polygamy and "images of harems [that] have captured the imagination of Western observers,"[21] polygamy is statistically insignificant in most Middle Eastern countries, outlawed in both Morocco and Tunisia and practiced by only a few, generally between 1 and 5 percent of married men, in other Middle Eastern nations.[22]

Love in Middle Eastern Marriage

Against this backdrop of a Middle Eastern feminist argument that Islamic personal status laws militate against strong and loving marriages, there is much evidence to the contrary, including within Islam itself. In the Islamic scriptures, marriage is considered a moral and legal mandate, and adultery is a major sin.[23] While allowing for divorce, Islam clearly extols the virtues of marriage, regarding it as *Sunna*, or the way of the Prophet Muhammad and as the "completion of half of the religion" (with worship and service to God completing the remaining half). Thus, Middle Easterners are among the "most married" people in the world,[24] with well over 90 percent of adults marrying at least once in a lifetime. Divorce rates are also relatively low, around 25 percent,[25] about the same as American couples who married in the 1980s, but only half the 50 percent U.S. divorce rate of the 1970s.[26] Among Middle Eastern Christian populations, men and women, once married, are generally forbidden to divorce. In fact, lifelong, monogamous marriage is a highly valued and normatively upheld institution throughout the Middle East, among *both* Muslims and Christians.

In addition, marriage is regarded as a "protection" for both women and men, especially against the desire for illicit sexuality and procreation. Within the Middle East, sex and childbearing are expected to occur with the confines of marriage. Remaining single by choice, especially to experiment with multiple sexual partners, is socially penalized for both men and women. Furthermore, cohabitation between unmarried adults of the opposite sex—a historically recent but increasing pattern in Western countries including the United States[27]—is rare among Middle Eastern adults of any social class or educational background. Given this propensity and pressure to marry, Middle Easterners in general take the call to marriage quite seriously, with most adults marrying at least once in a lifetime. As noted by Diane Singerman and Barbara Ibrahim in their path-breaking study of marriage economies in Egypt,

Marriage is an event infused with multiple meanings in the lives of Egyptians. It is a civil contract between two families with legally binding conditions on both parties. Marriage is a means for consolidation of social status, and in a conservative society, it also provides the only approved access for young men and women to sexual and reproductive partners. In the Arab world in general, and in Egypt in particular, marriage is considered a "social pinnacle and major turning point in the lives of both men and women," heralding the transition to full-fledged adulthood.[28]

As suggested by Singerman and Ibrahim, most marriages in the Middle East are typically arranged or at least semiarranged through family intercession, even among educated elites. Love is expected to emerge *after* marriage through the intense experience surrounding the birth and parenting of children. Middle Eastern societies are decidedly pronatalist: they highly value children for numerous reasons and expect all marriages to produce them.[29] As a result, few Middle Eastern newlyweds postpone marital procreation through the use of contraceptives, and most hope to achieve parenthood within the first conjugal year. In short, children are usually desired from the very beginning of marriage and are loved and cherished once they are born.

In this social setting of expected marital procreativity, the notion of a married couple living happily without children is unthinkable. Marriages are deemed inherently fragile and unstable until children are born. The absence of a culturally constructed notion of the couple is particularly problematic in infertile marriages, because in social structural terms, a husband and wife without children do not constitute a socially recognized, definable unit. Infertile couples are socially scrutinized and are usually under intense family pressure, especially on the part of husbands' relatives, to realize their procreative potential.

Yet, despite all this, infertile marriages in the Middle East are often quite successful and may be even more successful than fertile marriages with children. Why? A number of factors seem to be important. First, what might best be called the *romantically companionate marriage*—in which marital partners look to each other for love, emotional intimacy, friendship, and sexual fulfillment—is clearly emerging as the ideal form across the Middle East.[30] Scholars have found clear historical precedents for companionate marriage throughout the region, a pattern that appears to be intensifying over time.[31] According to Lila Abu-Lughod's studies of Egypt, for example, the idea of companionate marriage is endorsed today by both liberal secularists and Islamists in the country, the latter of whom are "framing an ideal of companionate marriage in Islamic terms."[32]

As I have argued in my own work on Egypt, most infertile marriages are characterized by *conjugal connectivity*.[33] I have derived this term from anthropologist Suad Joseph's important insights on *patriarchal connectivity*—or the ways in which Middle Eastern patriarchy operates through both male domination and loving commitments.[34] According to Joseph, socialization within Arab families places a premium on "connectivity," or the intensive bonding of individuals through love, involvement, and commitment. Extending Joseph's analysis, I suggest that the loving commitments of patriarchal connectivity, which are socialized within the Arab family, also operate in the marital sphere. Both men and women, including poor men and women, are negotiating new kinds of marital relationships—relationships based on the kind of loving connectivity that is experienced and expected in families of origin but has heretofore been unexpected and unexamined within the conjugal unit. That conjugal connectivity is true even among *infertile* Middle Eastern Muslim couples attests to shifting marital praxis and the importance of love, mutual respect, and the sharing of life's problems even in the absence of desired children. Despite widespread expectations within the Middle East that infertile marriages are bound to fail—with men necessarily blaming women for the infertility and divorcing or replacing them if they do not produce children, especially sons—such expectations may represent indigenous stereotypes based on the aforementioned features of Islamic personal status law.[35] As I would argue instead, the success of so many infertile marriages in the Middle East bespeaks the strengthening of conjugal connectivity at the expense of patriarchy, legal or otherwise, that is being undermined.[36]

As shown in the story of Hatem and Huda, Middle Eastern couples may experience an even more intense conjugal connection as a result of childlessness. Why? On the one hand, couples without children come to know each other better and to appreciate each other for their virtues apart from parenting. Although parenting, in and of itself, may be a very joyous and rewarding experience for couples everywhere, children are also a major responsibility for a husband and wife, who may focus more on the children than on each other. That childcare and childrearing may detract from the marital relationship itself has been shown in a wide variety of North American studies.[37] But this may be especially true in the Middle Eastern region, where childbearing occurs almost immediately after arranged marriage, at a time when a new husband and wife are only beginning to know each other.

Among couples who are unable to conceive within the first years of marriage, feelings of conjugal connectivity may be more likely to emerge over time, because a husband and wife are not distracted from their marital relationship by children. Infertile couples do not have to worry over childhood sicknesses and troubles in school. Infertile couples are not required to feed and economically support children in the context of serious economic constraints. And infertile couples do not feel the diminished marital intimacy that comes from exhaustion, breastfeeding, and little ones in the bedroom. In short, children do not come between infertile partners, who instead look to each other for love, affection, and support. The actual improvements in marital intimacy that may occur among infertile couples have been reported in the United States and European countries such as Denmark, where romantically companionate marriages are a widely held ideal.[38] However, the fact that infertility may strengthen marital intimacy elsewhere, including in the purportedly patriarchal and loveless societies of the Middle East, is an underappreciated reality.

In my earlier studies of infertility in Egypt, the vast majority of couples had achieved long-term, relatively stable marriages, and they openly professed their feelings of love and enduring marital commitment. Among the urban poor, such marital success was not what I—nor my informants—expected; but it was one of my most important and surprising findings.[39] In my later study of Egyptian elites, such love and acceptance was manifest in the sheer length of infertile marriages.[40] To wit, 20 percent of couples in my 1996 study had been married fewer than five years; 45 percent had been married six to ten years; 22 percent had been married eleven to fifteen years; 11 percent had been married sixteen to twenty years; and 3 percent had been married over twenty years, with the longest childless marriage lasting twenty-eight years. Overall, the average length of childless marriage was nine and a half years, or nearly a decade.

Many Egyptian women, including those who were themselves infertile and those married to infertile Egyptian men, told me that they had strong marriages to loving husbands. They considered their husbands to be their friends, whom they would never leave over infertility, and who they believed would never leave them either. I was struck by the tremendous amounts of love and commitment displayed by both Muslim and Christian Egyptian women to their long-term infertile husbands. Husbands whom I interviewed with their wives, usually at their wives' bedsides in Egyptian IVF clinics, also commented on the strength of their marriages, often holding their wives' hands or caressing their hair during interviews.

MIDDLE EASTERN MEN'S INFERTILE MARRIAGES

I was equally impressed when I had my first opportunity to interview Middle Eastern men alone, which occurred in Beirut, Lebanon in 2003. As noted in the introduction, 120 of the men in my Lebanese study were infertile, while 100 of them were fertile but married to infertile wives. They

hailed from three countries, Lebanon, Syria, and Palestine. In my reproductive life history interviews, I asked basic questions about marriage (e.g.,
How long have you and your wife been married?). But I did not prompt
men to comment on the quality of their marriages, nor did I ever ask if they
loved their wives. Nonetheless, in my interviews with these men, I was
literally inundated with *hubb*. Over and over, both fertile and infertile men
volunteered that they loved their wives, and would never consider divorcing them, even if it meant living a life without children. When I asked men
routinely,"Is this your first marriage?" the most common response was"the
first *and* the last," with some men adding emphatically, "I love my wife,"
"she is a good person," or"I would marry her again."

Interestingly, slightly more than half of these men (55%) said that
they had married"for love," either because a"love story" had developed at
school or at work or because they had met a woman to whom they were
extremely physically attracted,"falling in love" with her, sometimes at"first
sight." As in Hatem's case, seventeen men (8%) agreed to marry younger
cousins for this reason. Even among the hundred men (45%) who said
that their marriages were arranged by their families—usually with cousins, neighbors, or family friends—few men felt forced to marry. They often
agreed to these marriages because of physical and emotional attraction to
their prospective spouses. As some of these men explained it,"It was a'traditional' marriage, but now we're in love," or"We're lucky, because we're in
love now." In short, both"love" and"arranged" marriages among these men
were generally romantically motivated. And, for the majority, love continued well after marriage—often growing in intensity—despite the problems of marital fertility. Many men expressed a veritable outpouring of love
during interviews when the subject of marriage was broached (table 5).

Interestingly, marital research conducted in the United States suggests
that men's willingness to openly express their love, affection, and"fondness" for a spouse is one of the best predictors of marital strength and stability against divorce.[41] The fondness expressed by men about their wives,
as reflected in table 5, suggests that many Middle Eastern infertile marriages are much stronger than predicted, even by the infertile themselves.

Furthermore, in interviews where wives were also present or entered
the conversation at least briefly, men were often openly solicitous and
affectionate, kissing their wives, holding their hands, putting their arms
around them, or stroking their hair. When I asked men privately about
their sex lives, most men told me that they were faithful to their wives, with
only nine men (five fertile, four infertile) admitting to infidelities. Most
men were quite emphatic about their marital fidelity. They explained that
they may have had other girlfriends or casual sexual partners before marriage, but never afterward. Not only is adultery considered a form of *zina*,
or illicit sexuality in all of the major religions of the Middle East, but most

TABLE 5. Men's comments about love and marriage

Country	Fertility Status	Comments
Lebanese	Fertile	Not all men feel this way. But about my marriage, in our case about me, I don't care if she did or didn't have children. I love my wife. That's it. But every case is different.
Lebanese	Fertile	She loves me more in an emotional way. She shows her love more than I do. But I love her more with my mind. I understand her, and when there is understanding between partners, it's better than just love. As long as we're able to support each other, we have no problems. I would never consider divorcing her when she has this problem [infertility], because she might die [of heartbreak]. That is *haram* [forbidden]!
Lebanese	Infertile	We were in love and I went to a doctor and knew [about his infertility problem]. I tried to convince her not to marry me, but she refused. She doesn't care if we have children or not. She doesn't care if she gets pregnant or not. We've been married four years and there is a *strong* love. If there is love and logic, it will never affect our marriage.
Lebanese	Infertile	If you ask me about our problems, if this [infertility] is a problem, I say we have no problems. If I married another time, I'd take my wife. She's my baby.
Lebanese, living in USA	Fertile	I love her. Even if I married a second woman, I'd keep her. But I'm not going to marry a second woman. She's been good to me. I'm not going to dump her!
Lebanese	Fertile	[Is she your first marriage?] The first and the last!
Lebanese, living in Brazil	Fertile	I came back to Lebanon to try for a second IVF child, because I'm in love with her. I love her very much. That's why I'm in this country.
Syrian	Infertile	I hate the thought of babies because of her. I love her and I hate to see her suffer because of this.
Lebanese Armenian	Infertile	If I can only get one child, I'd like a girl. The girls, it's not that they're more loving than boys, but if life was under the hands of girls, it would be better! This is why I like my wife *so much!* She doesn't think of hurting people.
Lebanese	Fertile	We've been married twelve years, and if I had not been comfortable in the situation we've been going through, I would have left her a long time ago. But my marriage is good, *hamdu-lillah* [praise be to God]! Maybe from her outer appearance she's not beautiful, but from inside, she's beautiful.
Lebanese	Infertile	[Is this your first marriage?] It's the end! I love her! Our marriage is very good—no, excellent!
Lebanese	Fertile	We have understanding between us. We've spent so many years together that it would be difficult to leave her.

TABLE 5. Men's comments about love and marriage *(continued)*

Country	Fertility Status	Comments
Lebanese Armenian	Infertile	I'm doing ICSI for her. I'm not obliged to have kids except for her. She's a human being, and she needs to become a mother.
Palestinian	Infertile	I quit smoking because she has asthma and I love her very much.
Lebanese	Infertile	We have a very good marriage—I hope forever.
Lebanese, living in Venezuela	Infertile	[Is this your first marriage?] Hopefully, the last!
Lebanese	Infertile	My wife, she's good. We are a couple; we are company for each other. We have no discrimination between the man in the house and the woman in the house. She's my friend. My society is like that. I'm not exclusively like this with my wife. Eighty percent of the people I know are like that, including in my family.
Lebanese	Infertile	Love comes as a result of marriage. Before marriage, you discover common areas, attraction develops. But when two people unite [in marriage], they become more understanding of each other and love develops. Based on my age, forty-one years old, I think in a different way as compared to younger men. I'm more concerned about knowing her and understanding her than loving her, because when I become more and more understanding of her, I will give her as much as possible.
Lebanese Armenian	Fertile	I have a good wife. Why do we need children?
Lebanese	Infertile	She's my hashish [i.e., intoxicant]!
Lebanese	Infertile	So many times I've tried to comfort my wife, to let her know that not having children is not a big problem for us. But you know the Oriental woman, she thinks if we don't have children, maybe I'll divorce her. But I would never do that. I try always to convince her that I love her and this is not a problem.
Lebanese	Infertile	I care for her feelings more than I care for myself. She is a human being, and she has the right to say that "I need children."
Lebanese, living in Cote d'Ivoire	Infertile	Before marriage, I used to love my girlfriends, but I couldn't stay with only one. But after marriage, I became stable, because I love her very much, both her nature and her body. I love her a lot, and I consider her not just a sex partner like before [with other women].
Lebanese	Fertile	I don't have a problem, because I love my wife. We understand each other. My wife, she loves kids, and so this [IVF] is for her.
Lebanese, living in USA	Fertile	Infertility affects us, but not our marriage. Actually, it got stronger because of going through this together.

TABLE 5. Men's comments about love and marriage *(continued)*

Country	Fertility Status	Comments
Lebanese	Infertile	We are living a nice couple's life, and we have a lot of things we like to do together. You have to consider that we fell in love ten years ago. And in [Lebanese] Christianity, marriage is never just a way to get children. And that's why, with or without children, the relationship between the couple is unquestioned. Not having a family or staying together as a couple, not having children doesn't threaten marriage.
Lebanese	Fertile	After nine years of marriage and five operations [IVFs], it must be love!
Syrian	Fertile	I am protecting her because I love her, of course. People would tell me to marry again if they knew [she was infertile], and I don't want to. She's beautiful to me; her conduct is beautiful.
Lebanese	Fertile	I love my wife, and she loves me. Our marriage is *very* good. I love her, and she loves me.
Syrian	Infertile	It was love at first sight!
Lebanese, living in USA	Fertile	She is more than good! I still believe I can't find anyone better.
Lebanese	Infertile	The last four years, it was a good marriage, and it's still a good marriage!
Syrian	Infertile	I love her so much! We have an excellent relationship, and always will, *insha'Allah* [God willing].
Lebanese, living in Saudi Arabia	Fertile	I keep supporting her, because I very much appreciate the effort she's going through, because it *is* an effort [to do IVF across borders]. I'm supporting her the best way I can, because I love her.
Lebanese	Fertile	I'm happy with my wife. We have a perfect marriage. She has a career she likes. I have a career I like. We don't feel something is missing. Why don't others accept this?
Yemeni, living in USA, but wife in Yemen	Infertile	My marriage was totally arranged by our families. But now I love her. She's my lover.
Iraqi refugee, living in USA and married to another Iraqi refugee	Infertile	We were both refugees in Saudi Arabia. I met her, and I loved her. I did a lot of things to get married to her. And I still love her.

men in my study considered it to be disloyal to the wives they loved. As one man simply put it, "No way! I love her too much."

In fact, I asked all 220 men in my Lebanese study a series of questions about their sex lives. Nearly one-third of these men (30%) had never had another sexual partner other than their current wife. A few men seemed slightly embarrassed to admit marital virginity, or as one man put it, "Maybe you won't believe this, but it was when I got married. She was the first." However, others were proud of their lifetime monogamy, fidelity, and morality. For example, one man stated emphatically, "No girlfriends! No sexual relations!" while another man answered my question, "When did you first have sex?" by saying, "On my wedding night. Never before, and with no one else after!"

Eight percent of men in my study had had only two sexual partners, either because they had divorced and remarried or because they had one serious girlfriend before marriage. Exactly two-thirds of the men in my study (66%) reported sex with fewer than ten lifetime partners. These were mostly men who had lived their entire lives in Lebanon or Syria, where premarital sexuality does occur, but in a limited fashion compared to the West. As one Lebanese man explained, "It is very rare in Lebanon to have multiple partners, or sex before marriage." Another put it more whimsically, "In Lebanon, because of religion, you have to take sex like a thief! Lebanon is not sexually open like America, which is why all Lebanese men want to go there! "Virtually all of the men who reported more than ten sexual partners had spent their youths outside the Middle East, in either West Africa, Europe, Latin America, or the United States. This was particularly true of the 30 men (17%) who claimed to have had more than 100 sexual partners, or "so many" that the numbers were "uncountable." As we will see in later chapters, not all of these men were proud of their sexual pasts, sometimes openly regretting the dissipation of their reproductive potential.

Moreover, not all of these men were in their first marriages. Of the 220 men (both fertile and infertile) I interviewed in Lebanon, 27—or 12 percent—had been married before, as had 5 (2 percent) of their wives. These divorce rates are significantly less than those found in the United States, where 50 percent of those married in the 1970s have divorced (although divorce rates in the United States have significantly declined).[42] Interestingly, of the thirty Middle Eastern–born infertile men whom I interviewed in Arab Detroit, Michigan, ten of them—or exactly one-third—had divorced since arriving in the United States. After talking to these men, it was my general impression that "divorce, American-style" was easier to obtain than in the Middle East, not only for husbands but also for wives, several of whom had left their husbands over male infertility.

In the Middle East, in general, divorce is socially frowned upon by Muslims and is generally unavailable to Christians of all denominations. A

Lebanese Sunni Muslim man, who was living in the United States and had recently divorced his American wife, agreed shortly thereafter to an arranged marriage with a Lebanese woman. He explained, "Over here [in Lebanon], divorce is like a disaster! It's *not* a disaster, but over here, it's like the end of the world!" Most Christian men in my study described their marriages as being "for life," as divorce is religiously prohibited to them. When I asked one man, a Syrian Catholic, if this was his first marriage, he quipped, "If I were able to marry for a second time, I wouldn't be here doing IVF!" But then he explained, more seriously, "Among Christians, there is no divorce. All of them—Catholic, Orthodox, and Protestant. In the Arab world, you're allowed one only, and if she's infertile, you are not allowed to marry a second time."[43]

Of all of the divorces I encountered in my studies in Lebanon and Arab Detroit, most were after brief first marriages, either with foreign women or with cousins, which were incompatible and did not produce children (table 6). With only a few exceptions, these men had remarried and were

TABLE 6. Histories of divorce

Country	Husband or Wife Divorced	Their Fertility Status	Circumstances of the Divorce
Lebanese	Husband	Fertile	He divorced his first wife, who is his cousin, after 29 years of marriage and eight children (seven girls, one boy); cited many marital problems; remarried a woman who is infertile because of her age (42).
Lebanese	Husband	Fertile	Lebanese refugee to the USA, with two brief green-card marriages; he married a third wife (Lebanese American) "for love, the American way!"
Lebanese	Husband and wife	Infertile husband, fertile wife	He married a fertile woman, had ICSI twin daughters, divorced her and kept the twins; he remarried a divorced fertile woman whose first husband kept their twins (a boy and girl); in short, two women lost their twins to their ex-husbands.
Lebanese Armenian	Husband	Infertile	His first wife wanted to move to the USA with their two daughters, but he did not; he remarried an Armenian woman and discovered he is now infertile.
Lebanese	Husband and wife	Both infertile	He had two brief, one-year marriages, the first "for love" and the second to a divorcée with four children; both ended because of "family interference"; he is married to his third wife, who was divorced by her first husband over infertility; their current marriage is infertile and unstable; he is contemplating divorce.

Table 6. Histories of divorce *(continued)*

Country	Husband or Wife Divorced	Their Fertility Status	Circumstances of the Divorce
Syrian	Husband	Fertile	He married his first cousin but divorced her because of her infertility; he remarried and had two daughters, but divorced his second wife when his first wife wanted to return to him; he is currently married to his first wife, though he sees his daughters regularly.
Lebanese	Husband	Infertile	His parents pressured him to divorce his first wife, who is his first cousin, even though he is the cause of the infertility; he remarried, but she did not.
Lebanese	Husband	Infertile	He married a Palestinian woman during his war refuge in Switzerland; she wanted to remain there but he did not, so they divorced.
Lebanese, living in Cote d'Ivoire	Husband	Infertile	He had a brief, incompatible marriage to his cousin, which ended mutually after one year; he remarried a teenaged woman, ten years his junior.
Palestinian Lebanese, who lived most of adult life in USA	Husband	Fertile	He married an American Jewish woman and had a son; she asked for a divorce after five years because of financial problems; he sees his son twice a year; he remarried a 43-year-old Lebanese woman, a neighbor, who is infertile.
Lebanese	Husband	Infertile	He had a brief marriage to his cousin, which ended after four months; he fled to Switzerland as a war refugee, marrying an older, divorced, alcoholic British woman to obtain citizenship and receive her care; after eight years, he divorced her and married his third wife, also a cousin, producing ICSI twin sons with her.
Lebanese, living in the USA	Husband	Infertile, both husband and wife	He divorced his American wife after twelve years over infertility and cultural differences; they remain friends; he remarried a Lebanese woman who is also infertile because of her age (40); he questions whether he made the right decision.
Lebanese	Husband and wife	Unexplained infertility	He divorced his first wife after ten years because of infertility; he remarried a widow with three children and has been married for twelve years; he has threatened to divorce her or take a second wife if she does not bear his own children.
Lebanese	Husband	Infertile	His first wife divorced him after three years because of infertility and pressure from her parents; he remarried his first cousin and had an ICSI son with Down syndrome, who passed away at eight months.

TABLE 6. Histories of divorce *(continued)*

Country	Husband or Wife Divorced	Their Fertility Status	Circumstances of the Divorce
Lebanese	Husband	Fertile	He divorced his cousin after one year of marriage and the birth of a son; he remarried an infertile woman and has custody of his teenaged son.
Lebanese	Husband	Infertile	His first wife divorced him after four years of marriage because of his infertility; she was young and pressured by her family to have children.
Lebanese, living in Nigeria	Husband	Infertile	He had two brief marriages to Europeans (a Belgian for six months, a German for three years) while living in Dubai; he remarried a Lebanese woman.
Lebanese, living in Senegal	Husband	Fertile	His first marriage lasted five months, and he paid $25,000 to divorce; he is now married to an infertile woman.
Lebanese	Husband	Infertile	He was married briefly to a Latina while living in the USA as a student; she got pregnant and had an abortion; they divorced on friendly terms.
Lebanese, living in Netherlands	Husband	Infertile	He had a two-year"passport marriage"to a Dutch woman; he remarried a Lebanese woman.
Lebanese	Husband	Infertile	He had a nine-year marriage with two children and is on"good terms"with his ex-wife; the children live with him and his second wife; he has developed an infertility problem.
Lebanese	Husband	Fertile	He divorced his first wife and has custody of their two daughters; he remarried in order for his daughters to have a stepmother, but is unhappy in his second marriage; he and his first wife secretly see each other.
Lebanese	Wife	Fertile	His wife was divorced with a small son; he married her and has been a father to the child, who now works with him.
Lebanese	Husband	Fertile	He divorced his first wife after eleven years of marriage and the birth of two girls; his teenage daughters live with him and his new wife, who is infertile because of her age.
Lebanese	Husband	Fertile	His brief first marriage of three years was a"bad story."
Lebanese	Husband	Fertile	His American wife divorced him after two years of marriage, when he returned to Lebanon during the war and did not/could not communicate with her.

TABLE 6. Histories of divorce *(continued)*

Country	Husband or Wife Divorced	Their Fertility Status	Circumstances of the Divorce
Lebanese	Husband	Fertile	He had a brief, incompatible two-year marriage to his cousin.
Syrian	Husband and wife	Fertile husband, infertile wife	He divorced after eight years of marriage without children; he remarried a divorcee with a disabled daughter; he is unhappy in his second marriage.
Iraqi refugee living in USA	Husband	Infertile	His first wife of eight years divorced him because of his infertility and impotence; he remarried his first cousin, bringing her to the USA from Iraq.
Lebanese, living in USA	Husband	Infertile	His wife of seven years divorced him because of his infertility; they parted "on friendly terms," but he is still not remarried.
Lebanese, living in USA	Wife	Fertile	His wife was married to her first cousin for five years; she sought a divorce because "he didn't touch her— no children, no sex, not even hi's and bye's."
Lebanese, living in USA	Husband and wife	Both infertile	Both had fifteen-year marriages to first cousins; his wife divorced him because of azoospermia; her husband died of lymphoma; they remarried in their 40s.
Lebanese, living in USA	Husband	Infertile	He had a brief first marriage in Lebanon during college, but she "fell in love with someone else and my heart was broken"; he remarried a Puerto-Rican American woman and adopted two sons; he fell in love with a Venezuelan woman and divorced his second wife; his ex-wife and sons are angry at him.
Iraqi refugee, living in USA	Husband	Infertile	He divorced his Egyptian American wife of twelve years, who has custody of their three teenaged children; he is remarried to an Iraqi woman and has a number of health problems, including infertility.
Lebanese, living in USA	Husband	Infertile	He had a brief, two-year marriage to his American girlfriend; they divorced and he remarried a Lebanese woman.
Iraqi refugee, living in USA	Husband	Infertile	His Iraqi refugee wife of three years divorced him over his azoospermia; she remarried and has three children; he still talks to her on the phone and hopes to remarry a woman with children.
Yemeni	Husband	Infertile	He has been married to his first wife for 26 years; he took a younger second wife for three years in order to have children, but he divorced her because of his love for his first wife; the second wife has remarried and has children.

TABLE 6. Histories of divorce *(continued)*

Country	Husband or Wife Divorced	Their Fertility Status	Circumstances of the Divorce
Lebanese, living in USA	Husband and wife	Infertile husband, fertile wife	He was married for eight months to a Lebanese-Canadian woman but divorced her; she was unhappily married with three sons; they were in love as teenagers and "rediscovered" each other at an Arab American festival; the wife divorced her abusive husband and married her former sweetheart; they are hoping to have children together.
Lebanese, living in USA	Husband	Infertile	He had an unhappy, three-year marriage in Lebanon; he divorced her and is not yet remarried.

happy in their second marriages, despite facing current or ongoing infertility problems.

In general, men in this study were happily married. As shown in table 7, only two men were in current polygynous marriages, two men had ended brief polygynous marriages out of love for their first wives, and five men described themselves as being unhappily married, for reasons that varied. In short, not all Middle Eastern men in my study were in "fairy-tale" marriages, but the majority of men were quite happy that they had married their current wives, using the *hubb* word to describe their present conjugality.

The Middle Eastern IVF setting is imbued with *hubb.* In the IVF clinics I attended across the region, scenes of love and affection were readily apparent, as men accompanied their wives to the operating theater, uttering words of encouragement and catering to them at their bedsides. The deep feeling of love, loyalty, and commitment experienced by many Middle Eastern couples, including *both* husbands and wives in childless marriages, is ultimately the major factor behind the tremendous growth of IVF clinics in this region of the world. In fact, love is propelling the booming Middle Eastern assisted reproduction industry forward. Simply put, there would be no IVF clinics in places such as Egypt, Lebanon, Iran, and the Arab Gulf if Middle Eastern men did not love their wives and were therefore unwilling to pursue these costly reproductive technologies. When reproduction is delayed, Middle East men in love with their wives are usually willing to contribute in the ways that they can to mutually agreed-upon reproductive goals.

Table 7. Unstable and polygynous marriages

Country	Husband or Wife Unhappy	Fertility Status	Circumstances of the Marriage
Lebanese	Husband	Fertile	He married an older woman, who is a colleague, to "escape" his feelings for his girlfriend from a "disallowed" religious group; he does not love his second wife, is not sexually attracted to her, and is contemplating divorce.
Lebanese	Husband	Infertile	He knew he was infertile, but did not tell his "traditional" wife, whom he did not marry for love; he is having an extramarital affair with a "modern" Lebanese woman, while attempting ICSI with his wife.
Palestinian, living in Kuwait	Husband and first wife	Fertile husband, infertile second wife	He fled Lebanon during the civil war, leaving his childhood sweetheart, who is his first cousin, behind; he married another woman and has three children, but has been unhappy; he had a lover for ten years, but decided to take his childhood sweetheart as his second wife; she was a 41-year-old virgin and is infertile because of her age.
Palestinian, living in Lebanon	Husband and first wife	Infertile first wife	His first wife bore a stillborn child and suffered from an infection that rendered her infertile; after eighteen years of marriage, he took a young second wife in order to have children, but he is now impotent and they are trying ICSI; his first wife is unhappy and would still love to be a mother.
Lebanese	Husband	Infertile	He is married for four months and is blaming his wife for not becoming pregnant; he does not accept his poor sperm results; he has given her a "deadline" and has discussed taking a second wife.
Lebanese	Husband	Fertile	He is in a miserable second marriage to an ill-tempered, infertile woman, and wishes he had not divorced his first wife, mother of his two daughters; he secretly sees her in Syria but cannot remarry her according to Druze religious law.
Lebanese, living in USA	Husband	Infertile	He is in a miserable arranged marriage and wants to divorce his wife; he is azoospermic, with a serious chromosomal anomaly and will use this information as a justification for divorce.

Moreover, no matter the cause of the couple's infertility, men often express feelings of profound conjugal empathy. In this study, both fertile and infertile men felt sorry for their wives' embodied suffering, including the deleterious effects of artificial hormones (i.e., the multiple injections, weight gain, and concerns about future reproductive cancer), the risks of repeated IVF and ICSI surgeries, and the physical and emotional suffering of pregnancy loss, as seen so vividly in the case of Hatem and Huda's loss of IVF twins. Men often felt uncomfortable watching their wives wince in pain at various points in the IVF or ICSI cycle. "It's hard on a woman's body," as one man put it. Another man, feeling guilty that his wife had to suffer over his infertility problem, lamented to me, "I'm worried for her, of course. She has to go through too many pricks. We have to try ICSI, but this makes me so sad. Our life is hospitals and doctors."

Nonetheless, because men in the Middle East desire children *with the wives they love*, they are usually willing to try IVF or ICSI—often repeatedly—to achieve this. This is true regardless of which spouse is infertile. In my study, fertile men married to infertile wives tended to have slightly longer marriages (7 years on average) than infertile men (6.3 years on average). Indeed, fertile men such as Hatem who were married to infertile women tended to have the longest marriages (5–20 years) in the study.[44] This would suggest that fertile men are generally so committed to their infertile wives that they do not exercise their socially sanctioned options of divorce and remarriage—a key finding of this study in Lebanon, as well as my earlier studies in Egypt.

In Lebanon, infertile men sometimes expressed guilt about depriving their wives of the essential feelings of pregnancy and motherhood. Accordingly, in at least a few cases, they offered to release their wives from infertile marriages, offers that were usually refused. Similarly, infertile wives sometimes suggested to their fertile husbands that they remarry. But, as in Hatem and Huda's case, the men I interviewed were mostly adamant that they would never do this. As one man explained,

> She told me I should divorce her and remarry. She did this because she loves me a lot. I told her, "Forget about it!" I have two kinds of love—for her and for God. And if I was the cause [of the infertility], she would stay with me.

As the eldest of several brothers, another man described his wife's extreme guilt over depriving an eldest son of his rights to fatherhood. As he explained,

> There is a problem in that she is nervous, nervous, nervous! It's *just* her, not me, because I don't care about having kids. She tells me to "Go marry," and not, "If you want," because she can't have babies. She is suggesting this, not even asking me! She feels guilty that she can't have a baby. But I tell her, "Never mind! If I had wanted to do this I could do this without even asking you. But I won't do it, so just

throw away the idea from your mind!"Would I take a woman only for children? Certainly not, because I have a good marriage.

To ease infertile wives' suffering, many of the fertile men in my study made valiant efforts to share in a wife's infertility problem. In some of my interviews, fertile men attempted to misclassify themselves as infertile, blaming either themselves, their testicles, or their sperm for the problem. For example, men who had been told by physicians that their sperm were "okay," sometimes misinterpreted this as a sign of male infertility. As one man put it,"I'm okay, but not super, super."In addition, some men covered for their infertile wives, denying or downplaying female infertility problems. For example, wives who did not routinely ovulate were described by their husbands as having"a little weakness"in their ovaries. Finally, fertile men were often extremely willing to put their own bodies "on the line," undergoing all manner of infertility diagnosis and treatment in order to share in their wives' embodied suffering.

Stories of *Hubb*

That men and women together share the trials and tribulations of reproduction should become abundantly apparent in the love stories that follow. In my view, the best way to show Middle Eastern men's love for their wives is to narrate their stories, as conveyed to me during interviews. The four stories below are only a fraction of the hundreds I have collected. However, these four have been chosen to demonstrate men's conjugal commitments, often in cases of long-term, intractable infertility. Furthermore, these stories reflect the robustness of conjugal love across differences in social class, regional and religious backgrounds, and male versus female infertility. The solutions these couples pursue—often in the midst of considerable adversity and moral uncertainty—should serve to demonstrate the degree of conjugal connectivity found among many infertile couples in the Middle East as they consider their difficult options. These stories highlight the fact that love and strong attachment are common among infertile couples in the Middle East, as they search for ways to overcome their childlessness. It is *hubb*, love, that leads many infertile couples to assisted reproductive technologies, and it is *hubb*, love, that keeps them together when these technologies fail, as they often do.

Ibrahim and Mayada

I interviewed Ibrahim on February 23, 2003, in a private Beirut IVF clinic serving a largely working-class, southern Lebanese Shia clientele. Ibrahim himself was Sunni, the eldest son of a Lebanese father and a Palestinian mother. He was pulled out of school in third grade to work in his father's carpentry shop and to help support the other eight children. Having come from a "huge" family, Ibrahim deeply desires his own children, explaining to me, "There is no family without children. I want children *a lot, a lot, a lot*! I'm the eldest, and I raised my brothers and sisters. And the eldest is supposed to have children. It is the traditional way." Thus, it grieves the handsome, olive-skinned, green-eyed Ibrahim that his beautiful wife of eight years, Mayada, has been unable to have children.

Over the course of their marriage, Ibrahim and Mayada have visited many doctors. "Some said the problem is hormones, and some said her ovaries are not so good," Ibrahim explained. Like many men married to infertile women, Ibrahim also accepts partial responsibility for the childlessness, insisting that he once suffered from a low sperm count for which he was given pharmaceutical treatments. However, his current semen analysis is perfectly normal, and his physician is convinced that Ibrahim is both healthy and fertile.

Like many infertile women in the Middle East, Mayada feels responsible for depriving Ibrahim of his rightful children, and she has encouraged him to divorce her. As Ibrahim explained, "She told me, 'If you want to get married [again], please go.' But I said, 'No, never! And don't speak like this anymore. This is our *nasib* [destiny] from God, and if God gives us a child, okay, and if not, okay, too. I want only you. I have both love and faith.'"

Mayada's friend delivered a beautiful IVF daughter after many years of childlessness and told Mayada that she and Ibrahim should come to the Beirut IVF clinic. Mayada asked Ibrahim if he wanted to do this and he agreed. According to Ibrahim, "We came directly." However, the $5,000 required for one cycle of IVF was an exorbitant amount for a poor Lebanese carpenter. During the interview, Ibrahim kissed the back of his hand and then placed it on his forehead to show his gratitude to God. He explained how his large Lebanese family rallied to raise the necessary money, and how Mayada's brothers helped them financially as well. "All of them know, on both sides," he explained. "If we didn't tell them, all the family will be upset, asking, 'Why didn't you tell us?' So we cut the road short. Like any operation, it's a little expensive, and we needed their help. But I will pay them back."

When I asked Ibrahim if he had any religious concerns about IVF, he answered immediately, "In the religion, it [IVF] is *halal* [permitted]. God allowed us to do it, because it is from the husband and the wife. But I would refuse to take sperm from another man—*never*! Nor egg donation. Why take something from a strange body to put it inside my wife?"

Ibrahim is hoping for twins from their first IVF cycle, and claims that he ultimately wants "a football team!" However, he has not ruled out adoption, even though he knows it is "against the religion." As he explained, "If there is no way to get her pregnant, and she wants to have [an adopted child], I would do it for her. Only if *she* wants to have a child to raise it, then I will do it for her."

Fortunately for Ibrahim and Mayada, their first cycle of IVF was more than they had ever hoped for. When I left Lebanon, a very pregnant Mayada was on bed rest at a university hospital in Beirut, being carefully monitored with triplets.

Karim and Mona

At the same Beirut IVF clinic, I met Karim and Mona, a truly attractive, self-ascribed "career couple" who, as Lebanese migrant-entrepreneurs, owned a successful graphic design company in West Africa. Mona's family had migrated there during the Lebanese civil war, following an explosion that cost Mona the three middle fingers of her right hand. Karim's family, concerned for his safety in a country where most young men were being recruited into warring militias, sent Karim to the United Arab Emirates to wait out the war years. There, Karim was very sexually active and entered two brief and unsuccessful marriages with European women. As an educated, secular Shia Muslim, Karim says he feels no particular guilt about his early sexual exploits and heavy drinking, although he does worry that too much sex with several hundred women affected his sperm count. Karim has severe oligozoospermia, or a very low sperm count, which makes it quite unlikely that he can impregnate Mona, who has been proved fertile through a variety of diagnostic tests.

As Karim explained, "Actually, we have in our tradition, if we don't have kids, they always look to the woman. They blame the woman. So the first thing I did, when I got the news, was to tell my mom. 'We may have kids, we may not. But it's *me—my* problem.' As always, she prayed to see my kids, but she died last August. "Tearing up, he added, "For me, it's very sad, because we were *very* close."

On his part, Karim ardently desires children, saying he has wanted a family most of his life. "I adore kids," he stated. "I really love kids. Even when I was a young boy, I always took care of kids. I always liked to play with them."

As for Mona, she says that she is "not caring" whether she and Karim have children. "If it happens, it happens," she explained. "Really, we work, and we're very busy. *Maybe* if I'm sitting at home doing nothing, I'd feel differently. But to be frank, if it doesn't happen, it doesn't happen. Even when I have my period, I am never crying or getting depressed. I'm not going to kill myself. We've been married for six years, and we love each other, and we have a good life. That's enough for me."

At this point, Mona left the room to meet with their IVF physician, who had already seen them through two unsuccessful cycles of ICSI. Altogether, Mona and Karim have undertaken four cycles of ICSI, including two that succeeded but were followed by miscarriages. Karim continued the interview, stating "Honestly, I told [the doctor] if this time it didn't happen, I wouldn't be capable of doing it again. It's not a matter of money. When we travel, we come [to Lebanon] on a holiday. But we spend the month here between doctors and injections. We became tired and exhausted, really. So, from my end, I would say, yes, I would stop with this one. But I don't know what Mona thinks. I know she wants kids, but she's not trying to let it even bother her. But deep inside, I'm sure she's thinking about having a baby."

When I asked Karim about adoption, he responded readily, "Adoption, that's one solution. We did actually think about it. We said if we don't succeed [with ICSI], we should go for adoption, here most probably [in Lebanon]. I mean, we know it is not really something they would advise or agree on in our religion. You should not give the kid your name, and at a certain age, you should inform the child [about the adoption]. But it's a possibility for us if this time [ICSI] fails."

Two weeks after the interview, I saw Karim and Mona at the IVF clinic, where a post-ICSI pregnancy test revealed a negative result. Calm and collected, they were about to return to Africa, where the future of their loving marriage seemed certain, despite their ongoing childlessness.

Kamal and Nura

On a Saturday morning, in a crowded hospital IVF clinic run by Lebanese Christian physicians, I met an unlikely figure, a Lebanese Druze *shaykh* named Kamal, who was waiting for his wife Nura to emerge from her appointment with the doctor. The Druze are a Shia Muslim subsect who tend to live in the mountainous regions of central Lebanon. Over the centuries, they have fought bloody wars with Christian Lebanese, which is why I was surprised to find Kamal and his wife attending an IVF clinic run by Christian physicians. Although I had met other secular Druze patients at this IVF clinic, Kamal and Nura were "religious," dedicating themselves to their religion and serving as senior religious figures in their mountain community. Kamal wore black pleated pantaloons, a long-sleeved black shirt, and a white skullcap. Nura wore a long black dress and an enveloping, intricately pleated white headscarf, which was pulled diagonally over her entire face. These distinctive outfits symbolized Kamal and Nura's Druze faith and religiosity.

Having never before interviewed a Druze *shaykh*, I assumed that Kamal might be reluctant to speak with me. But, contrary to my assumptions, he was friendly and forthcoming, clarifying for me during the process of our interview many of the fine points of Druze attitudes toward marriage, divorce, assisted reproduction, and gamete donation.

As Kamal explained, he and his second cousin Nura have been married for eighteen years. Throughout their marriage, Nura has suffered from blocked fallopian tubes, requiring IVF to achieve a pregnancy. Securing the money to undertake IVF has been difficult for Kamal. He receives no compensation for his duties as a cleric, instead making about $500 a month as a truck driver who delivers horse feed to local stables. Accruing the savings to pay for IVF has been a great challenge for Kamal. Nonetheless, out of his deep love for Nura, he has managed to do this four times, spending approximately $40,000 to $50,000 in the process. (He shook his head and whistled as he conveyed this huge sum of money to me.) Only once has Nura become pregnant, but she miscarried after one month.

Having totally run out of money, Kamal is financing the current IVF cycle through loans from family and friends in his mountain community. As Kamal explained,

> After eighteen years, I now have no money, because I've spent all of it on doctors. We are borrowing from other people to do the operation [IVF]. [Who?] Mostly from friends. Our friends know we're doing the operation, and so do both of our parents. Her sister is with us. She has the same problem as my wife, and her husband divorced her after six years.

At this point, I stopped Kamal to ask, "Is divorce allowed in the Druze religion?" He answered, "Yes, there is divorce, but a Druze man cannot marry two [wives] at the same time. He must divorce and remarry." I then asked, "Have you considered doing this?" Looking wistfully at his small, thin wife, who was seated at a distance with her sister outside the doctor's office, Kamal explained,

> I've not gotten to that point. I keep on waiting and waiting with patience, in case we have success. Our marriage is very good, but of course, I'm feeling somewhat uncomfortable because every time I see a child, I want one for myself. And all of my colleagues and friends have them by now. I would like to have kids. So if there were no possibility of ever having children, possibly I would divorce her. But I love her.

I then asked Kamal if he would consider egg donation or adoption. He said,

> Donation, no. It has to be from the husband and the wife. But adoption is okay, and maybe I'll do this. For example, I have a niece who can have children. Both my niece and her husband, they agree that

they can give us a child. Because I don't want to divorce her [Nura], and my niece and her husband agreed to this for the sake of me not leaving my wife. My niece, she has a daughter and a son. She said she would get pregnant a third time just for us, to bring a child for us.

Kamal also admitted that he has thought of "escaping" with Nura to Canada, where his paternal uncle has lived for more than twenty years. "I would love to travel away from here," he said wistfully, "because I'm not feeling comfortable in my family and my community. My uncle would provide for us."

Turning to Kamal's uncle or niece may be necessary. At age forty, Nura responded poorly to hormonal stimulation at the hospital, producing only one egg for her final IVF cycle. The cycle was canceled, with no hope in sight.

Muhammad and Nafisa

Whereas Kamal was thinking of "escaping" his country with the wife he loved, Muhammad had already done this when I met him for the first time in the same Beirut-based hospital clinic. Muhammad was a small man from Aleppo, Syria, who, like Hatem, hailed from a large Sunni Muslim family. In his early twenties, Muhammad spotted a pretty teenaged neighbor on the street. Returning home, he told his mother about her, and his mother went to her mother, asking for the girl's hand in marriage. Her name was Nafisa, she was sixteen, and she agreed. "I didn't know her before marriage," Muhammad explained. "We didn't see each other again except on the wedding night. That's our tradition. But, *hamdu-lillah* [praise be to God], we liked each other."

On his wedding night, Muhammad discovered that Nafisa did not have a woman's breasts. According to Muhammad, Nafisa had suffered a strong shock at age fourteen, when her brother accidentally scared her while playing. The shock made Nafisa's breasts stop growing, and they did not fully develop until four years of marriage. In addition, Muhammad discovered that Nafisa had never had a menstrual period. What Muhammad described as "a little weakness," Nafisa's IVF physician described as hypopituitary failure, a form of premature menopause.

In a series of responses to my questions, Muhammad described how he keeps this information about Nafisa's serious infertility problem secret from his family:

ANTHROPOLOGIST: Does your family know?
MUHAMMAD: I tell my family that *I* am the one receiving treatment, *not* my wife. I'm protecting her, of course. I love her, of course, and they would tell me to marry another if they knew. But I don't want to.

ANTHROPOLOGIST: Your wife must appreciate this.

MUHAMMAD: She appreciates this, of course. She's beautiful; her conduct is beautiful.

ANTHROPOLOGIST: Are there many men like you in Syria?

MUHAMMAD: There *are* men like me, but very few. Usually, there, a person who is married for two or three years and doesn't get kids, he remarries. The longest I know of, other than me, is twelve years. But I'm the longest—seventeen years. Very, very few people—maybe ten out of a million—would be like me and not remarry. Because, naturally, men prefer to remarry in order to have kids and to show off in front of others.

ANTHROPOLOGIST: For their manhood?

MUHAMMAD: Yes, for their manhood. Because those who do *not* have kids in Syria face humiliation. They ask, "Why are you working? You don't have kids. Why are you living without kids?" They hurt you with words. Yes! Men do this to each other, among themselves. Even I was hurt. They started questioning me. "Why are you building up your future? Why are you working?" For men there, having children brings some sense of manhood.

Muhammad proceeded to explain how he "escaped" to Lebanon to avoid this community scrutiny and censure. A self-employed housepainter, he worked in Beirut for a decade, before saving up enough money to start a home in the city with Nafisa. For the past four years, they have lived in Beirut together, away from their families and the social pressure. Furthermore, in Beirut, they have been able to try IVF four times. Muhammad described their treatment quest in this way,

> All of our marriage, we've been looking for treatment. There is IVF in Syria, but we didn't do it there, because in Syria, there is no good medicine compared to Lebanon. The first IVF we did was a long time ago in Jordan. But we didn't benefit there, and they refunded us half our money. When we went to Jordan and saw the kind of treatment there, from then on, we preferred [this hospital in Lebanon]. It has a good reputation, and they work in the correct way. We've been with the same doctor for four years. Each year, we try one more IVF.

Muhammad explained that one cycle of IVF costs minimally $2,000, which is impossible for him to afford on his painter's salary. Thus, Nafisa's parents have been financing their annual IVF cycles, sending $2,000 from Syria once a year. According to Muhammad, this money is actually inherited from Nafisa's grandparents, who were affluent landowners. The use of this inheritance to fund Nafisa's treatment is not generally known within the family, where it would be frowned upon. Muhammad explained,

No one knows except her parents and her sister and her two brothers. Not all of the family, because there are some of her family who think "tubes" [IVF] is *haram* [forbidden]. They are narrow-minded, and there are still a lot of people like this in Syria. Over here in Lebanon, we're more psychologically comfortable with the treatment and the doctors. It's a much higher level of awareness in Lebanon than in Syria. I mean, there are really narrow-minded people over there. So I can't even tell my family. Not even my mother! [Really?] No, no, no, no, no! Because it is possible that they would doubt; they would think the egg is from someone else, or that this is something commercial, and maybe *haram*. And so I just don't tell them.

Like so many other men married to infertile women, Muhammad asserts that he "doesn't care" whether or not he becomes a father. His love for Nafisa is sufficient.

It's much more difficult on her. She's very affectionate, and she likes children. For me, I have no problem, because for me, children are for the purpose of continuity in life, but are not a basic thing in life. As opposed to her, she's very affectionate and loves the sense of motherhood. Psychologically, I'm not affected, because I regard it as something from God. If God gives, he gives. I would *never* consider marrying another. [Really?] No, no, no! Because I have hope in God. We're doing as much as we can, and the rest is up to God. If there is *rizk* [God's bounty], that is good, and if not, no problem.

When I asked Muhammad how many children he would like, he laughed, holding his hands upward toward God, "If we get even one tubes baby, no more! Her body is tired of the treatments, so if one baby, a boy or a girl, no problem." Concluding our interview, Muhammad reiterated, "She wants to be a mother—*a lot*! I'm doing this *for her*. It's much more important to her than for me."

CONCLUSION

Although Muhammad considers himself to be one of the rare Syrian men devoted to his infertile wife, I met many other Syrian men like Muhammad in Beirut IVF clinics. We began this chapter with another Syrian love story—of Hatem and Huda—and we also heard the stories of infertile Lebanese couples from three different Muslim backgrounds, Sunni, Shia, and Druze. In each case, the common theme was enduring love and commitment. As I have argued, conjugal love is a common pattern in the contemporary Middle East, even in childless marriages. Furthermore, the notion of love is not new to the region; it is one of the most important sentiments in everyday life, as it has been for centuries. Romantic love pervades popular culture and is what most couples hope for in their marriages, whether or not they are able to achieve it in actual life. Romantically companionate relationships of love, affection, and admiration are part of men's affective vocabularies, whether they are poor or rich, rural or urban, unschooled or educated, infertile or fertile. Not just women, but men, too, can be deeply tender and caring in the context of infertility, contrary to popular stereotypes.

Most of the men I interviewed were happily married and were not afraid to convey their loving sentiments to their wives and to the inquiring anthropologist. The majority of men told me that they married "for love," or at least "fell in love" within the context of arranged marriage. As I have noted, romantically companionate marriages are the emergent ideal. The exact historicity of this emergence is unclear. According to Western historians, companionate marriage and love are of fairly recent historical vintage in the West.[45] In the Middle East, however, historians have identified a notion of companionate love, at least among elites, dating back many centuries.[46] In his work on early Muslim biographical dictionaries, Cambridge historian Basim F. Musallam describes how the ideal of a monogamous, permanent, and loving marriage was a social norm across the Muslim Middle East.[47] According to Musallam, "Love between men and women was widely celebrated; the Arab love story of Layla and Majnun was arguably more widely known amongst Muslims than that of Romeo and Juliet in Europe. . . . 'Women are above men in many things,' declared the ninth-century man of letters al-Jahiz, 'it is they who are wooed, wished for, loved, and desired, and it is they for whom sacrifices are made and who are protected.'"[48]

In my own work—now spanning four decades rather than fourteen centuries—the ideal of companionate love continues to be expressed and is not dependent upon social class or educational level. I found as much marital love and companionship expressed by lower-class Egyptians as I did among elites, maybe even more so. Furthermore, the desire for, and expression of, a romantically companionate marital ideal is found as widely among men as among women. Men in the Middle East today are claiming their love for their wives—speaking expansively and fondly about their marital partners, even when recounting their struggles over infertility.

It is these mutual feelings and expressions of loving conjugality that fortify marriages when they are tested by infertility. In the Middle East, a clear pattern of *sharing the infertility problem* is emerging. As seen in this chapter, some men such as Muhammad protect their infertile wives by publicly proclaiming a male infertility problem. Other men deemphasize their wives' reproductive problems, even when these problems are intractable. Many men are willing to spend their life's savings to seek repeated cycles of IVF and ICSI. Most men in infertile marriages undergo scores of semen analyses, even "going under the knife" in search of a solution for the childlessness.

In short, emergent masculinities in the Middle East bespeak both conjugal love and enduring commitment. All of the stories in this chapter have shown that husbands and wives often love each other deeply and usually remain together in long-term marriages even in the absence of children. Divorce is not the necessary consequence of infertility that it is assumed to be, especially in the contemporary era of IVF and ICSI. These technologies are giving infertile couples hope that their infertility problems can be overcome, thereby cementing sentiments of conjugal love and loyalty. Significantly, this is true for both female and male infertility. From the "demand" side then, it is conjugal love that has created a flourishing market for both IVF and ICSI in the region. Even in relatively "closed" societies such as Syria, love means taking the plunge into the brave new world of assisted reproductive technologies.

CHAPTER 4

Consanguineous Connectivity

ABBAS AND THE FAMILY "LINE"

When I arrived in Beirut in January 2003, Abbas was the first man to volunteer for my study. As it turned out, he had lived in the United States for seven years, felt favorably toward America, and wanted to practice his English skills with an American anthropologist. That Abbas volunteered to participate proved to be an auspicious beginning for me in Lebanon. In our interview, which took place in both Arabic and broken English, Abbas proved to be a lively, even jolly interlocutor, who nonetheless wanted to share his deep heartache over aspects of his life that were beyond his control, including his medical condition.

Abbas was a tall, robust, sandy-haired man with a large moustache, which, along with his weathered skin, made him look much older than his thirty-four years. A Shia Muslim from a tiny, tobacco-growing village in southern Lebanon, Abbas came from a family of eleven children, as had his father before him. Abbas considered the latter fact quite remarkable: his grandfather, though missing a testicle, had still managed to produce nearly a dozen healthy offspring, thereby continuing the family line.

Abbas and his siblings loved their large family and the peaceful life in their small hometown, until the Lebanese civil war broke out in 1975. Then, Abbas, still a sophomore in high school, was drafted into the Lebanese marines. He was lucky to survive his two-year period of conscription. When he was released from the military, he first took refuge from the war in the neighboring island of Cyprus, then in America, where he worked at odd jobs in New York City. In the United States, Abbas found many young American women who were willing to help him with his English and to explore his as yet untapped sexuality. Abbas bragged that he had had many girlfriends in "*Amrika*," but he was careful to use condoms to prevent an unplanned pregnancy. Meanwhile, through messages sent back to Lebanon, he began to court a respectable young woman, Fatima, his *bint 'amm*, or his father's brother's daughter (FBD). Not only did she fulfill the ideal category in Middle Eastern practices of first-cousin marriage, but Fatima was also Abbas's love interest, and he was happy that his affections were reciprocated.

At the age of twenty-five, Abbas returned to Lebanon, where he married Fatima within a year. However, no pregnancy occurred within the first two years of marriage. The young couple consulted several gynecologists. Whereas Fatima was deemed to be healthy and fertile, Abbas was shown to be azoospermic, without any sperm in his ejaculate.

Multiple, painful testicular biopsies proved that Abbas was producing sperm in his testicles. But the sperm were trapped inside, because Abbas was lacking a vas deferens, the testicular vessel involved in sperm transport. Abbas described with painful eloquence how he felt when he learned this shocking news,

> We asked the doctor about what I can do, and he explained to me that there's nothing I can do. Everything else is okay, wonderful. I have sperm inside, and I "come" [ejaculate] when I make love with my wife and it's wonderful. It's "the line" [vas] I don't have. It's not only me; it's my brother and one cousin. I asked the doctor why this happened. The doctor explained to me, "It's biology. It's coming from your mother and father. It's coming to the men in your family."
>
> This problem changed my mind, my life, my prayers. I asked God, "Don't leave me to be like this, never to have children." It broke my life. I want to have my own children too much. I thought about divorce many times. My brain "moved" a lot [he motioned to his head, circling his hand around it]. I thought about my life, my wife, and it was a very, very dangerous period [i.e., he suggests that he was suicidal].
>
> But the first and last is my God. He sees everything. And I decided to leave that to God. If he wants to help, he'll help, but I can't do anything. It's not between your hands or in your brain. This is God's will. I prayed to my God, and I stayed to myself [during this period], even though my wife and I talked and talked, all night some times.
>
> Nobody can know how I felt. . . . you don't know how I was feeling inside. Anybody who has this problem, he can feel it. [Addressing the anthropologist] You're a doctor, so you can feel it. But other people have no idea how it feels [to be faced with this problem].
>
> About myself, about me, I'm okay now. I looked to my God, and this is what happened to me. I realized that there was not anything wrong with me. I was born with this. Not from a disease. There was nothing I did wrong, and nothing I can do. I am Abbas. I don't need it [a vas deferens] or children. You have to believe in yourself. You have to take care of that first. When you feel like this, then nobody will act differently toward you. I realized that it's not my problem if I don't have the "line."

> All my family knows [about his medical problem]. I can't keep it from them. Everybody was crying with me when I told them. Everybody thought about this problem and tried to help me. We sold land, 2,000 square meters, and I spent all of that for treatment.

The "treatment," Abbas came to realize, was ICSI. ICSI can create children for men with a congenital absence of the vas deferens through extraction of sperm directly from the testis. Nonetheless, ICSI can also perpetuate genetic disorders into the next generation, particularly among male offspring. Congenital absence of the vas—the condition that Abbas, his brother, and cousin all carry—is a definitive marker of the autosomal recessive cystic fibrosis gene. If their wives, who are relatives, carry this familial gene as well, then their children face the threat of cystic fibrosis, an inherited condition of the mucus glands, which leads to debilitating lung and digestive problems and death in early adulthood. When absence of the vas deferens occurs alone without these other symptoms, it is considered to be a mild, genital form of cystic fibrosis. For his part, Abbas was never told about his cystic fibrosis carrier status, or if he was counseled, he failed to understand the seriousness of this genetic threat to his future offspring.

With the help of ICSI, Abbas and his wife were able to bear a son, who was nine months old at the time of the interview. Abbas proudly described him as a "special boy," highly intelligent even though he was still too young to talk. Furthermore, when I met Abbas at the IVF clinic, he was in the process of helping his younger brother, now a resident of the Netherlands, to obtain ICSI in Lebanon. Abbas was profoundly grateful to the Beirut IVF clinic for giving him the gift of an ICSI son, and he wanted to share this blessing with his younger brother. Yet, Abbas was not aware of the debates surrounding ICSI, a technology that "assists" reproduction, while at the same time "reproducing" genetic disorders in the next generation.[1] If both Abbas and his brother are lucky, their ICSI offspring will be spared from painful deaths via cystic fibrosis. However, their sons will share the genetic destiny of their fathers—namely, serious male infertility, linked to cystic fibrosis, the likely consequence of generations of consanguineous unions, or cousin marriage.[2]

THE IMPORTANCE OF FAMILY

Abbas's story speaks to the importance of family—not only Abbas's desire to create a family of his own but also the support he receives from his natal family members in his darkest hour of need. Like so many other young Middle Eastern men, Abbas chose to marry his female cousin Fatima out of love and affection, as well as family expectations. Cousin marriage—known more formally as consanguineous marriage—is a common practice across the Middle Eastern region, from Morocco to Iran. However, consanguineous unions may perpetuate life-threatening genetic conditions such as cystic fibrosis, and may be the single-most important reason why male infertility rates across the region are so high, as we shall see.

Abbas is beset by a particularly intractable form of male infertility—what he understands as the absence of a crucial "line" to carry the sperm out of his body. The notion of a "missing line" has multiple meanings in Abbas's life. On the one hand, Abbas cannot perpetuate his family line if he does not reproduce. Yet, assisted reproduction through ICSI to overcome Abbas's missing "line" (vas deferens) means that male infertility and potentially cystic fibrosis will be carried to the next generation.

Most men in the Middle East ardently desire children, not only to fulfill dreams of fatherhood but also to carry on the "family line." When impediments to achieving this goal occur, families are often called upon to assist reproduction through various kinds of material and emotional support. This is perhaps especially true when an infertile couple is in a consanguineous union. In these cases, the extended family has a vested interest in ensuring the couple's future reproduction. I use the term *consanguineous connectivity* to signal the importance of these kinds of consanguineous, or "blood" ties—not only between married cousins but also between extended family members invested in a couple's fertility. The term derives from *patriarchal connectivity*, which, as noted in the preceding chapter, was coined by anthropologist Suad Joseph, the leading theorist of Middle Eastern family life.[3] In order to understand what I mean by consanguineous connectivity, it is important to examine what Joseph meant by patriarchal connectivity in her original formulation.

In an attempt to index the ongoing strength of family bonds in the Middle East, Joseph has argued persuasively that love and emotional commitment exists *within* patriarchal power structures. Patriarchy is evident when senior men (i.e., fathers, uncles, older brothers) exert their dominance and authority over women (i.e., wives, sisters, nieces, daughters), as well as junior males (i.e., sons, nephews, cousins) in the extended family. However, such gendered and aged patriarchy is not antisocial. As Joseph shows in her ethnographic research from Lebanon,[4] Middle Eastern men are socialized to be deeply enmeshed in family structures. Fathers love and care for their children, sons show lifelong commitment to their mothers and sisters, and men love, protect, and marry their female cousins, even if these males are also expected to demonstrate relations of dominance over the women in their lives. According to Joseph, socialization within Arab families places a premium on connectivity, or the intensive bonding of individuals through love, involvement, and commitment. As Joseph writes,

I use connectivity to mean psychodynamic processes by which one person comes to see himself or herself as part of another. Boundaries between persons are relatively fluid so that each needs the other to complete the sense of selfhood. One's sense of self is intimately linked with the self of another so that the security, identity, integrity, dignity, and self-worth of one is tied to the actions of the other. Connective persons are not separate or autonomous. They are open to and require the involvement of others in shaping their emotions, desires, attitudes, and identities. . . . The concept of connectivity is useful in characterizing the social production of relational selves with diffuse boundaries who require continuous interaction with significant others for a sense of completion.[5]

Joseph notes that connectivity can exist independently of patriarchy and probably occurs in most cultures in which individuation, autonomy, and separation are not valued or supported. In such cultures, family members are generally deeply involved with each other, expecting mutual love, exerting considerable influence over each others' lives, prioritizing family solidarity, and encouraging subordination of members' needs to collective interests. Persons are thus embedded in familial relational matrices that shape their deepest sense of self[6] and serve as a source of security when the external social, economic, and political situation is uncertain.[7]

Joseph developed her theory of patriarchal connectivity through long-term ethnographic engagement in Lebanon, the site of my own masculinities research. There, patriarchal connectivity has served as a kind of ballast against the politics of uncertainty, in a country that has undergone more than thirty years of civil war and external military occupation. Abbas's story is a case in point: mandatory conscription into a devastating civil war disrupts Abbas's education, turns him into a refugee, delays his marriage, and renders him undereducated and hence economically vulnerable. As a long-distance trucker, Abbas makes only $500 a month—not nearly enough to cover the costs of an ICSI cycle, which at $5,000, is ten times his monthly salary. Only by turning to family is Abbas able to afford the ICSI procedure. With a large and deeply emotionally connected family at his side, Abbas is able to pursue ICSI through his family's willingness to convert valuable, communally held farmland into cash. The result is the birth of Abbas's precious son—the tangible continuation of the family line.

Given the importance of family, fertility rates across the Middle East have tended to be high, especially in the generation of Abbas's parents and grandparents.[8] Like Abbas, most men in my study came from large—even huge—families, with an average of six children. A full 84 percent of men in the study came from families with at least four children. Almost half (47%) of families comprised four to six children, and more than one-third (37%)

comprised seven or more children, with twenty being the largest sibling set. Only 16 percent of men came from families of one to three siblings, either because they were Christian Orthodox or Protestant (whose natality rates are lower than those of Muslims and Catholic Maronites), or because parents had died, divorced, lost children through neonatal mortality, or experienced fertility problems. Families with only one or two children were relatively rare (only 7%) and were virtually all due to reproductive disruptions and deaths.

Men in the study tended to speak of their families—and especially their parents—with great respect and fondness, telling me how their families had sacrificed to invest in their educations or to spirit them out of the country during the civil war. Men's geographic and professional mobility were often the direct consequence of familial investments. For example, although men in this study were from virtually all social strata, the majority of them were educated—with at least a junior high or high school diploma—and many had advanced degrees (fourteen years of education was the mean). Reflecting Lebanon's relatively high literacy rates compared to other Middle Eastern countries, nearly all of the men in this study were literate in Arabic, and some in English as well, a finding that is unusual for the region as a whole. Exactly one-third of the men in the study were highly educated professionals, mostly engineers and architects (16% of all men in the study), but also health care workers (physicians, dentists, nurses, psychologists); educators (professors, principals, teachers); and economists, journalists, and diplomats. Reflecting Lebanon's entrepreneurial spirit, the majority of men in the study were in some form of business (39 percent), and of these, nearly 40 percent owned their own businesses, from small shops to large factories in West Africa. Government civil servants, including those in the police and military, made up 10 percent of the total sample. The rest were blue-collar workers (17 percent), including many drivers, construction and factory workers, electricians, and mechanics. Finally, a small number of men in the study were farmers or shepherds and one was a cleric. The wide distribution of occupational categories is reflected in table 8.

Although most of the men in the study were gainfully employed, salaries were actually quite low, reflecting the postwar economic crisis in a country where currency devaluation has been coupled with crippling rates of inflation. At the time of my study in 2003, Lebanon faced debts estimated at $32 billion, or 180 percent of gross domestic product (GDP)—a budget deficit to GDP ratio reaching 16.6 percent.[9] In 2002 unemployment figures ranged between 12 and 25 percent, making at least one-third of the Lebanese population at risk of poverty. According to a United Nations development report,

TABLE 8. Men's occupations, N (%)

Educated professional	71 (32)
Businessman	50 (23)
Blue-collar worker	38 (17)
Business owner	31 (14)
Civil servant	23 (10)
Farmer	6 (3)
Cleric	1 (1)
Total	220 (100)

Lebanon witnessed during the last few years additional pressures due to a dramatic drop in economic growth, which reflected negatively on the class structure by a widening of the social gap: a destitute majority, a very small class of the extremely wealthy and a dramatic reduction in the middle class. Studies indicate that around 61.9% of the Lebanese households fit in the low-income bracket, and that 12.9% are in the below 70 U.S. dollar per capita group. The decline of the middle class is due to economic stagnation and soaring unemployment. Studies indicate that unemployment rates reached 21% in the year 2001.[10]

Although none of the men in my study claimed absolute impoverishment, economic distress and accompanying psychological stress were abiding themes of men's narratives. I questioned all the men in my study about their monthly income levels. If we assume that their reporting was accurate, most men in the study made between $1,000 and 2,000 per month, with annual household salaries of significantly less than $20,000. Like Abbas, many men were making significantly less than $1,000 per month, resulting in annual incomes of less than $12,000. Even "middle-class" educated professionals in my study were "low income" compared to their counterparts in the United States. For example, most of the engineers and physicians reported monthly salaries of less than $2,000—low earnings that have been confirmed by an American University of Beirut study, which shows that the average Lebanese physician makes approximately $2,000/month.[11] According to some of the doctors in my study, $2,000 per month was a "good" middle-class salary; some Lebanese physicians made half that amount.

Men in my study criticized the increasing class stratification of Lebanese society, the war-related devastation of a solid middle class, the dramatic postwar decline in economic security, and their overall distrust of the government. Their economic lamentations, especially in the context of high-cost ICSI demands, were a constant theme. For example, as soon as I sat down with Maroun, a Christian Maronite dental surgeon, he asked me what I thought of Lebanon. Before I could even formulate a response, he launched into a tirade about the politics of economic uncertainty, as follows,

> Fifteen to twenty percent are making $250 a month—that's one-fifth of the population. And forty percent of the population are even poorer than that, living below the poverty line. Some studies say that—published in the [news]paper one or two years ago. Sixty percent are just living; they just can afford to make a living. And then ten to fifteen percent are very, very rich. But those rich before the war are not the same as the rich now. Before the war, $1 U.S. was equal to 2.5 Lebanese lira. Now $1 equals 1,500 Lebanese lira. There was profound devaluation of the Lebanese currency. So if you were rich before the war, you lost all of your money. And the political situation is getting worse, bringing the economic situation down with it. People are tired from fifteen years of war, and the economy is very, very bad. People are feeling very, very low.

Maroun continued without pausing,

> I know one guy who has seven girls. All his daughters are leaving. Even girls now, for the first time in Lebanon's history, are leaving. [Is this because they can't marry?] It's not only because of marriage. It is mainly the economic situation. Imagine: doctors in some cases are making $500 a month. This is very, very stressful, especially the economic situation. You have to pay two bills for electricity, two bills for water, two bills for the phone. [Why two?] Because for electricity, you have to pay the government, but because of power failures, you have to have your own generator. For water, you have to have your own source. And a mobile phone. We have a lack of water and power and phones in this country. For phones, it is better now, but for water and electricity, it's still not there.

Another Lebanese man named Amer, who had left the country during the war to make a life in Egypt, described the Lebanese as "living in fear,"

> In Lebanon, *all* the people have problems with money. If you enter a hospital, you can't know how much you will have to pay once in-

side. If you have a good income, you can end up paying more than $20,000. But if you don't, there is no humanitarianism. So there is a fear in Lebanon of these things. You always live in fear of any emergency. For example, in America, if your income is cut for some reason, your country will pay for you at least to live. But there is nothing like that here. There is no subsidized medicine here. It is something like trade. Medicine here is trade. And it's not *only* medicine, everything here is trade. *This* is the problem.

Amer continued by telling me a story of his friend, a Lebanese army colonel,

They wouldn't let his wife enter the hospital, because "our hospital doesn't have a contract with the army." She was an emergency case, and they didn't take her inside! Even for primary, immediate care, they didn't admit her. Because *this* hospital has no contract with the army, and he's a colonel in the army. Even though she was bleeding to death from an accident, they would rather let her die. If he's a colonel in the army, just think about simple people: How are they going to get care? All of Lebanese society is always living in fear of this.

As shown by Joseph and others,[12] throughout the war years and in war's aftermath, Lebanese have tended to rely heavily on family networks to sustain them through hardship. When individuals are ill, family members often rally to the cause, pooling resources needed to pay for health care. Family aid constitutes a vital resource in Lebanon, literally rescuing family members in times of acute medical need. A cell phone shop owner named Mahmoud, whose family members had mostly migrated to Michigan during the war, described the "Arab family" in this way,

In Lebanon, in the Arab family, everyone cares about someone else. In Europe, when someone becomes eighteen, he makes his own decisions. Here in Lebanon, it's different from there. The whole family cares for each other. For example, I am age thirty-six, but I go every day to my father. He has depression until now, because my two brothers died [in the war, when they were kidnapped and killed in Beirut]. For the first one to two years, he was really in a bad depression, and he's still depressed. He takes medication. Every day, if he doesn't take the medicines, he has nervousness. So, every day I go and I kiss his hand. I go straight from work and get his medicines. Children do take care of their parents here and are important for that reason, I think. In America, if I want to go to the hospital, I don't pay money. But in Lebanon, there is no safety net. If someone is not there for you, you die.

Both Amer and Mahmoud are correct in their assessments. It is estimated that approximately 40 percent of the Lebanese population lacks any
form of medical insurance, and that health care provided by both private-
sector physicians and nongovernmental organizations such as the Red
Cross and Red Crescent is beyond the financial reach of more than 80
percent of the Lebanese population.[13] Furthermore, public health care facilities were either destroyed or left to deteriorate during the war period.
Although there are nineteen government hospitals in different districts
of Lebanon, most of them are completely inactive. According to a recent
United Nations (UN) report, "In some cases, public hospital services have
deteriorated to such an extent that they lack all basic supplies and equipment as well as the necessary staff."[14]

Health care staff also left Lebanon in large numbers during the war
years. Although there has been some return of qualified personnel, particularly physicians, during the new millennium, salary levels remain so
low that many doctors are forced to seek extra employment in the private health care sector.[15] As a result, Lebanon now has among the highest
ratios of private doctors per capita in the region. Although this partially
offsets the erosion in the public health sector, "it has not contributed to a
meaningful improvement in health care in general," according to the UN
report.[16]

Given this context, most of the men in this study were not covered by
any form of health insurance, relying on out-of-pocket payments mostly to
physicians in the private sector. Only three groups of men in the study—
namely, engineers, lawyers, and government employees (including teachers, police, and men in the armed forces)—had access to health insurance
as part of their employment status or through membership in professional
syndicates. For example, all government employees in Lebanon are entitled to *daman,* or health insurance provided through the National Social
Security Fund (NSSF). But this coverage often restricts employees to Ministry of Health or military medical facilities. A former teacher, who used to
be covered by the NSSF, complained about the lack of coverage for ICSI,
although his complaints were tinged with humor,

> There are three things that are not covered by insurance, including
> the Ministry of Health and Social Security: dentistry, IVF, and brain
> surgery! IVF is not covered by insurance, like teeth! For example,
> there are certain types of injections not covered, because they know
> these injections are for IVF. If they see these types of medicines on
> your account, they would tear the paper and not pay for them. So
> I'm paying by myself. It's about $1,000 or so for ICSI, and the medi-
> cines are also $1,000, so altogether it's about $2,000. I'm just accept-
> ing the price. We're not buying vegetables, so I can't complain about
> the price!

The thirty-five engineers and architects in my study, all of them belonging on a mandatory basis to the Order of Engineers and Architects, were happy with their medical coverage in early 2003, as they received up to $3,500 per year for infertility treatment, including the costs of IVF or ICSI. Any excess costs, including in some cases the expensive hormonal medications, which can cost $1,500–2,000 per cycle, were to be covered out of pocket. However, by mid-2003, reflecting economic decline in the country, the engineers'/architects' benefit was reduced from $3,500 to only $1,000 per year. This left members frustrated. As one of them said, "I benefited last year, because with $3,500, I was able to do ICSI twice. So I was surprised to hear that our Order of Engineers reduced the fees this year. I wrote to the president of the Order to say that this is ridiculous. It is more honest to just stop the coverage, because it covers so little."

The cost of private health insurance—at about $2,000 per year for a husband and wife—was roughly the cost of one ICSI cycle in some clinics. Having private health insurance was seen as useful for hospitalizations and medical emergencies. But the few men in the study who could afford private health insurance noted that it did not cover most of their exams, blood analyses, or ultrasounds, all of which are routine parts of an IVF or ICSI cycle. Thus, in Lebanon, as in most of the Middle East,[17] individuals must pay out of pocket for health care, including for ICSI.

ICSI: A Family Affair

Given this background, it is no surprise that infertile men such as Abbas must turn to their families for help. Investing in IVF and ICSI is one of the ways in which families in Lebanon and other Middle Eastern societies care for each other. ICSI has become a "family affair"—a way to demonstrate love and concern for infertile family members through financial contributions and emotional succor. In Abbas's case, his family first "cried with him," then rallied to sell off prime farmland to finance his ICSI cycle. In the preceding chapter, we saw that Ibrahim and Mayada had borrowed money from both of their families—money that Ibrahim swore he would pay back and which fortunately led to a triplet pregnancy. Similarly, Kamal and Nura had received financial aid from both family and friends in their tight-knit Druze community. Kamal's niece had also offered to become pregnant and deliver an infant simply to overcome Kamal and Nura's eighteen years of childlessness. Muhammad and Nafisa, who had escaped the social pressure of their childlessness in Syria, were receiving annual gifts of $2,000 from Nafisa's Syrian parents, who had taken this money out of an inheritance from the grandparents' generation. As bad as the situation is in Lebanon, it is worse in neighboring Syria. The twenty men in my study who had come across the Syrian border to pursue IVF or ICSI in Lebanon had monthly salaries ranging from $150 to $4,000 a month. If the five Syrian men making more than $1,000 per month were eliminated from this group, then the average monthly salary was $318, even among highly educated professionals. As one Syrian engineer put it, "ICSI is $5,000, but the average salary in Syria is $150 a month. I'm an engineer, and I make $150 a month. Obviously, money is my main concern." In short, for ordinary, working-class Middle Eastern couples in Lebanon, Syria, and beyond, ICSI is well beyond their financial means, making resort to families a necessity.

I asked more than 150 men in my study whether their families knew they were undertaking ICSI and whether they were receiving any form of familial support. The level of family involvement was striking. Nearly 30 percent of men said that "all of the family"—their own and their wives'—knew about the infertility and the ICSI quest. An additional 60 percent had informed at least one family member, usually a mother, both parents, or siblings. Twenty-four couples in the study were receiving financial aid, either from parents or from siblings and cousins, especially relatives living overseas. Even when families were too poor to provide financial aid, they were heavily involved in "encouraging" their sons and daughters to try ICSI, often seeking information about local physicians and IVF clinics. Eighteen families had physician relatives, upon whom they relied heavily for medical information, physician referrals, injections, and general monitoring of their cases.

Female relatives did the "accompanying." In IVF clinics across the region, waiting rooms are packed with female relatives—mothers, mothers-in-law, sisters, sisters-in-law, aunts, female cousins, nieces, and occasionally IVF daughters. In Lebanon, whole waiting rooms are sometimes turned into "grandmothers' space," as worried mothers wait for their daughters and daughters-in-law to emerge from "the operation." There were days in my study when waiting rooms were draped in black—full of elderly widows veiled in black from head to toe. At other times, I mistook "youthful" grandmothers clad in Western fashions and coiffed blonde (dyed) hair as men's wives (much to the amusement of their sons). Furthermore, when men sat with their mothers-in-law in waiting areas, they were often sitting with their own aunts—who, by virtue of arranging a cousin marriage, had become both "auntie" and mother-in-law to these men. These female-intensive waiting areas were sometimes stressful spaces for men, as we will see in the next chapter on masturbation and semen collection. But, in general, female accompaniment during ICSI procedures was seen as comforting and supportive to men's wives.

To reiterate, ICSI is now a family affair. The "coming out" of male infertility as a problem to be overcome by ICSI has drawn the Middle Eastern family in. The deep stigmatization, secrecy, and moral taint that I found in my mid-1990s research are no longer so prevalent.[18] The majority of

Infertile couples today are disclosing their problems to family members, who encourage them to head directly to an IVF clinic. The acknowledgment of IVF as a solution for female infertility has softened families' patriarchal pressure on sons to divorce their infertile wives, which has always been a lamentable problem across the Middle East.[19] In cases of both male and female infertility, families are now encouraging infertile couples to undertake IVF or ICSI, often paying for these expensive technologies and praying for their success. In doing so, they demonstrate their loving connectivity toward their kin.

CONSANGUINEOUS CONNECTIVITY

An additional reason for this high level of family involvement is consanguineous connectivity, or the tendency to marry "blood" relatives as a signifier of familial closeness. Abbas's family story is an example par excellence of consanguineous connectivity—namely, a large extended family bound together by love *and* by generations of interfamilial marriage. However, Abbas's family story also exemplifies the embodied consequences of consanguineous connectivity. Three issues are of particular significance: First, infertility sometimes occurs in consanguineous unions. Second, male infertility cases may co-occur in intermarried families. And, third, consanguineous unions may be a risk factor for male infertility in the Middle East.

Consanguineous unions occur in 16 to 78 percent of all Middle Eastern marriages, according to a variety of recent studies (see table 9).[20] Between 8 and 30 percent of these marriages are first-cousin marriages, or the closest form. Of all of the Middle Eastern countries reported, Lebanon has the lowest rate of consanguineous marriage, particularly among the Christian population. Nonetheless, nearly one-third of all Lebanese Muslims and nearly 17 percent of all Lebanese Christians marry consanguineously (even if technically forbidden by some Christian sects).

In my own study of 220 Lebanese, Syrian, and Palestinian men, exactly 20 percent were married to their cousins. Rates of consanguineous union were much higher in the parental and grandparental generations. Fully two-thirds of Muslim men and one-fifth of Christian men in the study were the product of first-generation (parental) or second-generation (grandparental) consanguineous unions or both, indicating the intergenerational pattern of this practice in many families.

Significantly more of the *infertile* men were the offspring of prior consanguineous unions, suggesting that this form of marriage may produce infertile male offspring (table 10). Many infertile men in the study also had infertile brothers, and some had other infertile male relatives, as in Abbas's case. More than 40 percent of infertile men in my study could

TABLE 9. Rates of consanguineous marriage in the Middle East (%)

Country	Consanguineous Unions	First-Cousin Unions
Algeria	36.4	—
Bahrain	32	—
Egypt	29–39	11.4
Iran	23–78	—
Jordan	51.3	32 (declining)
Kuwait	35–54.3	26–30.2 (declining)
Lebanon	29.6 Muslim, 16.5 Christian	17.3 Muslim, 7.9 Christians (declining)
Libya	46.5	—
Mauritania	60.1	—
Oman	54	34 (stable)
Qatar	46	—
Saudi Arabia	54–57	31.4–41.4
Sudan	65	—
Syria	38	Declining
Tunisia	40.2	—
Turkey	21.2	—
United Arab Emirates	50–54	30 (increasing)
Yemen	—	32 (increasing)

identify other known cases of male infertility in the immediate family, particularly among brothers, first cousins, uncles, and, in some cases, fathers.[21] In addition, infertile men with the most severe cases of oligozoospermia and azoospermia were significantly more likely to be the offspring of first- and second-generation consanguineous unions (see table 11). Among this "most infertile" subset, nearly half of all men were born from consanguineous marriages among parents, grandparents, or both. Clearly, these findings suggest that consanguineous marriage over generations may lead to familial patterns of male infertility.

Not surprisingly, a growing literature suggests that genetically based sperm defects cluster in families and may be linked to ancestral consanguineous unions. For example, recent studies conducted in Italy show that consanguineous unions are highly correlated with rare genetic sperm defects.[22] These defects include a range of syndromes that impact sperm morphology and motility and may be transmissible to male offspring. The researchers conclude that male infertility may be heritable and may cluster in families and communities, depending upon the level of consanguineous marriage in the general population.

TABLE 10. Men's consanguineous marriage status and familial infertility

	Infertility Status	
	Infertile, N (%)	Fertile, N (%)
Consanguineous marriage with wife		
Wife not related	101 (84.2)	73 (75.3)
Wife: maternal cousin	8 (6.8)	16 (16)
Wife: paternal cousin	10 (8.5)	7 (7)
Wife: both paternal and maternal cousin	1 (0.9)	1 (1)
Consanguineous marriage of men's parents and/or grandparents		
None are related	66 (54.1)	60 (62.5)
Parents or grandparents are related	34 (27.9)	28 (29.2)
Both parents and grandparents are related	22 (18)	8 (8.3)
Infertility problems in men's families		
Male factor (brother, cousin, uncle)	42 (35)	11 (11)
Female factor (sister, cousin, aunt)	5 (4.2)	6 (6)
None	70 (58.8)	83 (83)

TABLE 11. Consanguineous marriage and family clustering of male infertility

	Severely Oligozoospermic and Azoospermic Men, N (%)
Distribution of consanguineous marriage	
None	33 (50)
First or second degree	19 (28.8)
Both first and second degree	13 (19.7)
Distribution of male infertility problems among close relatives	
None	38 (57.6)
Male factor	5 (37.9)
Female factor	2 (3.0)

As a result of advances in the field of genetics, it is now realized that male infertility cases, particularly those that are severe, are often due to genetic abnormalities. Indeed, "a virtual explosion in the identification of genes affecting spermatogenesis has occurred" in recent years.[23] A variety of abnormalities in both the Y and X chromosomes, as well as genetic abnormalities of the hypothalamic-pituitary-gonadal axis involved in the production of reproductive hormones, are now well-established causes of male infertility.[24]

Probably the most frequent genetic cause of infertility in men involves microdeletions of the long arm of the Y chromosome, which are associated with spermatogenic failure.[25] In men with such Y microdeletions, the spermatozoa will always be infertile, because these genetic alterations are incurable and will be present throughout a man's lifetime.[26] Such deletions are manifest in a variety of sperm defects, including defects of the sperm head (e.g., round heads, heads with craters) and sperm tail (e.g., stunted, immotile, or detached tails).

According to a recent overview of genetic mutation research, Mediterranean populations, and Muslim Mediterranean populations in particular, rank highest in the world in terms of increased frequency of congenital malformations and recessive disorders linked to consanguineous marriage.[27] As shown in *Genetic Disorders among Arab Populations*, Arab populations have high frequencies of autosomal recessive disorders, homozygosity of autosomal and X-linked traits, and a plethora of new genetic syndromes and variants, the majority of them autosomal recessive.[28] In clinical settings in the Arab world, consanguineous unions may lead to offspring with congenital malformations, mental retardation, blindness and deafness, sickle-cell anemia and thalassemia, cystic fibrosis, congenital hydrocephalus, Down syndrome, and specific metabolic diseases.[29] Recent studies have also linked consanguineous unions to a range of poor child health outcomes, including neonatal diabetes mellitus, low birth weight, and apnea (cessation of breathing) associated with prematurity.[30]

Although male infertility has never been definitively linked to the practice of consanguineous marriage in the Middle East, genetic studies of this condition are beginning to emerge from the region.[31] As seen in the previous chapters, male infertility cases make up 60 to 90 percent of the patient case load in many IVF clinics there. Furthermore, men often present with severe oligo-, astheno-, and teratozoospermia, as well as azoospermia of nonobstructive origin. According to nearly all of the Middle Eastern IVF physicians I interviewed, a genetic etiology, probably linked to consanguineous marriage over time, is the primary cause of these frequent and severe male infertility problems. As one physician explained it,

> Scientifically, of course, the relationship between azoospermia and severe oligozoospermia and Y deletions is well proven. The problem here is that there are a lot of interfamilial marriages, especially among certain sects. The Druze want to marry a Druze. The Maronites want to marry Maronites. You must only marry within one sect. And most

of Lebanon is made up of small villages, where people tend to marry their cousins, their first cousins. This has really increased the prevalence of Y microdeletions. The increased risk of male infertility is due to this, I think.

Another physician who worked in an IVF clinic that served primarily Shia Muslims said,

> Here, male factor infertility by itself is at least 50 percent—*at least* half of cases. Plus we see *very severe* cases—severe oligozoospermia, severe asthenozoospermia, maybe 13 percent of men with nonobstructive azoospermia. Definitely the nonobstructive [azoospermia] cases are high here, and most recent studies show that nonobstructive azoospermia is due to Y microdeletions. So it's a genetic factor here.

An embryologist who worked in the same clinic added her thoughts about the many azoospermia cases,

> We have a lot of cases of men with no sperm, so we have to do testicular aspirations. For example, today, there were two. One had no sperm, and in one, we found sperm. But he was a repeater, and this is the first time we've ever found any sperm. Most of these cases are nonobstructive azoospermia, where the testicles are small and hard to aspirate. I don't know if it's something familial, but, if you ask, other men in the family also do not have babies.

The tendency of male infertility to run in families is an observation made by both patients and clinicians in the Middle East. Whereas clinicians attribute the problem to genetics (specifically Y microdeletions) and consanguineous unions, patients invoke *wiratha*, "heredity," without linking the problem to consanguineous marriage per se. Instead, consanguineous marriages are socially accepted across the Middle Eastern region, as shown in table 9.

The Middle East does not stand alone in this regard. Consanguineous marriage is a socially sanctioned institution throughout much of the non-Western world, and is supported by many major religions. For example, in the primarily Hindu states of South India, marriages between close relatives occur in 20 to 45 percent of all cases, with uncle-niece and first-cousin marriages, usually mother's brother's daughter (MBD), the preferred form.[32] Before World War II, MBD first-cousin marriages were also quite common among the Han of China, who make up about 90 percent of the total Chinese population. Similarly, Buddhists, Christians, Jews, Parsees, and Druze living in Asian countries frequently marry their kin. Anthropological and ethnographic surveys have also reported cousin marriage rates of 35 to 50 percent across sub-Saharan Africa.[33] Contemporary Western nations have generally prohibited consanguineous unions, particularly with first cousins, either religiously or legally. However, it is noteworthy that 0.5 percent of North Americans and Western Europeans marry their cousins,[34] and legal statutes in many American states disallow first-cousin marriage but allow consanguineous unions with other relatives of varying degrees.[35]

Among the world religions, consanguineous marriage finds it highest level of support within Islam, with the Prophet Muhammad having married his daughter Fatima to his first cousin Ali. In Middle Eastern Muslim societies, first-cousin marriages—especially patrilateral parallel, that is, father's brother's daughter (FBD) marriages (*bint 'amm*)—are the preferred form, a preference that is unique to the Middle East. In such cases, partners have at least one set of grandparents in common, and sometimes two.[36] In the various regions of the Muslim world, including North and Sub-Saharan Africa, the Middle East, Central, South and Southeast Asia, 20 to 55 percent of all marital unions are consanguineous, with even higher rates (> 75%) in some regions.[37]

But consanguineous marriage is not simply a reflection of Islam, given that the practice is found in Middle Eastern Christian populations as well. A wide range of deeply rooted historical, sociocultural, and economic rationales support consanguineous marriages in these societies. It is often believed that consanguineous marriages offer a range of social and economic advantages, including better compatibility between husband and wife and their respective families (who are known to each other rather than being "strangers," often within the context of arranged marriages); maintenance of wealth, property, and inheritance within the family; superior prenuptial negotiations vis-à-vis reduced bridewealth payments; reinforcement of familial and tribal affiliations; strengthened affective ties between the relatives who marry their children to each other; and fewer of the complications and uncertainties inherent in marriages with nonrelatives.[38] Furthermore, it is believed that the family is the main source of personal identity and security; thus, only through endogamy (within-family marriage) can a family's strength and family members' personal security be assured. For women in particular, marrying a cousin facilitates the transition of a wife to a husband's family in a "soft" manner, without the disruption of existing family bonds or even household arrangements.[39]

As I have argued in my earlier research from Egypt,[40] cousin marriages may also serve as a buffer against divorce in cases of marital infertility. Familial loyalty seems to play a role in securing such marriages, since male cousins often tend to feel protective toward their female cousins in general, and female cousins often feel an obligation to "take care of their husband's name" (i.e., to protect his and the family's reputation) in cases of male infertility. In addition, it is widely believed that fertility may be *enhanced* in cousin marriages, because of the salubrious mixing of the "same blood." In a pronatalist setting, the belief that cousin marriages produce more and better offspring may be a major impetus for perpetuation of this practice.

In my Egyptian research, more than one-third (35%) of all marriages were between cousins, but particularly among nonworking women of lower educational backgrounds. This finding is similar to studies across the Middle Eastern region, which show that poorer women tend to be married to their cousins.[41] However, among men in many Middle Eastern communities, the higher the educational-occupational status, the higher the rate of consanguineous unions. One plausible explanation for this pattern is that the "best males" are pressured to remain "within" the family by marrying a cousin. Such males, especially eldest sons, are regarded as valuable assets, who should be conserved within sociofamilial boundaries. This "best males" hypothesis has been forwarded in studies conducted in Yemen and Jordan but has been questioned as a cause of cousin marriage in studies conducted in Lebanon,[42] as well as in the Gulf states of Kuwait and Saudi Arabia.[43]

As noted earlier, Lebanon has among the highest educational and literacy levels in the Middle Eastern region, and among the lowest rates of consanguineous marriage. Nonetheless, consanguineous marriage practices in Lebanon remain strong, with 30 percent of Muslims and 17 percent of Christians marrying their cousins. One recent study suggests that consanguineous marriage in Lebanon may be increasing over time, perhaps because of the fracturing of society by years of civil war and ongoing political violence.[44] Many demographic disruptions occurred in Lebanon as a result of the civil war, including delayed age at first marriage; decreased family size; an increased proportion of unmarried adult women as a result of high male outmigration and mortality; reduced employment opportunities; and shortages of safe, affordable housing. Because of the dearth of wage-earning males, Lebanese women increased their levels of educational attainment and involvement in the labor force. The influence of higher educational attainment among women has further affected their postwar lives, resulting in what has generally been referred to as a "celibacy trap": namely, the postponement of marriage to the late twenties, coupled with the dearth of marriageable Lebanese men, has resulted in an increased lifetime expectancy of celibacy (what used to be known as "spinsterhood") for many Lebanese women.[45] As a result, Lebanese women have become more tolerant of less socially desirable marriages, including to either younger or much older men, men with lower educational levels, and cousins whom they might not have preferred to marry otherwise.

To illustrate some of these issues, it is useful to turn to the cases of two infertile Lebanese men, one whom I will call Hussain and the other Waleed. Like Abbas, both had difficult male infertility problems, and like Abbas, both volunteered to participate in the study after reading an advertisement that I had placed in the clinic's waiting area. Both men offered compelling accounts of their severe male infertility problems, although neither attributed these problems to consanguineous marriage per se. Moreover, both men had met familial expectations by marrying cousins, even though these cousin marriages were fraught with sadness.

HUSSAIN AND THE DEATH OF AN ICSI SON

Hussain was an unlikely volunteer. A tall, hulking Lebanese army commando with tobacco-stained teeth, Hussain was dressed on the day of the interview in camouflage gear and army boots, with a closely shaved head and massive arm muscles bulging out of his uniform. As a devout Shia Muslim, he would not shake my hand when I extended it.[46] Nonetheless, he was amazingly candid and forthcoming during the interview, perhaps experiencing some catharsis through the telling of his painful story.

Hussain was thirty-seven years old and had spent twenty years of his life in the Lebanese army. As a career soldier, Hussain was "on the front line" throughout the fifteen-year civil war, experiencing "everything," including participation in combat and living through periods of intense bombing. He does not attribute his male infertility problems to the stresses of the civil war, as many other Lebanese men in this study did. In fact, although he saw many frightening scenes of war and carnage, he said that he never felt fear while participating in actual combat.

Hussain had been married twice. His first marriage occurred when he was only a teen (aged seventeen) and did not produce any children. His mother-in-law blamed him for the infertility, and so he went to a doctor for a semen analysis. According to Hussain, the semen analysis was normal, so he took the report to his mother-in-law, telling her, "The problem is not from me." Although the lack of pregnancy was not the ultimate cause for the divorce, Hussain blamed "family interference" and now doubts the accuracy of his initial semen test.

In his second marriage, Hussain took the safer route by marrying a woman named Najat. Najat is Hussain's double first cousin—both his father's brother's daughter (FBD) and his mother's brother's daughter (MBD). Hussain himself is the product of multiple generations of consanguineous unions. His grandparents on both sides were cousins, and both sets of grandparents were related to each other (i.e., the grandfathers were brothers). His mother and father are first cousins (FBD). Hussain has never considered consanguineous marriage as an important factor in his life or health, since cousin marriage is so"normal"in his Shia Muslim community in southern Lebanon. He said that his marriage to Najat, a tall, attractive, veiled woman, is"happy enough,"although they have had ongoing sexual problems throughout their marriage. Hussain admitted that he is"hyper" and suffers from premature ejaculation virtually every time he and Najat try to have sex. He has been told that the problem is"psychological"but has never been treated for the sexual disorder.

Instead, Hussain has focused all his of efforts on overcoming his male infertility problem. In the interview, he went on to relate a painful seventeen-year history of male infertility punctuated by hundreds of semen analyses, multiple hormonal injections, four unsuccessful intrauterine insemination attempts (using his sperm), and an unwarranted varicocelectomy, which is commonly performed in Lebanon as a moneymaking surgery by unscrupulous urologists. Hussain said that"only God knows" why he is infertile in his second marriage. To his knowledge, there are no other known cases of male infertility in his family, as all of his five brothers (and six sisters) have children. As he explained,"I went to all *good* doctors, specialists and professors in Beirut, but not one of them said,'You have *this* problem that causes your infertility.'"

Finally, through a loan from the army in the year 2000, Hussain gathered together enough money to undergo one cycle of ICSI. The ICSI procedure was performed, but Hussain lamented that"the doctor, he didn't do his best for us." Hussain was elated to learn that Najat was pregnant for the first time after ten years of marriage. But his happiness lasted only through the delivery, when the nurse came to tell him that a baby son had been born. Minutes later, the nurse reappeared and, according to Hussain, "told me he is a Mongol"(i.e., a baby with Down Syndrome).

"I had a strong shock, and I threw up," Hussain recalled."I stayed for one month crying. My wife also felt so bad. But I believe in God, and this is what God wants. So *hamdu-lillah* [praise be to God]. If he had lived, we would have raised him. But I felt so bad when he died [eight months later, from a heart defect]. I cried and cried. He was so intelligent. Even though he was a Mongol, it wasn't a'strong case.'"

Although Down Syndrome is one of the genetic disorders attributable to consanguineous unions in the Middle East, Hussain has not considered this possibility and is instead trying to mobilize the financial resources for a second ICSI cycle. His father is helping him to pay for treatment but has not been informed about the ICSI, which Hussain and Najat are keeping "top secret."They believe that an IVF or ICSI child would be ridiculed in their conservative Muslim community. "Because all my family have children, perhaps in the future they'll say to my child, 'You are an in vitro child.' Not all people understand IVF, what it means. Perhaps they will think bad things about it, like that we've used other people's sperm."

As Hussain explained at the end of the interview, "The child, he completes the family, and no marriage is complete without the child. Because they are fun, children make for a nice family life, with happiness and humor. We *must* have children to be happy. No couple is happy without them. My wife and I are happy now, but to complete our happiness, we must have children."

Given his history of long-term, severe male infertility and the birth of an ICSI child who died from a Down Syndrome–related heart condition, repeating ICSI may not be advisable. However, genetic screening and counseling are not well-developed specialties in Lebanon, or in other parts of the Middle East, for that matter. At the time of Hussain's interview, only one geneticist was known to be working in Lebanon, and no genetic counseling clinics or educational materials were yet available to advise ICSI patients. Therefore, Hussain and Najat did not receive any information about their genetic risk factors. At the time of the interview, they were getting ready to embark on their second cycle of ICSI, hoping, *insha'Allah*, that they would be blessed with a healthy child.

WALEED AND THE DEATH OF A FAMILY

Two weeks after my meeting with Hussain, Waleed volunteered for my study, bringing with him a thick medical file. At age fifty-seven, Waleed seemed old and defeated. The war years had been hard on Waleed, who had fled with his family from their mountain homestead to the Shia slums of Beirut at the outbreak of the civil war. Waleed described the "horror" of living through the conflict. His mother died within the first year of the family's exile, and Waleed and his siblings spent many months in basement bomb shelters, where he developed a phobic fear of rats. Nearly thirty of his family members were killed during the war, but Waleed was lucky to escape with only a bullet graze to his forehead. Because he could not sleep during the bombing raids, he began using anti-anxiety medications, eventually developing an addiction. Everything about Waleed's life was disrupted: he barely managed to finish high school, he could not afford to go to college, and he felt responsible for supporting his motherless siblings, putting off his own marriage in the process. Eventually, as the war receded, he was able to open up a small photography studio in Beirut, where he met many "beautiful women." He estimates that he slept with at least fifty of these women during his "bachelor years" from the ages of seventeen to forty Waleed's need to divulge the dark secrets of his sexual life was clear, for he began his interview like this,

> When I was young, I was really shy and blushed around girls. When I was seven years old, I used to masturbate *a lot*. At age seven, I was already thinking bad thoughts. Then, at age seventeen, I started going out. It was then that I caught a *microbe*. I had an infection, and I took an antibiotic. I had these [sexually transmitted] infections more than two times, maybe more than three to four times. I took antibiotics. But I think the problem [male infertility] comes from the diseases I got from the girls. My sperm went down to 25 percent active after I got infected, and then when I took antibiotics, it returned to 45 percent. But I think this [the sexually transmitted infections] is the direct cause.

Because Waleed had raised the issue so directly, I asked him if he felt guilty about his earlier sexual encounters. He denied feelings of sexual guilt, because "it's normal, it's natural" for young men to have sexual desires. Furthermore, Waleed was forced to delay marriage on account of the war and his family situation. He was already aged forty at the time of his first marriage, choosing a second cousin out of a sense of familial loyalty and obligation. However, this cousin marriage was ill-fated and short-lived. When his new bride discovered that Waleed had an infertility problem, she divorced him, even though Waleed underwent a preemptive varicocelectomy operation on her behalf.

Waleed remained celibate for another two years, then, at age forty-two, decided to marry a pretty, twenty-three-year-old woman named Yusra, who was not his relative. This was in 1988, three years before ICSI was discovered in Belgium, five years before the first Lebanese IVF clinic opened in Beirut, and six years before ICSI made its way to the Middle East. These were "wasted years" for Waleed and Yusra, who were aging, reproductively speaking, without producing a desired child. During this period, Waleed underwent a second varicocelectomy, which was the only purported "treatment" for male infertility at the time. But Waleed now regrets this decision, calling the second varicocelectomy a "mistake." He explained,

> They did something wrong in the second operation. My testicle became swollen on the right side, *very* swollen for two months. I went to a doctor, and he said that there were 5 cc's of water on the right and on the left, 2 cc's of water in the testicle. He did another operation to drain the testicles. And on this last operation, they told me that it "killed the [sperm] cells." But there was an infection, so they had to drain. In Lebanon, for the past twenty-five years, anyone who

has a problem having a child, they immediately tell them to do a vari-cocelectomy. The doctors here say you have to do it. But before the operation, my percentage [of sperm activity] was higher, and after the operation, it went down. It wasn't useful.

After two unsuccessful varicocelectomies and nearly a decade of child-lessness, Waleed admits he began losing interest in sex. According to Waleed,

> In the beginning, I made love to my wife every other day, to try to get her pregnant. Even if I didn't feel like doing it, I would have sex with her if her eggs were good. For the last five to six years, my psychological state isn't good. I have problems in my erection and in my excitement. I'm getting older, and I'm not feeling good in my situation, and sex feels routine. About 15 percent of the time, I have "weakness," I can't get an erection, but I don't want to take, for example, Viagra, because I love natural things.

Despite his sexual troubles, Waleed became an active ICSI patient once the new technology was introduced to Lebanon in 1996. He underwent ICSI three times to no avail in another Beirut IVF clinic, before switching to the clinic where I met him. There, he had undertaken ICSI four times, achieving two pregnancies with Yusra. However, both were ectopic (tubal) pregnancies, which had to be treated by a medication called methotrex-ate. This information was available in Waleed's medical chart, which he had brought to the interview. But it was clear from Waleed's descrip-tion of what happened to Yusra that he did not understand—or chose to misrecognize—the nature of the ectopic pregnancies. They had occurred because of the particular way in which the IVF physician had transferred the embryos to Yusra's fallopian tubes.[47] Instead of blaming the physician, Waleed blamed Yusra and her family for the pregnancy losses. "You haven't asked me if she has anything wrong," he said. "Does she?" I asked. He then launched into the following story,

> She has a problem—a small uterus. She is small like a girl of twelve or thirteen. She did two times a surgery to make it bigger, but, of course, it returned to its small size. Dr. [name] did one operation, and Dr. [another name] did the other. I don't know if she can carry a pregnancy to term. You would have to ask the doctor. But her sister has the same problem, a small uterus. She miscarried three to four times when the baby was three to four months. Then she had two girls, who are nine and four years old, then she had a boy. This is Yus-ra's younger sister. When she was married for only two months, she got pregnant, but then she miscarried. She couldn't have children back then. She would get pregnant, then miscarry. But now she's

pregnant, and she's getting sick all the time. They definitely have a pregnancy problem in their family. Her husband, he has no problem. He has 55–60 percent active [sperm], and he was like Toro!

As Waleed proceeded to talk, it became clear that none of the men in his own family could be described as "Toro-like." Waleed eventually admitted that his older brother, too, was infertile, with three failed marriages as a result. Waleed asked if he could have a piece of paper from my notebook, and he proceeded to draw a detailed genealogy of all of the men in his family, circling five men who were infertile (i.e., Waleed, his older brother, his paternal cousin, and two paternal uncles). Waleed went on to complain about his younger brother, age fifty-one, who had still not married. Waleed was extremely critical of his younger brother's "free" lifestyle, eventually breaking into tears of frustration as he spoke,

> Both me and my older brother, we tried our chances and we couldn't get children. So why is the third one not trying his chance? He is working, and he has money. He's happy the way he's living. He travels; he went to America and stayed three months. But we hardly see him in Lebanon. He's in Germany still.[48]

It took Waleed several minutes to regain his composure. I offered him some tissues, and tried to console him. He apologized to me profusely, saying that he needed to be "stronger" but that my questions had "brought everything out." At this point, a veiled woman popped her head into the interview room, and it turned out to be Yusra. At first, she scolded Waleed for being "late," but then looked perplexed when she saw that he was crying. Waleed told Yusra that he would be with her shortly, and she disappeared from the doorway. He then told me, in hushed tones,

> My wife is really nice, and it's *haram* [forbidden] that I go with another woman to see if she can get pregnant. Yusra is so nice; I can't leave her. But I think about it. Would it work to get married to someone else if I hope to have children? Maybe to do it in secret, without her knowing? Not to get married, but just to "test" my fertility in a secret way. But to have a girlfriend, I would have to pay money that I don't have, to set up such a thing. And I love my wife, but at the same time, I want kids.

Waleed estimates that he has spent at least $25,000 in his quest for conception, and has no extra income to support a mistress, if he could find one. "All the money I made," he bemoaned, "instead of going out and having fun, I've kept for the operation."

Realizing he should end his interview, Waleed wiped the tears from his eyes, saying, "We are three brothers with no children. One is not married, and two cannot have children. I am the 'hope of the family.' If I don't have children, the family will disappear."

Over the next four months, I followed Waleed and Yusra's case, happy to learn that she had become pregnant during their eighth ICSI cycle. However, two months later, Yusra miscarried again, which the clinic staff attributed to her "advanced maternal age" and the subsequent poor quality of her eggs and embryos. In short, Yusra, now thirty-nine, was "reproductively elderly," having given up her peak fertile years for her infertile husband, Waleed. Yet, Waleed did not truly appreciate Yusra's great sacrifice for the man she loved. On my final visit to the clinic, a tearful and agitated Yusra came to find me. She told me that, following her miscarriage, Waleed decided that his need to continue his family line outweighed his love for her. He had told Yusra that he wanted a divorce.

THE CHALLENGES OF CONSANGUINEOUS CONNECTIVITY

It is important to include these tragic stories, as well as infertile love stories with happy endings. Not all infertile marriages are everlasting, nor is ICSI a technological panacea. Two decades after its discovery, ICSI still cannot provide a guarantee that male infertility will be overcome or that a healthy baby will be born. As I have argued in my earlier research from Egypt,[49] ICSI has ironically increased the potential for divorce among Muslim couples, as seen in the sad story of Waleed and Yusra. ICSI is a technology to overcome sperm deficits, but it requires high-quality oocytes (eggs) to be successful (figure 8). As a result, the wives of many infertile men, who have "stood by" their infertile husbands for years, even decades in some cases, may have grown too old to produce viable oocytes for the ICSI procedure. As we will see in part II, egg donation is not accepted by the majority of Muslims in Lebanon, as elsewhere. Without it, reproductive "elderly" infertile couples such as Waleed and Yusra face four difficult options: to remain together permanently without children; to remain together in a polygynous marriage, which is rarely accepted by women themselves; to legally foster an orphan, which rarely occurs, for reasons to be explored in chapter 7; or to divorce so that the husband can attempt to have children with a younger wife. Some Muslim men like Waleed *are* choosing to divorce or take a second wife, believing that their own reproductive destinies lie with younger more fertile women. Although Waleed was the only Lebanese man in my study to initiate a divorce during the period of my fieldwork, clinicians in Lebanon told me that divorces do happen among Muslim couples who do not accept egg donation.

In fact, on the first day of my research, a Lebanese Christian embryologist explained to me, "In Lebanon, infertility is *the* problem. Everyone loves

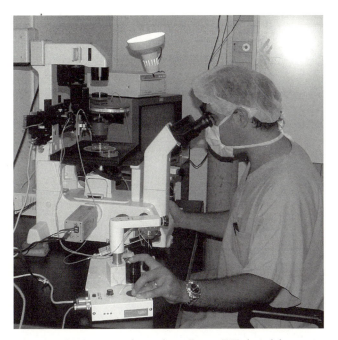

FIGURE 8. ICSI being performed in a Beirut IVF clinic laboratory

having children. Among Muslims, even if *he* is infertile, he comes back to the clinic with a new wife. There are high rates of divorce. Among Christians, it's *very* difficult to divorce. Both Orthodox and Catholics consider marriage to be for life." Another Shia Muslim staff member at the same clinic urged me study these "social things," because "men *do* leave their wives because of infertility. Sometimes women come to the clinic alone saying that they want to do IVF without their husbands' knowledge, because their husbands will leave them if they don't get pregnant." He added, however, "We tell them that they can't proceed without their husbands. This would be very dangerous." In fact, this clinic had organized a systematic egg donor program partly because of the clinic director's desire to prevent male-initiated divorce. Egg donation—and the religious debates surrounding it—are the subject of chapter 8. Suffice it to say here that when egg donation is not a possibility and repeated ICSI does not work to overcome a male infertility problem, then older wives such as Yusra are at risk.

The stories in this chapter also speak to another tragic outcome of ICSI—namely, the high percentage of pregnancy losses and infant deaths. In the Middle East, ICSI has the potential to perpetuate severe male infertility into future generations, as well as other genetic disorders such as cystic fibrosis. Although it remains to be seen whether Abbas's precious son will suffer an early adult death from cystic fibrosis, Hussain's ICSI son lived only briefly, a life that was bittersweet for his first-cousin parents. Waleed, too, experienced the challenge of Yusra's life-threatening ectopic pregnancies, although he blamed these losses on Yusra in the momentum toward his divorce. Although the experience of pregnancy loss and child death does not lead to marital demise in most cases, it can nonetheless be a devastating and profoundly disruptive experience, especially after the high financial and familial investment in the ICSI outcome.

The impact of ICSI loss and death cannot be overstated. In my study of 220 men, there were 146 pregnancy losses or perinatal deaths, including the death of 7 ICSI babies (including two sets of twins); the stillbirth of 11 ICSI infants (including four sets of twins); the loss of one set of ICSI quadruplets (following a medical intervention); 10 ICSI ectopic pregnancies; 55 miscarriages following ICSI, IVF or IUI; and 60 spontaneous miscarriages, 4 of which were ectopic pregnancies. Men often described these reproductive events with great dismay, especially if they attributed the loss to medical error. Men also described the naming and burial of their dead infants. Particularly moving was my interview with Issa, a Christian Orthodox engineer from Syria. Issa told me about his "half-arranged" marriage to a second cousin, then immediately asked if consanguineous marriage within his family could have led to his ICSI baby's congenital heart defect, which had led to her postoperative death only six months earlier. Upon learning of the heart defect, I asked Issa if his baby had been born with Down Syndrome. "No. She was very beautiful," Issa said. "Do you have a picture?" I asked. He pulled out his wallet, showing me the photo of his gorgeous newborn daughter, bringing tears to both of our eyes. I expressed my condolences for the baby's death, sharing with Issa my own loss of stillborn twin daughters exactly a decade earlier.

Yet, Issa was one of only two men in my study who questioned whether consanguineous marriage could, in any way, have led to his baby daughter's medical condition. In general, questions about cousin marriage evoked little response among the men in my study, because the practice is so common across the region. Furthermore, "genetic thinking" is not part of the cultural milieu in Lebanon, Syria, or most parts of the Middle East. Instead, religion is often invoked to explain genetic diseases as manifestations of God's will, as seen in the stories of Abbas and Hussain. Furthermore, consanguineous marriages are common, while genetic conditions are relatively rare. Thus, community members are often unwilling to link consanguineous marriage to genetic disorders, particularly when there are strong religious, sociocultural, and economic incentives for marrying cousins.[50] Besides Issa, only one other man in my study, also a Christian, had anything to say about cousin marriage and genetic health risks. "We

Maronites can marry cousins if we like," he explained to me. "Before, it was more common, especially in our grandparents' generation. But now we don't like to so much, because there are some problems in the children, coming from the 'same blood.' Even in England, the royal family is known to have boys who died at fourteen years because of this."

Genetic counseling and premarital screening programs are just beginning to emerge in the Middle East, and are now mandatory among some religious communities (e.g., Catholic Maronites, Armenian Orthodox), in some countries (especially in the Arab Gulf, where rates of consanguineous marriage are quite high), and for some genetic conditions (e.g., thalassemia, a Mediterranean hemoglobin disorder like sickle-cell anemia). Glossy brochures and well-designed Arabic-language Web sites are beginning to be developed, often portraying attractive Middle Eastern families and couples. The need for culturally sensitive, Arabic-language genetic counseling programs and materials has been noted by a number of scholars working in the region.[51] However, to my knowledge, no efforts have been directed at the infertile population per se, including men who are infertile because of consanguineous marriage in previous generations, and who may pass their familial male infertility onto their own male offspring via ICSI. Only one Turkish study—which showed relatively high frequencies of both chromosomal abnormalities and Y-chromosome microdeletions in a genetic survey of 1,935 Turkish men—has suggested "the need for genetic screening and proper genetic counseling before initiation of assisted reproduction treatment."[52]

Furthermore, preimplantation genetic diagnosis (PGD), which is now being used in Western IVF clinics to detect genetic disorders in eight-cell embryos,[53] would be useful in preventing the births of disabled ICSI offspring in the Middle East. For example, had PGD been available in Lebanon in the year 2000, it might have been offered to Hussain and Najat. The embryo that eventually became their ICSI son would likely have been discarded, and a child with Down Syndrome and a life-threatening heart defect would never have been born. Like ICSI itself, PGD brings with it profound ethical and moral conundrums, which are just beginning to be debated in the Middle Eastern region.[54] As of now, PGD programs are firmly in place in only three Middle Eastern countries—Egypt, Jordan, and Saudi Arabia. However, this technology is being learned and incorporated by embryologists in many neighboring countries, and will likely be widespread within the next decade. I predict that PGD will have major clinical impacts in the context of widespread, consanguinity-related Middle Eastern genetic disorders. Should PGD and genetic counseling programs reach Middle Eastern IVF clinics in the coming years, they will need to be incorporated in ways that do not condemn consanguineous marriage per se as either "backward" or "dangerous." Rather, the links between consanguineous marriage, male infertility, and genetic diseases in children will have to be explained to couples through culturally tailored messages that are neither frightening nor offensive.

MEN'S CRITIQUE OF CONSANGUINEOUS CONNECTIVITY

Although men in the Middle East may not be questioning the health effects of consanguineous marriage per se, they are questioning consanguineous connectivity, or the perceived need for family bonding, loyalty, and enmeshment in each others' lives. I heard five major forms of critique on the part of my male informants: against war, against government, against religious divisions, against poor quality health care and providers, and against families. This last critique—against families—was aimed at three facets of Middle Eastern family life: first, the "family pressure" on a couple to conceive, which takes its toll on men and women in different ways; second, the family's "interference" in a couple's marriage, sometimes leading to divorce, even among cousins (see tables 6 and 7 in chapter 3 for proof of this) ; and third, the "burden" on men to support their extended families, especially aging parents, unmarried sisters, and any relatives in need.

Men talked quite openly about these familial pressures and their own forms of resistance. For example, a small percentage of couples (15%) were keeping their infertility and IVF or ICSI treatment seeking entirely secret from their families. Men explained this secrecy in one of three ways: fears of moral ridicule, especially for those who were using donor eggs or sperm; fears of *hasad* (envy, or evil eye), which might lead to a poor pregnancy outcome; and fears of raising family expectations, which would have to be addressed if the IVF or ICSI procedure did not succeed.

In general, men in my study invoked the need for "privacy" in their marriages, or the need to build a protective wall between themselves and their prying family members. Hassan, a Lebanese engineer who had received his PhD in the United States, felt sorry for his wife, who suffered from a severe case of endometriosis, which he called "the silent invader,"[55]

> I feel bad for her. It's not been the smoothest year. We're not stressing that much, but now it's always on the back of our minds. Our parents *desperately* want grandchildren. But we haven't told them, so that they don't get worried. Eventually, if it takes long enough [to get pregnant], we'll have to tell. But now, we're not telling them, so they don't get worried, and frankly, we don't need the stress. But sometimes they ask, "When am I going to be a grandmother?" They put a lot of stress on us, because I'm an only child. But this is "the

normal" here. At work, people you barely know ask, "When are you going to get a baby?" "Are you hiding something?" Like you're hiding a gift! "Are you going to surprise us with something?" Personally, I don't do this, and I don't like it, for two reasons: Either they don't want children, and asking them won't change it. Or they're having a problem, and you're reminding them of their problem. But here, it's normal. It's a social tradition. Everything should be fast. You have to finish school, get married, have a child. There's an "average" timeline. So if you're late, everyone starts asking you. If you're married, "Where are the kids? *The kids*!" It's a lot of pressure.

This sort of familial pressure and conjugal interference was a major theme of men's narratives (table 12). Clearly, at least some men in my study felt incredibly burdened by their family's expectations for involvement and disclosure of their reproductive lives. In a society where individualism is not valued, men craved privacy in their marital lives. This desire was usually shared by women vis-à-vis their in-laws. Some of my most memorable interviews were with infertile couples who, together, lamented the expectations for connectivity within the Middle Eastern family.

An educated, Lebanese Muslim career couple, Abdullah and Rana, talked to me about "family interference,"

RANA: Especially here in Lebanon, the family of the man asks the husband to divorce. The woman has to suffer more if the source [of the infertility] is the woman. She suffers more from the husband's family, and sometimes gets threatened with divorce. I felt in the early days, in the beginning of our marriage, I used to hear his mother talk. Each time we would visit, she would ask about children. Later on, she got silent, once she knew the reason [male infertility].

ABDULLAH: This is her idea [Rana's]. I think families try to help at first. They don't recommend divorce in Lebanon. They try to help. When we, a Muslim couple, want to divorce, they try to solve the problem at first, before recommending divorce. It's difficult, *very* difficult, to divorce.

RANA: We see things from a different angle. When a man knows his wife has a problem and needs lots of medication, the man will ask for divorce!

ABDULLAH: This happens little, little. My idea is that this happens little. In this region, Beirut, they don't recommend divorce. They try their best to prevent it.

RANA: Most women are often victims of family interference. When a couple has a problem [of infertility], I recommend that they solve their problem alone! But in Lebanon, with all of the family ties, they interfere, "For the sake of my child! My baby!"

TABLE 12. Men's stated desires for privacy

Country	Fertility Status	Men's Comments
Lebanese	Infertile	It's personal for us. If it fails, we'll tell them, and if it succeeds, they'll know. But not right now, because I don't want the family to be obsessed about it. They can't push us, but they want to push us! But they can't, even though they're nearly pushing! But I've put light limits on this. I guess all parents are like this.
Lebanese	Infertile	I wouldn't tell anyone what we're doing. You know, in Lebanon, I wouldn't tell anyone, not even my family. This society obliges you *not* to tell! It doesn't make sense to keep telling stories to the family, but we have to do something to help ourselves, without their involvement.
Lebanese, living in UAE	Infertile	Social pressure can be a big problem. It depends on the family. There are some families who say, "My child *will* go to a doctor." But I'm the kind of person, in the end, I don't grant anybody access. "To hell with them!" Whether we're happy is not their problem. It's personal.
Lebanese, living in Cote d'Ivoire	Fertile	I returned to Lebanon to avoid the family problems. Even my parents don't know [about IVF], because when a wife can't have children, his parents will nag and say he should divorce her. And I don't want this thing. Only her relatives know, her parents, but my parents, no. Because my parents have interfered a lot, and encouraged me to divorce her. But I love her.
Lebanese	Infertile	There is social pressure, but we don't allow anyone to interfere. We keep all of this private. A major problem here is family interference. But we tell them, "It is our life and don't interfere, please!" So no one knows. This is *completely secret!* We don't tell, because we don't want people to talk, "What's happening?" We say, "It's our problem; don't ask!" There is no privacy in Lebanon, so from the first time we went to the doctor, we said, "Don't ask!" They don't know what our problem is, even when she had surgery. We keep things to the two of us, as a couple. This is to lower the pressure, because if our families knew, they would say, "Do this! Don't do this! Go to this doctor! Don't go to this one!"
Lebanese	Infertile	You get, from time to time, questions like, "What's happening? Where are you going? Is your wife pregnant?" It happens once every two months, maybe. It's not heavy pressure, but it is pressure, on the other hand. I just tell them, "Actually, I have the problem," and then they become quiet.
Lebanese, living in Cote d'Ivoire	Infertile	I have no time for these family obligations. This is a "black spot" in my life that I don't fulfill these obligations. But I prefer to abide by my own life schedule. There's still time for me to have kids. So I'm staying in Abidjan [the capital of Cote d'Ivoire] because I want a good life with my wife, and I could never have this in Lebanon! *All* of them, including my relatives, are motivated by self-interest. I don't trust *anyone* in Lebanon. But I know I love my wife very much.

TABLE 12. Men's stated desires for privacy (continued)

Country	Fertility Status	Men's Comments
Lebanese	Infertile	We asked Dr. [name] to start ICSI immediately, because we wanted to speed up the process of having kids, just to avoid the gossip, people's talk. "Why don't you have kids yet?" From the first week [of marriage] the family asks this! We traveled to Egypt for two weeks, and when we came back, the family immediately started asking. In general, within one month maximum, people start asking. So we preferred the fastest way possible, and asked for ICSI. [Does anyone know?] It's the two of us only, to avoid questions and answers. Not even our sisters or mothers know.
Lebanese	Infertile	Social pressure? *A lot!* They ask questions, people from outside the family, and relatives on both sides. They ask, "Is there anything? Do you have anything? Shouldn't you visit doctors?" This is the Middle Eastern way. But we just say we're postponing having children.
Lebanese	Fertile	The generation before us, they make pressure. My parents, if I only have one child, they will say, "*Mais non?*" [But, no?] I usually don't submit to such pressure. Up until now, my parents don't affect my decisions in any way. I try to be nice to them. I always visit them every weekend. But such decisions I usually take on my own. My wife is more sensitive to her parents and my parents. In the last two months, I think she felt bad [about her infertility], and I try to support her. I make it clear, in front of my parents, that if I don't have kids, for me, it's not a crisis. But, sometimes, her parents *and* my parents talk to her. I tell her, "You should not listen to them!" The problem is, they don't say it to me now, because they know that this will not be the reason for me to have a kid. I will have a kid because I like kids, not because of their pressure.
Syrian	Infertile	It's a common question. All my [doctor] wife's patients ask, "Do you have children?" "No, not yet." It's a common question she gets every day, from patients, from her parents, my mother. For us, just the questions are the problem. We're not feeling it's a problem. If we have children, it's okay, and if not, it's not a problem. But my mother and mother-in-law, they don't ask directly, but we can see it in their eyes that it's their wish. Two to three months ago, my mother asked me very privately, "I wish to see your children." I always answer, "It's up to God. We are doing our best." I give her no details, especially my mother, because my mother is very curious about this, and she's an old woman, 73, with an older mentality. It's a total secret, because even though she can understand, she's a mother. So I just tell her, "It's from God."
Lebanese	IVF doctor	Here, it's a *family* life more than a *couple* life. It's not only you and your children, it's you, your cousins, your parents. Personally, I like it! It's like a small mafia. But *a lot* of divorces happen because of families. Because marriage here is not purely based on love and the will of the couple to live together. It is mainly based on what families want, including getting children.

Whereas Abdullah and Rana did not see eye to eye on the level of family intervention, Jad and Michelle, an educated Lebanese Christian couple who had been happily married for fifteen years, agreed that their families were their only major source of stress,

JAD: We have a bit of pressure from the family.

MICHELLE (LAUGHING): My family! They like him very much so it's his fault that they are pressuring me to have a child for him.

JAD: Her whole family lives in the same building. It's nice, but we don't have our privacy always, and it's a bit difficult.

MICHELLE: We got used to a quiet, very organized life together. We have many things in common in our characters, me and Jad, but they don't understand that. It's a hectic social life in Lebanon—of family.

JAD: They don't leave you any space.

MICHELLE: This is what bothers me.

JAD: At the beginning, there was a bit of pressure. "Come on! Bring a child!"

MICHELLE: It used to be a little bit depressing. But, *khalas*, now it's over. But they still want to know everything!

JAD: They mind *your* own business, not *their* own business! Every minute, "Where are you? What are you doing? Where are you going? What are you dressing? What are you eating? What are you going to have for dinner?"

MICHELLE: "Do you have people over? Who are you inviting tonight? How come you didn't tell us?!" It's stressful, believe me!

JAD: That's why we always travel. We run away! Just for weekends to Cyprus, just to escape from the family, believe me!

MICHELLE: We didn't tell them about my hysteroscopy, because they would all be here. At home, they would have to wait for me! But I'm tired, I don't even want for them to know. So we told them I'm at the bank doing a little business with my husband. Believe me, I'm always tense, unconsciously, because of these stories.

JAD: They want to know *everything* about you.

MICHELLE: We want to go to the States or Canada, where everybody minds their own business. We've thought about it, I don't know, but not seriously.

JAD: We could, though, because we're a career couple.

MICHELLE: Here, before they ask you your name, "How many children do you have?"

JAD: One month after marriage, they asked, "Are you hiding something from us?" It means, "Do you have a pregnancy?" The mentality here is that you got married just to have children. For many men, "Then why are you married to her?"

MICHELLE: There is no "couple" here. They always look at us, me and Jad, with pity. Now, they never ask us about children. If they did, we would say, "We are satisfied. We are happy. We have accepted the idea of being a couple without children."

JAD: Believe me, we have no problems in our marriage. We're just trying everything, just for no regrets.

MICHELLE: I'm forty-two, I want a child, but I see it as a big responsibility. I feel the responsibility more than the joy.

JAD: We're afraid that the baby messes up our life. Either you are united in a good relationship or not. But here, the priority is for having children, not the marital relationship.

MICHELLE: Here, it's unacceptable not having children. No one would understand. They will think you're crazy.

JAD: But I'm "with" this idea. People ask me, "You don't have children? How are you living without?" And I tell them, "I'm happy with my wife. We have a perfect marriage. She has a career she likes. I have a career I like. We don't feel something missing." Why don't others accept this?

MICHELLE: They need time to change.

CONCLUSION

Although Michelle remains doubtful, I would argue that Lebanese society has already begun its change. As we have seen in this chapter, new ideas about family, responsibility, and the right to privacy, both individual and conjugal, are clearly emerging. Although men may love their parents and feel a sense of responsibility to their families of origin, they are also questioning the ethos of consanguineous connectivity, or the sense of hierarchical and duty-bound enmeshment within larger family structures.

In his article, "Closeness in the Age of Mechanical Reproduction: Debating Kinship and Biomedicine in Lebanon and the Middle East," anthropologist Morgan Clarke points to the importance of *qaraba*, or "closeness," which is the nearest equivalent in Arabic to a concept of "kinship."[56] Although *qaraba* is indicative of both family ties and a strong sense of Middle Eastern "sociability," Clarke's informants often complained of the claustrophobic, even oppressive nature of *qaraba*, or their too-close-for-comfort relations with family members.[57] In Clarke's research, his informants asserted not only the primacy of family relations but also the need for some distance. This was true in my research as well. While men were grateful for their families' aid in generating funds for an ICSI cycle, they also complained about "family interference." Family members, they explained, were often intrusive and even stressful in pressuring infertile couples to conceive, and in asserting their own rights to grandchildren and familial continuity.

Some men today are resisting these pressures, even rejecting familial demands outright. Michelle's husband Jad is a perfect example in this regard. He does not perceive a felt need to become a father or to reproduce for the sake of his family line. He expresses life satisfaction with his "perfect" marriage to Michelle and their dual careers. He views himself as part of a committed "couple," and he resents the family's interference in their marriage. To that end, he has considered emigration as a form of resistance—perhaps the only way he can experience conjugal peace and tranquillity away from prying relatives. Although Jad's emigration fantasies may never materialize, Jad is, in fact, like most of the Middle Eastern men in my study. Middle Eastern men today are seriously rethinking marriage, family life, and what it means to be a man in the twenty-first century— which may or may not include having children with the wives they love.

PART II

Islamic Masculinities

CHAPTER 5

Masturbation and Semen Collection

THE FORLORN AND FRUSTRATED SHAYKH ALI

Spring was just around the corner in Michigan when I ventured to Dearborn, the so-called capital of Arab America, on a still cold and overcast day in May 2005. Each Monday and Friday afternoon, I attended an Arab-serving IVF satellite clinic in Dearborn, where I met many infertile immigrant men of Lebanese, Palestinian, Iraqi, and Yemeni background. On this day, the clinic staff said that someone had come to the clinic to meet me, after reading the study ad posted in the waiting area. This volunteer was Ali, and as I was soon to discover, he was a religiously trained Iraqi Shia Muslim *shaykh*, whose life could only be described as sad, lonely, unfulfilled, and sexually frustrated.

This tall, substantial man—standing well over six feet tall in his black suit and white dress shirt, with a closely trimmed beard—was an imposing figure. Yet, as we sat together in a private space in the clinic, it became clear that Shaykh Ali was a broken man, with a life story that was quite tragic.

Shaykh Ali had been born in southern Iraq to a large family of six sons and six daughters. In the early years of Iraq's Baathist political regime, even poor Shia families were able to educate their children under the social welfare system. So Ali and all his brothers were sent to the University of Baghdad, where they earned master's degrees in engineering. However, before they attended college, Ali and his brothers had studied in a Shia *madrasa* (religious school) in the holy city of Najaf, where Ali had learned to read and interpret the Qur'an. He graduated as a Shia cleric in 1985, six years before the First Gulf War, an event that would change his life forever.

When U.S. troops invaded Iraq at the end of 1990, the U.S. government armed both the Shia Muslims in southern Iraq and the Kurds in northern Iraq, encouraging them to rise up against the regime of Saddam Hussein. Shaykh Ali's religiously trained family members did not fight but were caught in the postwar dragnet. Targeted by Saddam's regime for being "religious" Shia Muslims, Shaykh Ali and his two brothers were sent to prison. The two brothers—both shaykhs, both engineers, and both young fathers of two children—were killed, news that made their elderly father go blind instantly. Shaykh Ali survived his three years of imprisonment, but he was brutally beaten and tortured in a small, dark prison cell where he lived from 1991 to 1994. Upon his unexpected release, he fled to neighboring Syria, then Lebanon, where the large Shia Muslim community took him in on a temporary basis. Soon thereafter, he was granted political asylum in the United States and was resettled as a refugee in Arizona.

In Arizona, Shaykh Ali met his future wife, Nadia, also a resettled Iraqi refugee. Shaykh Ali and Nadia loved each other and were physically passionate, sometimes making love two to three times a day. This was partly intended to conceive a child, which both of them ardently desired. However, Shaykh Ali's undisclosed medical past caught up with him early on in marriage.

Namely, Shaykh Ali had been born with "undescended testicles," a condition that occurs in approximately 3 to 4 percent of full-term infants and more commonly in premature ones. In most cases, an undescended testicle will descend into the scrotum on its own during the first year of life. If not, early surgery (before two years of age) is highly recommended to bring the testis into the scrotum and to prevent irreversible testicular damage (from the body's relatively high internal temperature). Furthermore, undescended testicles are at higher risk for testicular cancer.

In Shaykh Ali's case, both testicles were undescended and remained that way until adulthood. Shaykh Ali's parents were aware of his condition but, like many other minimally educated parents in the Middle East, did not seek corrective surgery. Instead, once Shaykh Ali reached the age of twenty, his parents encouraged him to undergo semen analysis, to make sure that he was fertile. Unfortunately, semen analysis confirmed that Shaykh Ali was azoospermic. "That was in 1983, twenty-two years ago, when I did my first test in Iraq and they found no sperm," he said. "That day was very sad, very sad. The doctor explained, 'No, nothing!' and I cried." Shaykh Ali now blames his parents for forgoing the corrective surgery (called orchiopexy), which he did not obtain until age thirty upon his release from prison and escape to Lebanon. Following the orchiopexy, Shaykh Ali underwent a testicular biopsy, in which small samples of the testicles were removed in an attempt to find any existing spermatozoa. Again, no sperm were found.

Hoping that some future scientific discovery would "cure" him, Shaykh Ali went on to marry Nadia. For example, he had read about a football player in California who had injured his testicle but had undergone a supposed testicular transplant from his brother.[1] Shaykh Ali wondered if this was a common operation, for which he would be eligible.

Meanwhile, Nadia was becoming desperate to have her own children, given the scrutiny of her childlessness in the growing Iraqi refugee community in Arizona. Although she loved her husband, she loved children even more, telling him "I *need* a baby." Eventually, Nadia exercised her right to divorce within the American judicial system, leaving Shaykh Ali after three years of marriage. She remarried quickly, becoming the mother of three children. Out of love and compassion for her first husband, Nadia continued to call Shaykh Ali, letting her young children speak to their "uncle" on the telephone.

To mend his broken heart, Shaykh Ali moved to the much larger Iraqi refugee community (of nearly 80,000) in Arab Detroit. There, he knew no one, but he found easy employment as a clerk in a Lebanese-owned gas station. In his job, he earned $500 a week, barely enough to cover his rent ($700/month), his food ($300/month), his car payments and gasoline ($300/month), and the $200 monthly remittances to his elderly, disabled parents in Iraq. Ever since he fled Iraq, Shaykh Ali has not worked as either an engineer or a Muslim cleric, the two professions for which he was highly trained.

The only joy Shaykh Ali has experienced since his divorce six years ago was his two-month trip to "post-Saddam" Iraq. Back home, he visited his large, consanguineous clan, learning that there are thirty-four people in the family—including seventeen women and seventeen men—who are currently experiencing infertility problems. To his knowledge, he is the only one in the family who has suffered from undescended testicles. Instead, Shaykh Ali blames the familial infertility on consanguinity. "We are a *big* family, 10,000 people, and they all marry *in* the family," he said. "So this *is* the problem. But," he added, "because of Saddam, we stopped thinking of having children, because we are so poor and have so many problems."

One of Shaykh Ali's problems has been his inability to remarry. He went to Iraq hoping to find a new wife. "There are lots of women in Iraq," he said, "but they all want children. There is no Iraqi woman who does not want to be a mother." Shaykh Ali is not opposed to marrying a divorcée or a widow with children, but this kind of marriage would have to occur in the United States; the logistics of sponsoring a whole family out of Iraq would be too difficult. During our conversation, Shaykh Ali asked me if I was married ("Yes"), and then if I could help him to find an American wife. "My health is very good," he explained. "Every day, I wake up with an erection. I am *strong.* My sex drive is very good. But for the past six years in America, I've not used it. I *need* a wife. I need one *now.* Any wife, American or Iraqi, Muslim or not. It doesn't matter to me. Can you help me?"

I told Shaykh Ali that I would contact a friend, a widowed Sunni Muslim woman with children, who also hoped to remarry. Meanwhile, I asked Shaykh Ali if he was allowed to masturbate to relieve his sexual tension. "No, this is *haram* [religiously forbidden]," he explained. "I cannot do this." Instead, he told me, the semen was being released "naturally," through nighttime emissions, which were occurring once or twice each week.

Furthermore, during the afternoon's office visit, Shaykh Ali had been advised by a Lebanese Shia Muslim doctor to consider using sperm donation."It's difficult,"Shaykh Ali confided to me afterward."In Iran, Ayatollah Khamene'i says it's *halal* [religiously permitted]. But it's a problem. For example, if the [infertility] problem was from your husband, would you get donor sperm? It's hard. I love science, but it is very difficult for me to accept this [donor sperm]. After [the doctor] suggested this, my self-feeling was very bad. My psychological state is now very bad."

I left Dearborn on that cold spring afternoon feeling very sorry for Shaykh Ali and his plight. As promised, I contacted my widowed friend to see whether she would be interested in meeting Shaykh Ali as a prospective husband. However, as a devout Sunni Muslim woman, she could not imagine herself being married to a devout Shia Muslim cleric. She declined my offer of an introduction to Shaykh Ali, a self-described *miskin*, or"poor one,"in every sense of that term.

REPRODUCTIVE AND SEXUAL EMBODIMENT

Shaykh Ali's tragic story could be analyzed on a variety of levels. It is a story of a devout Muslim man struggling with his infertile body, his attitudes toward sperm donation, and his unrequited sexuality. Shaykh Ali suffers from a preventable form of male infertility—namely, uncorrected, undescended testicles—which have robbed his body of the ability to produce sperm. Shaykh Ali is now irrevocably sterile, and will never be able to produce his own genetic offspring. He has been offered the possibility of sperm donation, but, like the vast majority of Muslim men, does not accept this option for fatherhood. Furthermore, Shaykh Ali's azoospermia, which he failed to disclose before marriage to Nadia, led to a divorce, initiated by a young wife who otherwise loved her sexually passionate husband. However, Shaykh Ali's infertile body was an impediment to Nadia's own happiness, which included becoming a mother. With Nadia's divorce of Shaykh Ali, he is left single, socially adrift, and sexually starving. Iraqi women will not marry him, once they know of his sterility. For six years following his divorce, Shaykh Ali has remained completely celibate, given that sexual intercourse outside of marriage is a major form of *zina*, or illicit sexuality in Islam. Furthermore, as a pious Muslim, Shaykh Ali considers masturbation to be a form of *zina*. Thus, he does not masturbate to pleasure himself, nor can he easily produce a semen sample in this way. For Shaykh Ali, sperm must be withdrawn directly and painfully from the testicles—a kind of"medical torture" of testicular needlework—on a refugee body that has already suffered the embodied agonies of political torture and imprisonment.

Not all Middle Eastern men are as religiously pious as Shaykh Ali, nor have they suffered the same physical and emotional pain. Nonetheless,

Shaykh Ali's story speaks in a powerful way to many of the themes in part II, including the role of Islam in shaping the uses of assisted reproductive technologies; Muslim men's general unwillingness to consider third-party reproductive assistance, especially sperm donation, as a solution to male infertility; and emerging areas of dissonance and dissent to the prevailing religious discourse. For example, Shaykh Ali signals his willingness to marry a non-Muslim, American divorcée or widow with children, so that he can fulfill his fatherhood desires while engaging in a sexually active conjugal life. As a lover of science, Shaykh Ali also dreams of testicular transplantation—a futuristic scenario, which, like uterine or ovarian transplantation, has yet to be successfully achieved in the new millennium.

Shaykh Ali's story also speaks powerfully to the importance of sperm and ways of collecting sperm that involve both testicular needlework and masturbation. Islamic attitudes toward masturbation—and toward semen itself—shape the experiences of infertile Middle Eastern Muslim men. Male masturbation in IVF clinics is part and parcel of infertile men's experiences the world over. However, in Muslim IVF clinic settings, moral issues make masturbation particularly problematic. Sexual performance issues may also complicate clinic masturbation. Unlike Shaykh Ali, who is proud of his strong, daily erections, some infertile Middle Eastern men have sexual performance problems, which may impede semen collection, interfere with satisfying marital sexuality, and actually lead to marital infertility if a man's sexual problems interfere with impregnation. Although male infertility and impotence (erectile dysfunction) are two separate medical conditions, they do become entangled in the lives of some Middle Eastern men. The stories of Hussein and Najat and Waleed and Yusra in the preceding chapter were indicative of the problems of sexual performance that can affect the quality and outcome of marriage.

In this chapter, we explore Middle Eastern Muslim men's lives as reproductive and sexually embodied subjects.[2] Men experience their bodies in particular places, at particular historical moments, with particular culturally infused ideas about the ways that bodies should be handled and healed. As shown by Pierre Bourdieu in his *Outline of a Theory of Practice*,[3] bodily "hexis"—the very living *in* one's body—and "habitus"—the everyday habits and embodied practices of quotidian life—take specific, culturally regnant forms. According to Bourdieu, the smallest bodily practices, involving subtle nuances of posture, gesture, gait, and gaze, have powerful meanings. If this is true, then the bodily practices surrounding sex—with oneself and with others—may be symbolically, morally, and emotionally loaded.

In this chapter, I focus on hexis and habitus surrounding men's sexually reproductive bodies in the Muslim Middle East. I argue that the ICSI experience—inherently fraught for men because of the demands of

procreation—takes on additional complex meanings involving sexual performance, guilt, sin, and sometimes illicit pleasure. As seen in Shaykh Ali's
case, masturbation connotes illicit sexuality and is deemed by some men
to be the actual cause of their own male infertility. Furthermore, semen,
though life-giving, is also deemed polluting, a source of impurity that requires ablution before prayer. Given these ambivalences and ambiguities,
Muslim men in Middle Eastern IVF clinics may be especially conflicted
about delivering semen samples in the clinic. Furthermore, clinic practices may either exacerbate men's anxieties, when sexual privacy cannot be
guaranteed, or promote guilty pleasures, when illicit pornography is made
available as a mechanism of sexual stimulation.

Anxieties about semen collection via masturbation have been reported
from IVF clinics around the world. For example, in France, masturbation
and discomfort about it appeared as a central theme in interviews with
men attending Parisian IVF clinics.[4] In Israel, rabbinical (Halakhic) law
prohibits masturbation for orthodox Jewish men;[5] as a result, unique strategies to collect semen without masturbation via sexual intercourse using
perforated condoms have been reported for Israel.[6] Although the Catholic
Church also prohibits masturbation, given that sex should be for the purposes of procreation,[7] sexual anxieties and incumbent guilt over masturbation in IVF clinics serving predominantly Christian populations have not
been well documented by scholars. In my own work with Middle Eastern
Christian men, including Coptic Orthodox men in Egypt and Greek Orthodox, Armenian Orthodox, Catholic Maronite, and Protestant men in
Lebanon, anxieties surrounding masturbation were also present but were
less pronounced than among Muslim men in my studies. The role of religion in fueling men's anxieties over masturbation in IVF clinics is an important topic for further investigation.

Furthermore, the guilt and shame associated with semen collection reflect compulsory notions of sexual performance. Namely, masturbation in
the IVF clinic setting is premised on a man's ability to achieve an erection
and reach orgasm. However, IVF researchers from around the world have
described men's performance difficulties.[8] The sexual demands imposed
by infertility treatment in general, and clinic-based masturbation in particular, have been deemed a major source of "iatrogenically imposed impotence" by some scholars.[9]

In this chapter, I draw upon the provocative work of Middle Eastern
body theorists Fuad Khuri and Basim F. Musallam to explore Islamic attitudes toward masturbation, semen, and pollution,[10] including the defile-
ment that occurs when semen is released outside of, and onto, the body
through masturbation. Although some Islamic jurists have condoned the
practice of masturbation for "lonely persons" such as Shaykh Ali,[11] mas-

turbation is condemned by other scholars and continues to be viewed un-
favorably in many, if not most, Middle Eastern societies as an illegitimate
form of sexuality. Hence, some Middle Eastern men feel guilty and disturbed about their own youthful masturbation experiences and link those
experiences to their subsequent infertility problems.

Semen collection procedures in Middle Eastern IVF clinics can also be
viewed as a troubled site of sexual practice. Depending on the physical arrangement of IVF clinics, special rooms may or may not be designated for
men's semen collection, and may or may not be private and safe for the
performance of sexually explicit acts of masturbation. As a result, some
men in the clinic setting may fail to produce the imperative semen sample
because of temporary impotence or more long-term sexual dysfunction
problems.

As we will see, men's own discourses of semen collection expose their
anxieties and critiques of clinics' practices. Men themselves are often the
best interlocutors of their own bodily experiences in IVF and ICSI and
have much to say about how clinics could be reformed to promote male
reproductive health and sexual well-being. Their stories also reveal why
some Muslim men may actually look forward to clinic semen collection in
a region where public displays of sexuality are condemned and pornography remains an illicit form of male entertainment. Although many Muslim
men in IVF clinics are troubled masturbators, I would venture that many
are not. Masturbation is being viewed by at least some Middle Eastern
men today as a healthy, "natural" form of male sexuality, and part of the
emergent masculinities in the region.

ISLAMIC DISCOURSES ON SEMEN AND MASTURBATION

Before turning to Muslim men's lived experiences of their reproductive
bodies, we need to examine Islamic discourses on male bodies, including
those found in the Islamic scriptures (Qur'an and *hadith*) and the *shari'a*
(body of religious law). Basim F. Musallam in *Sex and Society in Islam*[12]
and Fuad I. Khuri in *The Body in Islamic Culture*[13] have provided excellent accounts of Muslim male bodies as described in the scriptures and by
medieval Muslim jurists. As noted by Khuri in the opening of his volume,
"I was bewildered by the frankness and openness in which sex and sexual
problems are discussed in Islam."[14] This would hold true for the practice of
masturbation, which has been openly debated by Muslim jurists throughout Islamic history.

In Islam, sex—"albeit *legitimate* sex"[15]—is considered a right and is not
bound by procreative purposes, as in Catholicism. As a result, masturba-

tion has been permitted by some Muslim jurists and schools of Islamic law, particularly as a means to prevent *zina*, or illegitimate sexual intercourse. Accordingly, these jurists have argued that masturbation is lawful "in the absence of a legitimate partner to satisfy sexual lust."[16] For example, Ahmad Ibn Hanbal, the founder of the Hanbali school of Islamic law, argued that masturbation is permissible for prisoners, travelers, and "indigent, lonely persons who did not have access to a lawful sex partner."[17] Furthermore, medieval jurists who agreed with this line of thinking argued that masturbation could, indeed, prevent death by releasing a harmful accumulation of semen in the testicles. Thus, male masturbation was likened to allowing a sick Muslim believer to break his or her fast in the case of a serious illness.

Having said this, such a permissive view toward male masturbation has remained a minority opinion in the world of Islamic jurisprudence. Perhaps because of an unverified *hadith* that states that "the [masturbator] will not be seen on the day of resurrection,"[18] a great number of both medieval and contemporary jurists have viewed the practice "with distaste and repugnance."[19] In one school of Islamic law, the Shafi'i, masturbation has been forbidden altogether, with most Shafi'i jurists regarding the practice as religiously unlawful (*haram*), unless performed by a man's wife or concubine.[20]

Clearly, part of the ambivalence toward masturbation involves ejaculation of polluting semen onto the male body. Although the "spilling of seed" has been acknowledged in Islamic thought as a natural, even necessary function of the male body for the purposes of procreation, semen itself is accorded no special sanctity and is officially regarded as a polluting substance.[21] According to Islamic *shari'a*, semen is a pollutant that, like menses and other bodily wastes, must be purified before prayer and the performance of other Islamic rituals. A person polluted by semen on the body is not allowed to "pray, fast, walk around al-Ka'ba, touch or read the Qur'an or the poetry recited in praise of God and his Prophet. He is also forbidden from entering or staying in the mosque."[22] As noted by one jurist: "Purification by washing the body after orgasm is an absolute requirement; the person who intentionally leaves a single hair unwashed will be doomed to fire."[23] Furthermore, this impurity occurs whether the semen is released through intercourse (inside a vagina), coitus interruptus (withdrawal from a vagina), masturbation, or through sleep (wet dreams). Furthermore, it makes no difference whether semen is released with or without lust or in small or large quantities. In short, semen constitutes impurity once released outside the body and must be removed with water or, in the absence of water, the use of earth or sand.

Because of semen's polluting character, lovemaking is inherently impure, leading many Muslim believers to ask for God's forgiveness before sexual intercourse, "as if he is committing an evil act."[24] Khuri concludes that, "while the literature on sexual life encourages marriage, play and laughter before intercourse, the desire for women, and to regard love-making as equivalent to alms-giving that deserves a divine reward in the afterlife, it simultaneously condemns the results of orgasm, the flow of semen."[25] He continues, "Like blood that flows for a noble cause, prayer and the appeal to God may help nullify the polluting effects of semen, thus rendering it an admissible instrument for the continuity of the human race. After all, children are the joy of this world's life."[26]

This ambivalence toward semen as simultaneously life giving and polluting, and toward masturbation as a defiling and repugnant release of semen onto the body, is seen in contemporary thought and practice in Middle Eastern Muslim societies. As I have shown in my earlier work in Egypt,[27] and as other anthropologists have reported from Morocco, Turkey, and Iran,[28] monogenetic theories of procreation still found across the region view men as creating human life, which they carry as preformed fetuses in their sperm and ejaculate into women's waiting wombs. This notion that men create life—and hence, that only fathers (and by extension, father's relatives) are the true "blood" relatives of their children in societies where bloodlines and lineage are profoundly important cultural concepts—certainly serves to give men, and not women, biological "ownership" of their children. It also provides strong ideological support for the nearly universal presence of patrilineal kinship systems in this region of the Muslim world.

Despite the ideological importance of semen in patrilineal kinship systems, bodily practices surrounding semen suggest that this substance is inherently defiling and should be removed from men's bodies as quickly as possible and especially before prayer. Furthermore, semen is seen as polluting to women's bodies as well. In Egypt, for example, women told me about the rather rigorous standards of genital purity that they maintained, including routine removal of all pubic hair (which is practiced across the Middle East).[29] Most poor urban Egyptian women undertook frequent manual vaginal douching, sometimes once or twice daily, sometimes before prayer, and usually immediately following sexual intercourse. As women explained, immediate internal washing of the vagina with warm water, using the first and second fingers, is imperative as a purifying method within the first half-hour after the sex act is completed. But because this practice also lessens the likelihood of pregnancy, infertility physicians must constantly remind Egyptian women to remain on their backs for at least thirty minutes, and to refrain from douching for as long as possible, ideally twenty-four hours after intercourse. The thought of remaining "unpurified" for up to one day with an inherently polluting sexual secretion from their husbands' bodies was a condition that many of my female informants found defiling and even repugnant. This revulsion toward semen also helped to explain why most poor Egyptian women were unwilling to perform fellatio on their husbands.

For Middle Eastern Muslim men, such ambivalence toward semen as a polluting substance is reflected in three ways: in the purification practices and required pre-prayer ablutions just described; in anxieties over masturbation as a form of sexual self-gratification; and in anxieties over semen collection as a routine part of infertility diagnosis and treatment. Furthermore, because the act of masturbation itself—in which semen is spilled onto the body—is viewed by many Islamic jurists as an illegitimate form of male sexuality, many Middle Eastern Muslim men are deeply conflicted about whether to masturbate and whether having masturbated in the past was wrong.

In short, masturbation is a complicated form of hexis, or bodily practice, for Middle Eastern Muslim men. These conflicted feelings about masturbation are reflected in the story of a man whom I will call Ahmed, who became my driver in the United Arab Emirates. Over six months of fieldwork in 2007, I spent hundreds of hours in the backseat of Ahmed's taxi, as he transported me to and from my home to IVF clinics in that country. Ahmed was not from the UAE. He was a rural Syrian, who, as a labor migrant, had spent the better part of a decade outside of his home country. His story reveals a great deal about Middle Eastern manhood, sexuality, and lives of quiet desperation led by male labor migrants in the globalizing, petro-rich Arab Gulf.

AHMED, A LONELY MASTURBATOR

Ahmed was a Sunni Muslim man, but, because of long hours spent driving, he admitted that he did not pray five times a day. Nonetheless, Islamic influences were all around him. For example, many of the Pakistani cab drivers in Ahmed's company were devout Sunni Muslims. So were Ahmed's five married Egyptian housemates. Ahmed and his housemates shared a cramped apartment with a single bathroom. Working fourteen- to twenty-hour days, Ahmed was rarely in the apartment with his housemates, including when they prayed. But he did return twice daily for brief periods of sleep, as well as for two hour-long showers.

One day, Ahmed picked me up for work and was visibly upset. When I asked him what was wrong, he told me that he had had an argument with his housemates, who were very "stingy." Apparently, they had accused Ahmed of using more than his fair share of the water; thus, they intended to charge him two-sixths of the monthly water bill.

Ahmed found this to be very unjust, especially since he underutilized some of the other utilities in the apartment (such as gas and electricity). Furthermore, he explained that, as a good Muslim, it was very important for him to be clean, and he described his methodical practices of scrubbing his body after a long day of driving in traffic emissions and sand.

But there were other "emissions" that bear mentioning in Ahmed's story. One morning, Ahmed asked me a rather startling question,

AHMED: *Duktura Marseeya,* as a professor of public health, what do you think about masturbation?

ANTHROPOLOGIST: Well, Ahmed, why do you ask?

AHMED: My Egyptian roommates tell me that this is a very bad thing, that it is *haram.* They say that it is better for this to happen "naturally" during sleep.

ANTHROPOLOGIST: Well, Ahmed, I know that masturbation is not looked upon so favorably by Islam. But, from a medical standpoint, it is a very healthy form of sexuality. It is good for a man's prostate. And, most important, it is certainly better to masturbate than to have sex with a prostitute and to catch HIV/AIDS or some other sexual disease. Do you agree?

AHMED: Yes, this is what I told them. It is better to masturbate than to have sex with a prostitute.

ANTHROPOLOGIST: Do any of them go to prostitutes?

AHMED: No, not my Egyptian roommates, because they are educated Muslims. But many of the taxi drivers do, and some of them even serve as, what do you call them . . . ?

ANTHROPOLOGIST: Pimps?

AHMED: Yes, pimps! They take these prostitutes to the homes of their clients. And then they make money from this.

This led us to one of our many discussions of prostitution in the UAE. Although prostitution exists to some degree in every Middle Eastern country, nowhere is it found in such great supply—or demand—as in Dubai. With its global workforce, its tourist economy, and its thriving nightlife, Dubai is teeming with prostitutes, many of whom are trafficked against their will.

In the course of his years as a cab driver, Ahmed had transported many prostitutes from many countries, and he often told me stories about them and about the men who were their clients. Furthermore, Ahmed had encountered a number of male prostitutes and transgendered "lady boys," some of whom had asked Ahmed to sleep with them for money.

Ahmed himself claimed that he had never slept with a prostitute. But when I told him that I never quite understood men's motivations in paying for sex, Ahmed explained, quite matter-of-factly, "It is for variety. You get tired of eating the same kind of food each day."

Ahmed also admitted that because he transported so many prostitutes, he could not "help but to think about these things." After our preliminary masturbation discussion, he told me that he himself masturbated at least every other day (one of the reasons for his long showers). Ahmed's frank revelation about feeling sexually aroused but also guilty about his masturbation practices was not surprising to me. In the course of interviewing hundreds of infertile Middle Eastern men, I knew that masturbation was a source of anxiety and guilt. I assumed that Ahmed was telling me about his masturbation, because he wanted a kind of professional "permission" from me—as a Western medical anthropologist and public health professor—to condone this practice on medical if not on religious grounds.

SEXUAL GUILT AND BLAME

Although Ahmed was not infertile (he was the married father of three children back in Syria), it is likely that he would have blamed any experience of reproductive difficulty on his excessive masturbation, about which he felt conflicted. Ahmed would not be alone in this regard. In interviews I conducted with infertile Muslim men in Lebanon, some men lamented their youthful practices of masturbation as the probable cause of their current state of infertility. These men told me that their own excessive premarital masturbation had, in effect, "used up" all of their good semen, leaving their bodies depleted of the sperm necessary to impregnate their often healthy, fertile wives. They also doubted that such masturbation was moral within their societies and religion. Such attitudes could be found among highly educated professionals, as well as among blue-collar workers in my study, and was found among both Sunni and Shia Muslims. For example, a highly educated, Sunni Muslim Lebanese pediatrician, who had trained in the United States and had had sex with only one woman, his wife, after marriage at age twenty-seven, described to me the various reasons why he believed he was infertile,

> Well, I did some reading, and some sources suggest that exposure to hot water in tubs, which I did while a teenager, could cause infertility. And then medications, and then toxic exposures, which I didn't have. So hot water was the only thing. And the other thing I was thinking about was that when I was a resident, I kept going with patients to the CT scan and x-ray; maybe this hurt me before I got married. I used to take small babies and give them sedation to go into the CT scan. This is the only explanation I have in mind.

But then, he added,

> And there's one other thing I had in mind. I very rarely mastur-
> bated when I was a very, very young child, even before puberty. But
> I felt numbness [when I did masturbate]. I can remember this. Even
> though this is normal, it has a bad connotation here. It's something
> which is a taboo. So I used to feel guilty about this for a long time.
> I think it's natural—the child discovers this. But I thought maybe I
> abused my reproductive organ and it affected my fertility, especially
> because I used to masturbate a lot as I got older.

Another Lebanese man, a Shia Muslim construction worker who had
been beaten and tortured in a southern Lebanese prison during the civil
war, framed his current sexual and infertility problems within an earlier
discourse about his childhood and adolescence and his lack of sexual education and knowledge. Very self-reflexively and critically, he explained how
his strict Muslim upbringing was linked to his current sexual and infertility
problems,

> Arabs don't have a reasonable attitude toward sex. The problem is,
> the mothers are always telling their children, especially in the Mus-
> lim community, "This is no good. *Hayda haram!*[30] [i.e., this is forbid-
> den]." Just to *think* about sexual matters is wrong. Ever since I was
> young, my mother used to "shush" me if I even brought it up. The way
> I was raised and the things I was taught may have affected my fertil-
> ity now. I had no education on sexuality. Everything was "no good."
> It was a big mistake that I wasn't taught. So, in cases where I would
> have an erection as a teenager, I wouldn't know what to do, because
> I wasn't taught . . . All over the world, every teenager goes through
> this experience, and at this age, they start masturbating. I'm asking
> myself, maybe due to excess masturbation, maybe this affected my
> sexual life and my fertility later on. Muslims say masturbation is *ha-
> ram*. If they have a pain in their "eggs" ["balls," or testicles], and they
> tell their parents, their parents will take them to the doctor and the
> doctor automatically does an operation on the testicles [a varicoce-
> lectomy]. In Islam, because masturbation is *haram*, some people who
> feel pain in their prostate or testicles actually end up in surgery!

Clearly, some men attribute their current male infertility problems to
premarital masturbation practices, especially when "excessive." Others attribute their problems to excessive premarital sex, encounters with prostitutes, and the contraction of sexually transmitted infections (table 13).
Furthermore, those men who had extramarital sexual partners, past or
present, often felt guilty about adultery, although they may have tried to
justify it as a result of sexual problems within marriage. It is important

to reiterate a point made in chapter 3: overall, one-third of men in my study had had sex only with their wives, and another third had had fewer than 10 lifetime sexual partners. Of the 17 percent of men who claimed to have had more than 100 lifetime partners, virtually all of them had spent significant periods of their lives outside their home countries, mainly in West Africa, Europe, North America, and Latin America. There, they had experienced youthful premarital sexuality, and, as shown in table 13, some deemed their current infertility problems to be the outcome, even God's "punishment," for their illicit sexual pasts.

To take but one example, Mohsen, a southern Lebanese Shia man who fled to West Africa in 1977 to escape the ravages of war in his home community, described to me—while literally hanging and hiding his head in

TABLE 13. Men's reported sexual problems and guilt

Country	Fertility Status	Reported Problems
Lebanese, formerly living in USA	Infertile	Too much premarital sex with approximately ten partners. "I thought probably that I exhausted myself before marriage. I let myself go. I let everything out before the right moment, and now I'm being punished."
Lebanese, formerly living in USA	Fertile	Sexual incompatibility with his wife, who is Catholic and almost became a nun. She is disgusted by sex and tells him to sleep with other women, as long as he uses condoms. Currently, he has girlfriends who perform oral sex on him, although he feels "it's bad to sleep with someone else after marriage, so I don't do intercourse." He reminisces about a passionate love affair with a married American woman, who was willing to divorce and marry him. "Ooohh, she taught me a lot. She was wild!"
Lebanese	Infertile	Assumes his infertility was caused by a sexually transmitted infection (STI) from premarital sex with about ten partners. "Here in Lebanese society, there are no open relations. So you have to take sex like a thief! It's this way because of the religion." Currently, both he and his wife have lost interest in sex but do it to conceive. "We want a baby a lot, so all of our concentration is on this."
Syrian	Infertile	Covering his face in shame as he spoke, he admitted to multiple sex partners and a history of STI, including during the last six years of marriage. He currently has a mistress. He attributes this to his marital infertility problem, which has caused him to suffer from impotence with his wife. "I feel like I make love with her because of pregnancy. I stayed with her without other [sexual] relations for about seven years. But with the infertility problems, I started to have other relationships." [Are you still attracted to her?] "Yes! I love her very much."

Table 13. Men's reported sexual problems and guilt *(continued)*

Country	Fertility Status	Reported Problems
Lebanese, living in Panama	Fertile	Considering himself "like a Panamanian with too many" sexual partners, he currently has one primary mistress and two to three other extramarital relations. He is impotent about half the time he tries to make love to his wife, so he uses Viagra. "The problem here is marriage. It's something psychological. I have a problem, and I have to talk about this problem. But the culture makes it difficult to talk about personal things. I don't like this. I'm not a medical person, but if someone explains this problem [of impotence], then we can learn about this." [Speaking to the anthropologist], "Maybe you will write a book, and I can read it and learn."
Lebanese	Infertile	Impotence problems since before marriage. He sees a urologist for monthly testosterone injections. "It helps a lot for my weakness."
Lebanese	Fertile	Occasional impotence. "If I'm stressed, I have a problem with my erection. Beginning the infertility treatment was a little stressful, because they used to specify the day I had to sleep with my wife, for example, the day of ovulation. This is stressful."
Lebanese	Infertile	Impotence and sexual infrequency. "My wife would like to have more sex, but I have psychological problems. I work two jobs and I'm stressed out. So I have impotence, yes. Mainly it's psychological, related to the ICSI procedures. I have a problem giving the [semen] sample. I'm 'sensitive' a little bit, and I'm always stressed. If things are happy or sad, I don't have control over my emotional state, and whenever I'm stressed, it affects my sex life." He took an Arabic traditional remedy for impotence. "The one who gave me this recipe told me I'd become a 'Superman.' But I didn't become a 'Superman.' I became worse."
Lebanese	Infertile	Covering his face in shame, he admitted to having "weakness" in sex and problems producing a semen sample. He attributes this to diabetes. He believes his infertility is due to participation in group sex with an African prostitute, which led to an STI.
Syrian	Fertile	Loss of libido. "I don't think so much about sex as I did at the beginning of marriage. I like to go out now and have lunch or dinner and smoke *shisha* [waterpipe]. It means more to me now than having sex. My wife and I have a very close relationship, intimate. But the sex part is not that important to me." He finds producing a semen sample difficult, "because it's like someone is ordering you, and you won't have the right mood."
Lebanese	Fertile	Married to his first cousin, with occasional impotence. "If I'm thinking too much about work, there *are* problems."
Lebanese, living in Gambia	Fertile	Married to his first cousin, and ejaculates too rapidly. "Now, when I have sexual relations, the sperm goes inside, but too quickly. It's something psychological. When I think too much, I have problems. I went to a doctor and he said 60 to 70 percent of people have some problem [sexually]. He gave me [a medicine], and it works well."

TABLE 13. Men's reported sexual problems and guilt *(continued)*

Country	Fertility Status	Reported Problems
Lebanese, formerly living in Russia	Infertile	Premarital sex with more than twenty-five partners in Russia, where he contracted two STIs. Blames his infertility on the STIs. "One friend, a doctor in Russia, told me to get married back then, because maybe these infections will cause long-term problems. I'm happy with my wife and my life, but sometimes I think, 'Why didn't I get married in Russia, so that I could have a child?' If I had gotten married in Russia, I'm sure I would have a child now."
Lebanese, living in Sierra Leone	Infertile	Married to his second cousin. Had premarital gonorrhea from an "uncountable" number of sexual partners. His virginal Russian girlfriend became pregnant and had an abortion. He believes his infertility is the "price he paid" for his sexual history. "Sexually, during the old days, I was enjoying life a lot when living in Africa. My girlfriend got pregnant and she had an abortion. After that, when I got married, these little things caused weakness. I enjoyed [sex] a lot, but I already spent my reproduction." [Do you feel guilty?] "Not guilty exactly, but too much of it [sex] brought some weakness. In my opinion, the problem is that any young guy living in Africa needs to receive the advice, 'Take good care of yourself.'" Currently, he lives apart from his wife in Lebanon, so has problems of quick ejaculation when he has sex with her after long periods of abstinence.
Lebanese	Infertile	Occasional impotence over the past eighteen years. Has taken injections and is currently taking an Arabic traditional remedy.
Lebanese	Fertile	Sexual intercourse is painful for his wife, which affects the quality of their sex life.
Lebanese	Infertile	Believes his infertility is due to a history of four to five STIs with more than fifty sexual partners. Now suffers from impotence and loss of sexual desire.
Lebanese	Infertile	Married to his first cousin and suffers from untreated premature ejaculation. "The doctors said it is a normal thing; it's psychological. But I feel 'hyper.' I always feel 'hyper.'"
Palestinian, living in Dubai	Infertile	One year of impotence, "maybe from diabetes and from being tired and sick. I am *so* tired from work [fifteen to seventeen hour days standing in high heat], I can't make love."
Palestinian, living in Lebanon	Fertile	Married polygynously to an infertile first wife and a fertile second wife. His sperm count is normal, but he is now impotent due to diabetes. He cannot ejaculate. "The first time I married, the problem was her tubes. The second time, the problem is from me, my weakness. My wife is not the problem."

Table 13. Men's reported sexual problems and guilt (continued)

Country	Fertility Status	Reported Problems
Syrian	Fertile	Sexual intercourse is painful for his wife, which affects the quality of their sex life. "Every time it hurts her. The doctor said maybe it's an infection, or the essential reason is psychological. But it's a *big* problem for me."
Lebanese, living in Nigeria	Infertile	Had several hundred premarital sexual partners in Dubai and Europe. Contracted genital herpes, which recurs when he is under stress. He experiences impotence "when I have to give sperm."
Lebanese, formerly living in USA, Europe, and Africa	Fertile	Had more than 100 sexual partners, especially in Africa, where he contracted five STIs. His wife suspects he is having affairs and asks him about this frequently. "She's very suffocating!"
Lebanese	Infertile	Has a serious mental health disorder and sees a psychologist. Attributes his problems of both impotence and premature ejaculation to hypertension. He is being treated with four medications, including two for anxiety.
Palestinian, living in Lebanon	Infertile	Married to the daughter of his first cousin. Has had impotence since before marriage, which he attributes to being beaten in the testicles by a youthful gang. He has been prescribed both Viagra and testosterone injections. "I didn't take the Viagra at that time, because it was killing people. People were having bad reactions, and I'm afraid of it." He does not have much sex with his wife. "She wants it sometimes, but I have no erection."
Lebanese	Infertile	Has had more than 300 sexual partners, never liking to sleep with a woman more than once. He told a doctor, who prescribed an antianxiety medication and an antidepressant. Since marriage, he has been overworked and has painful migraine headaches after sex, which has affected his desire. "When I have stress, I don't feel like it [sex]. And sex makes me feel tension, not relaxation. I have the drive, but no time, and I'm worried about a migraine after intercourse."
Lebanese	Infertile	Describes his problem as "weak ejaculation." He asked the anthropologist to prescribe medication for him, because "I don't trust the doctors here."
Lebanese	Fertile	Ejaculates too quickly (two to three minutes), which he attributes to smoking and overwork. "I suppose it's a problem for her, but we got preoccupied with these IVF things. But maybe in the future I'll get help if it gets worse."
Lebanese	Fertile	Occasional impotence, which he attributes to high triglycerides.

TABLE 13. Men's reported sexual problems and guilt *(continued)*

Country	Fertility Status	Reported Problems
Lebanese	Infertile	Started masturbating and having sex at age sixteen, contracting two STIs and eventually developing a problem with ejaculation. "At first, it was a very strong ejaculation, then it weakened." He attributes his infertility to "an excess of sexual intercourse" with more than 100 partners. "Having several women could weaken the sperm. It's like eating too many different foods at once; it makes you feel nausea, vomiting. So how about having several partners? I think this is the main cause. I had sex without condoms, and it weakened the sperm. Although I felt the desire to have intercourse at the time, maybe I do feel guilty now."
Lebanese	Infertile	Lack of sexual desire and rapid ejaculation. "I don't enjoy having sex. I like to exercise a lot; I prefer playing football over sex, and my whole life I was like this. If I had to choose, I would choose football. I would rather *not* have sex, because I ejaculate in three to five minutes, and my wife feels uncomfortable about that. She is nervous, and she nags and questions why this is happening. She's not getting satisfaction. But I can't control it." [Asking the anthropologist], "Are there any medicines?"
Lebanese	Infertile	Blames his infertility on excessive premarital masturbation. "I think the problem here in the Middle East with male infertility goes back to sexual problems that the individual goes through. Here, there aren't any normal sexual relations [premaritally]. So what this means is that guys who don't practice early sexual relations masturbate a lot. It tires or weakens the sperm."
Lebanese, formerly living in Switzerland	Infertile	Has extramarital sexual partners in Dubai and Europe when he travels for business. Blames his infertility on excessive youthful masturbation and early sexual activity. "I became sexually active at a very young age, fifteen onwards. I think a man should be sexually active at age thirty. [Do you feel guilty?] I don't feel guilty, but now there is no room any more for mistakes. If I make any mistake, this won't be acceptable because I'm a man." [Do you feel you are being punished by God for your past mistakes?] "Yes, sometimes, perhaps this could be it."
Lebanese	Fertile	Married to an older woman to whom he does not feel attracted. "It's not her mistake. I chose this, so it was my mistake. But we have very infrequent sex, because she isn't able to satisfy me in the right way. I don't feel so attracted to her, so sex is more of an obligation or duty than pleasure."
Lebanese	Fertile	Married to the daughter of his first cousin. Infertility treatment made him unable to ejaculate inside his wife. A doctor gave him antianxiety medication to relax. He also did his own "test" with a prostitute to see if he could ejaculate inside another woman. "There was no problem [with the prostitute], and I told my wife about it later." [Was she upset?] "She wasn't happy about it."

Table 13. Men's reported sexual problems and guilt *(continued)*

Country	Fertility Status	Reported Problems
Lebanese	Infertile	Infrequent sex. "Sometimes we go on for a very long time without. We have very few, *very, very* few sexual relations. [Are you attracted to her?] "It's not a problem of attraction, just exhaustion. We're too busy, I guess."
Lebanese	Fertile	Infrequent sex. "All the time, the man wants [sex]. It's our nature. But she doesn't want to, because she's upset about this problem [infertility]. She keeps thinking of this, and all the time she's nervous; it's affecting her mood."
Lebanese	Infertile	Had both Hodgkin's disease and a serious car accident which injured his spine. He is impotent. "I have some problems in my legs and penis and the right side of my back; I don't feel at all. My penis, I have to control by my head. With my hand, I can't finish, it is impossible." He took Viagra at the beginning of marriage, but stopped. "The doctor said the sensations of my penis will recover, but I think the doctor was a liar." He has suggested that his wife divorce him, "but she is young and won't leave me."
Lebanese	Infertile	He doesn't enjoy having sex with his wife, only with his mistress of two years. He experiences both impotence and very quick ejaculation with his wife, for which he was prescribed Zoloft, unsuccessfully.
Lebanese	Fertile	Fast ejaculation—"sometimes too fast."
Lebanese	Infertile	Fast ejaculation—"too fast, a minute."
Syrian	Fertile	Infrequent sex. "I want, but she no. It's a problem for me, *a lot!*" [Do you tell her?] "I don't tell her, because I don't want to overburden her. This problem has been since the beginning of marriage. I used to have sex a lot more *before* marriage than I do now. But I would never say this to her because I think that this is how much [sex] she can give. She's not a sexual person. I've tried to teach her, but I don't like to pressure her."
Lebanese	Fertile	Occasional impotence. "It's all psychological, based on psychological tiredness." He took Viagra only once, "which was a mistake."
Lebanese	Infertile	Occasional impotence, for which he took Viagra only once. Believes his infertility is due to excessive premarital masturbation.
Lebanese, living in Cote d'Ivoire	Infertile	Blames infertility on numerous STIs contracted during excessive sex (which he estimates as 10,000 different women) in Cote d'Ivoire between the ages of sixteen and thirty-seven. "In my opinion, the problem is when I didn't take injections for the infections for the first two months. I wouldn't go to see the doctor, because I was afraid of the injections, which were very painful. And sometimes I didn't feel the infection. But maybe these [sexual] infections, I think this is the problem. There is no other cause for my infertility."

TABLE 13. Men's reported sexual problems and guilt *(continued)*

Country	Fertility Status	Reported Problems
Lebanese	Infertile	Blames infertility on excessive premarital masturbation. "I used to masturbate every day before marriage, ever since I was fifteen years old." He experienced impotence while taking a locally produced cough medication.
Lebanese, formerly living in Venezuela	Infertile	Blames his infertility on his premarital masturbation, when he did not have a constant sex partner. "A doctor said to me that infertility is the consequence of *not* having constant [sexual] relations. The interruption. This is the only problem [for his fertility]." Even so, in Venezuela he had "for sure" more than 1,000 sexual partners, "or five to seven women every month." He contracted an STI, and was circumcised at age twenty-two "for cleanliness."
Lebanese	Infertile	Infrequent sex and rapid ejaculation. "My wife doesn't like sex, so maybe this is the problem. I ejaculate inside her, but sometimes too quickly, maybe one to two minutes. Before, with my girlfriend, I was having a lot more sex, so I could go much longer."
Lebanese, living in UAE	Infertile	Rapid ejaculation, and "sometimes she complains."
Lebanese	Fertile	Infrequent sex, due to his wife's painful endometriosis. "Maybe we go one to two months with no sex. This is hard for me! It has affected my sex life, but I love her too much, so we don't think about this."
Syrian	Infertile	Rapid ejaculation. "Every time, it lasts about one-half minute, which is a problem for her. I took a lot of medications, but with no success."
Lebanese, living in Saudi Arabia	Infertile	Loss of libido since living in Saudi Arabia. "Psychologically, I don't feel like it. I'm tired from work, the heat, the humidity, and our social relations are not good there. My wife wants [sex] more than me." He also went through a very painful premarital circumcision at age thirty-one [because Christians are not generally circumcised like Muslims]. "I got too much pain! I would not advise anyone to do it!"
Lebanese	Fertile	Married to a cold, sexually repressed woman, who has been under the care of a psychologist. "She isn't comfortable. She doesn't feel like having sex. Probably this has affected, psychologically, the infertility, because she's not relaxed during sex."
Lebanese	Fertile	He was sexually normal during the first year of marriage [as also confirmed by his wife], but has suffered from complete impotence for two years. Neither Viagra nor testosterone injections have helped. "I don't know, but I don't feel anything. Dr. [name] said it's psychological. Maybe this is stress related. But it is affecting our getting pregnant because there is not enough frequency." According to his wife, he is totally impotent, so they must undertake IVF to conceive.

TABLE 13. Men's reported sexual problems and guilt *(continued)*

Country	Fertility Status	Reported Problems
Lebanese	Fertile	Has untreated diabetic impotence since the first year of marriage (nine years).
Lebanese	Infertile	Blames his infertility on STIs. Lived with a Filipina maid/girlfriend for eleven years, and then with a woman from Mauritius. Both became pregnant and aborted. He contracted two STIs, including genital herpes. "I got sick with an STD from a woman, a bad woman, and I took injections. I had some herpes from the woman from Mauritius, the kind that comes on the mouth."

shame—that he and eleven other Lebanese refugee men had had group intercourse with a West African prostitute. Following this episode, he contracted a sexually transmitted infection, which was quickly resolved with an antibiotic. Nonetheless, both Mohsen and his close hometown friend who had also participated in the group sex had gone on to suffer from long-term infertility in their subsequent marriages, of fifteen- and twenty-year durations, respectively. In Mohsen's view, it was this illicit sex act that caused his infertility. He lamented, "Only God knows if this is the reason, but I think so. I feel guilty. But all of us were like this back in Abidjan [the capital of Cote d'Ivoire], because there were so many prostitutes there."

Although some men such as Mohsen disclosed having sex with prostitutes, no men in my study admitted to having sex with other men. I was frankly reluctant to ask this question in these "very married" IVF clinic settings where men were attempting to conceive with their wives. In retrospect, it would have been interesting to know more about homosexuality, which is considered in Islam to be a grave form of *zina*.[31] As shown in table 13, some men admitted having little interest in sex with their wives, and a few men were totally impotent within marriage. Men who desire men, but who feel forced by social propriety to marry women, may lack the capacity to undertake mandatory heterosexual sex.[32] Childlessness, in fact, may be the outcome of sexual problems induced by mandatory heterosexuality within the Middle East, in which enforced marriages are bound to fail "in the bedroom," if not elsewhere.

Although I failed to ask men about non-heteronormative sexual experience either before or after marriage, I did a better job of asking all men in my Lebanese study a series of questions about age of sexual initiation, numbers of sexual partners (past and present), histories of STIs, and current sexual problems. In doing so, I sometimes opened a veritable floodgate of emotional angst and haunted psyches. As in Mohsen's story, various forms of *zina*-related sexual guilt—over premarital sexuality, use of prostitutes, and STIs—were deemed by some men to be the cause of their current male infertility problems. Furthermore, male sexual problems, particularly erectile dysfunction (impotence) and problems of ejaculation, were affecting some men's marital lives for the worse. So were female sexual problems, including lack of desire and pelvic pain during intercourse, about which some men complained to me. As noted in table 13, some of these men were married to their cousins; consanguineous marriage in the Middle East has been reported to inhibit sexual function in infertile men.[33] However, most of the sexual problems described by men were not attributable to cousin marriage. In fact, exactly one-quarter of the men in my Lebanese study reported sexual problems and guilt feelings, even if they were otherwise happily married to their wives. This finding is similar to my earlier study of infertile couples in Egypt, where exactly one-third suffered from "sexual troubles."[34] In short, sexuality may be fraught for Middle Eastern men, most of whom are Muslim and who may suffer sexually for reasons of *zina* and sexual guilt.

Unfortunately, these sexual problems go largely unresolved. At the time of my study in 2003, there was one sexologist in Lebanon, a woman, just as there was one female sexologist in Egypt and in Saudi Arabia, according to media reports.[35] Whether Middle Eastern men feel comfortable seeking help from a female sex therapist remains uncertain. In my own studies across the region, I have never heard of a man seeking help from a sex therapist. Instead, the minority of men who seek help of any kind go to male urologists and andrologists, or they may ask a male IVF physician for treatment in the course of an ICSI cycle. Most men are told that their sexual problems are "psychological," yet are rarely directed to psychologists. Instead, Viagra or testosterone injections are the "magic bullets" for male sexual dysfunction.

In short, most cases of sexual dysfunction go completely unrecognized and untreated. In Middle Eastern clinical settings, a "don't ask, don't tell" policy prevails, rendering sexual problems invisible.[36] As one Lebanese Shia Muslim IVF physician admitted,

> This problem of sexual dysfunction is definitely much higher than what we discuss with our patients. Few volunteer this information unless we ask. It's definitely very common; at least one-third have some kind of sexual problem. Because in addition to our strict social community, where parents teach children that sexuality is bad, *haram*, there are strict religious beliefs. So this makes a higher percentage of sexual difficulties. And we doctors don't ask all the time. In fact, it's very, very common that we don't go further into these problems, of whether male infertility is actually due to premature

ejaculation or impotence. What we do know is that lots of patients can't produce specimens for semen analysis. So they end up undergoing sperm aspiration under anesthesia.

Semen Collection in Middle Eastern IVF Clinics

There are two common ways of retrieving sperm from the male body, through masturbation and through testicular surgery, and both are commonly employed in IVF clinics throughout the Middle Eastern region. Although masturbation is the most common method of semen collection, it sometimes fails, leading to the second more invasive option. Reasons for masturbation failure are varied but clearly reflect the anxieties and ambivalences over the practice of masturbation.

Furthermore, the IVF clinic itself is a site of bodily practice where infertile bodies are touched, poked, prodded, manipulated, sedated, and cut open. The very space of the clinic—and the conditions under which such bodily practices are performed—may either add to or mitigate patients' suffering, including in the act of semen collection through masturbation. Semen collection is a mandatory part of clinic routines. Semen is collected not only for the purposes of male infertility diagnosis (i.e., semen analysis) but also at the important point in the ICSI cycle when harvested eggs, or oocytes, are to be fertilized. For many men, "timed" semen collection on the day of egg retrieval is an inherently stressful event, but it may be made even more stressful because of clinic practices and conditions. Consider this scenario, which was described to me by an Egyptian IVF patient, whose husband failed to produce a crucial semen sample,

> Unfortunately, I told [the IVF doctor] that my husband has difficulty making a sample in the clinic, and I asked can we do it at home. He said, "No, it's better at the center and come on Friday [i.e., the Egyptian weekend]; you'll find no one there, and he'll feel free and feel so good." So, the doctor told us at the last minute, "Come on Friday, and he will do it [masturbate] easily." When he went there, he found many, many, many people. It was crowded even on a Friday. It was in September, so the weather was very hot. And it was a small, small bathroom right beside the nurse's office. And he started sweating and couldn't do it. After that, he was very upset and said, "I hate marriage."

She continued,

> My ovaries had started to work, and I took all the expensive medicine, and then there was no use, because he couldn't provide a se-

men sample. [The doctor] said, "Oh well, you can try next time." I was really angry, and I told him, "You are not a doctor. You are not honest. You're wasting the time and money of people. We are not people from a village to be told, "Come here. Do this. Do that." Really, these doctors are savage—against humanity.

Although this woman clearly blamed her IVF physician for her husband's difficulties—and the costly cancellation of her IVF cycle—the physical layout of the IVF clinic was at least partly to blame, especially because no special "semen collection" room was set aside for this purpose. Of the five IVF clinics in which I conducted research in Egypt and Lebanon, only two provided separate semen collection rooms in which men could masturbate fairly privately, and in only one of these was sexually arousing material, in the form of a pornographic videotape, made available to husbands. The latter clinic was the only one located in a private office complex. The rest were situated in either private or public hospitals. Because so many Middle Eastern IVF clinics are hospital based, policies of the hospital, including the prohibition on pornographic material (which is illegal in most Middle Eastern countries), may affect the nature of the site in which semen is collected. As noted in the Egyptian woman's testimony, her husband was expected to masturbate over a toilet in a clinic bathroom—probably the most common site of IVF semen collection in the Middle East (and perhaps in the world). Even if special rooms are set aside for semen collection, privacy may not be guaranteed, leading to profound performance anxieties for some husbands.[37]

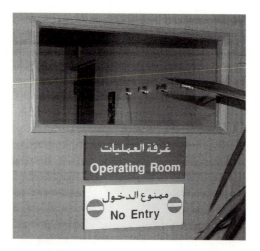

FIGURE 9. Door to an IVF clinic operating room

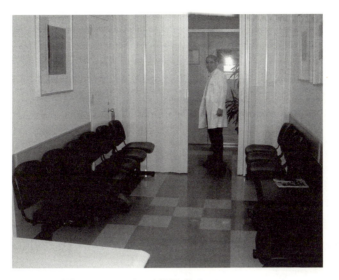

Figure 10. Waiting room in an IVF clinic

The description of an IVF clinic in one large teaching hospital in Lebanon illustrates the nature of semen collection through masturbation in many Middle Eastern IVF clinics. On the seventh floor of the hospital, there was a small cluster of rooms constituting the hospital's IVF clinic (figure 9). This hospital-based IVF clinic could only be described as "intimate." A hallway off the main ob-gyn outpatient department led into the IVF unit, where patients sat in a tiny waiting area with two rows of black leather chairs facing each other (figure 10). Beyond the waiting area was a screen door, which opened and closed as the doctors and patients entered the operating and recovery room areas. Thus, the IVF unit had an almost theatrical quality, as the screen to the secret "backstage" world of the IVF clinic regularly opened and shut.

While women who were undergoing IVF procedures were allowed to enter behind the screen door, the nervous husbands usually waited outside, trying not to make eye contact as they sat facing each other, often rubbing prayer beads, in the small waiting room. Occasionally, men in the waiting room did chat, asking each other how many times they had gone through this agonizing ritual. Men could be heard giving each other encouraging words of *insha'Allah khayr* (i.e., God willing, goodness will prevail).

For some men, the relative intimacy of this hospital-based IVF clinic was extremely uncomfortable. Not only was it obvious why they were there (i.e., to overcome an infertility problem, most commonly male infertility),

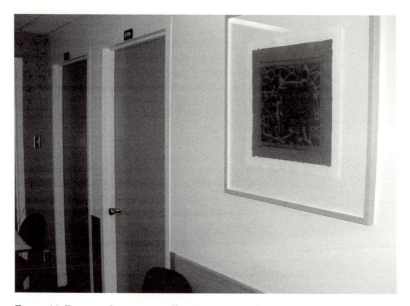

FIGURE 11. Door to the semen collection room within a waiting area

but they were asked to provide their semen in a small room, whose door was located directly *within* the waiting room area (figure 11). The semen collection room was small, with only a black leather settee, much like a psychiatrist's bed, on which men could recline while staring at two pictures of a sexy blonde (white) woman, wearing a provocative corset and garters, placed on the opposite wall. No other stimulating materials, be they magazines or videos, were provided. Before entering this space, men were handed a plastic cup by a laboratory technician and were asked, usually in full view of other patients, to enter the room for the purposes of masturbation. All those present in the waiting area, including in some cases elderly mothers and mothers-in-law, were fully aware of what was required, and they watched (and perhaps informally timed) the men as they went in and out of the semen collection room.

For many men, the public nature of this most intimate, even shameful act was deeply threatening, and performance anxiety problems, where men were unable to provide a semen sample, were not infrequent. For example, one patient, who happened to be a cardiologist, was visibly upset when he exited the semen collection room. He found the head nurse and complained to her, although in a joking fashion: "What am I, a donkey? I cannot do this in that room, where I feel like the others are watching me. I might as well do it in the waiting area in front of everyone! (He made the hand motions of masturbation.) It would be easier! I'm a cardiologist, and I say: What is this room?!" He stomped off down the hall to find his IVF physician in order to complain. Another physician with severe oligozoo- spermia was asked by the embryologist to return to the semen collection room to produce a second sample, since so few spermatozoa were found in his initial semen analysis. He was clearly distraught, asking the embryolo- gist if this was really necessary. She replied, "We found eleven live sperm, and that is good enough, but I wish you could give us a second sample." He then turned to me and stated, "Ejaculation is 'in the head,' it's some- thing psychological, and it's not so easy to produce under such clinical conditions."

Because these two men were physicians, they felt entitled to complain about semen collection to the IVF staff. They were told that little could be done. Chronic shortages of available hospital rooms meant that privacy could not be maintained in one of the most intimate acts—the collection of semen—that occurred within the hospital's walls. Less-educated men were often reluctant to register their complaints, fearing that this would affect the quality of the physician-patient relationship. One such man, a janitor with only five years of schooling, had taken out a large bank loan to fund his one and only cycle of ICSI. However, on the "big day" of egg retrieval, he complained to me about his worst fears,

> Now I have to do sperm collection. It's difficult to produce the sam- ple. I had to give a sample once in that room and it's not spacious. At home, I would feel more comfortable, and it would work immedi- ately. The doctor told me I could go home, but I would have to take the day off work, and this is a problem. It would eliminate a day from my annual vacation.

He continued,

> There is no video. I'm wondering how people manage to do this without help, without videos. Each man should be given a video when he enters that room, then return it immediately afterwards to the clinic staff. Then the whole procedure would take five minutes, so that someone can relax. [How about if they had magazines?] A video is nicer than magazines, and works better. Magazines are not enjoyable, but a video is. The posters in there are not helping; they are not effective.

Many of the men in my study who had either experienced or witnessed the travails of this hospital's semen collection room lamented the prob- lem of semen collection as the worst part of the embodied IVF and ICSI experience for men. Some were vociferous critics of clinic policies, insist- ing that clinics provide other avenues for successful semen collection. Two passages from lengthy interviews are illustrative of men's anxieties and critiques. In both of these cases, the men were educated professionals, who had returned to their home country of Lebanon from other Middle Eastern countries where they worked, in order to attempt a cycle of ICSI with their wives. Although they privileged the quality of Lebanese IVF clinics over similar clinics in their host countries, they were both deeply dismayed about their experiences of semen collection in Lebanon, which they considered highly fraught. One of these men, a Shia Muslim engineer who had already tried ICSI six times with his wife in Tunisia, had this to say,

> I think ICSI is better in Lebanon than in Tunisia, because there is a relationship between Lebanon and Marseilles, Paris, London. We have something good in Lebanon [medically speaking] with respect to the Middle Eastern area. Syria, Tunisia, Egypt—I think Lebanon is better. So, I decided in the end to do it [ICSI] in Lebanon. Six times in Tunisia, and we didn't succeed. I pushed my wife to do it this time [though] she didn't want to.

He continued,

> But ICSI affects sex. Psychologically, it's not good. In IVF centers, they say, "Give me the sperm now! After five minutes, I need your sperm. Now, now! Give me, give me!" This is not good. The male encounters problems when they do that. It's not good. I start thinking about when I will give the sperm, and I feel uncomfortable.

Pointing to the semen collection room in the IVF waiting area, he said,

> This room here. The first time I go to do it [masturbate], I find one chaise lounge chair. How will I do it? At least in the other center [in Tunisia], they give one room for me and my wife. It has a [pornographic] video film and a toilet. It is separate with a bed—a room for us, like a hotel. They tell you, "Stay, and try to give us some sperm." They help us to stay calm, and we'll do it easily. With my wife, it's better! We'd even pay extra for this. Give me one room, and we'll pay! Take $66 and give me one room. We pay for many things in ICSI, so why not this? Here, it's like a prison cell.

Similarly, a Sunni Muslim Lebanese-Palestinian man, who was a highly paid medical diagnostics salesman, began his interview with me by complaining,

> Do you want to know the problem? [My IVF doctor] asked me in front of everyone to give sperm. People [in the waiting area] were laughing, smiling. Old women sitting and smiling. And he told me, "Do it with yourself" [by masturbation]. I'm not fourteen years old!

You go into this room and there is one journal—with cars, not wom-
en! I can do it at home and bring [the semen sample] in, rather than
to enter that room again.

He added, jokingly, "Tell [the IVF doctor] I'll have to sue him!"

In fact, this man was unable to "produce" on the day in which his wife's
eggs were retrieved for in vitro fertilization, as happens to men who have
anxieties about the semen collection process. Thus, after his wife awoke
from anesthesia and after most of the waiting room had cleared (by 2:00
pm), she was asked by the IVF nurse to accompany her fretful husband
into one of the more private ultrasound rooms in order to produce a semen sample with him. Without his semen, the IVF cycle could not be completed, with significant loss of both valuable eggs and money.

It was not at all unusual for men in the IVF clinic to seek accompaniment of their wives for semen collection. The clinics I studied never refused
this, knowing full well that some men could not produce a semen sample
without the help of conjugal partners. Furthermore, one clinic in which I
worked catered to religiously pious Shia Muslim couples, including some
members of Lebanon's Hizbullah political party. All such "religious" couples were allowed to collect semen together, in a room specified for this
purpose. Tape was put over the door, with a "Do Not Disturb" sign. "Sperm
collection by intercourse" was noted in such patients' files. When I asked
one of the Shia Muslim IVF physicians about what went on in such rooms,
he said he had no idea, but he suspected that intercourse, followed by
coitus interruptus into the plastic semen collection cup, might be taking
place. Presumably, some religious wives also masturbated their husbands
to ejaculation, a practice permitted in some of the legal schools of Islam,
as described earlier.

In addition to catering to religious Muslim couples, this clinic was also
the only one in my study to provide a separate semen collection room
for men. The room was located on a separate floor for the purposes of
privacy and was fully equipped with a VCR and pornographic video designed to produce sexual arousal. According to the West African janitor (a
convert to Islam), who routinely took male patients to this room and then
retrieved their semen samples, male patients enjoyed coming to the clinic
precisely because of its semen collection routine. He theorized that Arab
men are sexually repressed, because Muslim society prohibits open dis-
play of or education about sexuality. Access to pornography is only available on the black market (and increasingly through satellite television).[38]
Thus, for most Lebanese men, semen collection at the clinic provided their
only opportunity to watch pornographic material, which, although guilt-
producing, was also distinctly pleasurable. According to him, most men
were able to produce semen samples quickly and easily while watching

the video. The only hitch: The pornographic movie was constantly being stolen, requiring frequent replacement!

One Shia Muslim man happened to be due for semen collection on a day when the video went missing. During his interview, he complained to me, "I had trouble giving the sample. The videotape is not downstairs, and it's difficult to do it without the video. Why did they take me down to the first floor if I could have stayed upstairs with my wife? Between you and me, I wouldn't go to the first floor if there wasn't a videotape."

Fortunately for this man, he was able to provide a semen sample, even without the videotape. But what happens to those poor souls, religious or secular, whose guilt and anxiety overwhelm them, militating against production of a timely semen sample? To take but one example, a man emerged from the semen collection room, pleading with a hospital orderly, "Can you tell them to stop the operation [egg retrieval from his wife]? I'm not having success." Because the success of semen collection is so crucial to ICSI success, some clinics opt to perform invasive, surgical sperm retrievals on such men, who suffer from clinic-based performance anxiety. Testicular sperm can be retrieved by different techniques, including testicular sperm extraction (TESE), which refers to a testicular biopsy to remove tissue with sperm in it; testicular sperm aspiration (TESA), which refers to methods by which sperm are aspirated with suction from the testicles; percutaneous epididymal sperm aspiration (PESA), by which sperm are aspirated with suction from the epididymis; and fine-needle aspiration (FNA), in which thin-gauge needles are used to aspirate sperm from the testicles. These techniques are performed under either general or local anesthesia. As a form of testicular "needlework," they are usually accompanied by significant pain and discomfort. However, they are required when men are unable to ejaculate sperm because of impotence or performance anxiety. Furthermore, a significant number of men are azoospermic, producing no sperm whatsoever in their ejaculate. As in Shaykh Ali's case, azoospermic men are automatic candidates for testicular sperm retrieval.

On the basis of my postoperative observation in Middle Eastern IVF clinics, the multiple testicular penetrations often required to extract sperm from the testicles are exquisitely painful for men who have suffered through these operations. In one of the clinics in which I worked in Lebanon, testicular aspirations were routinely being performed under general anesthesia. In the other clinic, testicular biopsies were being performed under local anesthesia by a urological surgeon, usually in one of the clinical consultation rooms in the IVF clinic. Men who were taken into these rooms for the purposes of testicular biopsy often emerged, walking slowly, with their legs spread apart. Their pained expressions and gait were telling of these testicular penetrations. Other infertile men in the waiting areas sometimes whispered about the "difficulty" of such "operations," probably feeling grateful that their own genitals had been spared.

In short, assisted reproduction has brought with it new forms of embodied agony for men, with new forms of male bodily penetration being practiced for the purposes of sperm extraction. Indeed, the need to obtain sperm "at all costs" in the IVF clinic leads to profound trauma for some men, who are unable to successfully ejaculate through masturbation, and may end up having their testicles poked and prodded.

CONCLUSION

We began this chapter with the story of Shaykh Ali, a man with a tortured "body history."[39] Shaykh Ali refused to masturbate out of religious piety. However, he believed in "science" and had undergone testicular aspiration in his quest to become a father. It seems imperative that we begin to ask Muslim men, pious, secular, and those in between, about their own reproductive and sexual bodies and listen seriously to what they have to say. My own scholarly forays into Middle Eastern Muslim IVF clinics suggest that Muslim men, both fertile and infertile, are excellent interlocutors of their embodied experiences. Many men are willing to talk at great length about their reproductive and sexual problems, if they are encouraged to do so. But, because so few Middle Eastern Muslim men are asked—by either doctors or scholars—a great deal remains unknown about sex and reproduction as aspects of male embodiment throughout the Muslim world.

As I have shown in this chapter, ambivalence toward masturbation and semen collection is the result of Islamic religious mores, which regard masturbation as disdainful and semen as defiling. Religiously based injunctions against masturbation as a legitimate, healthy form of male sexuality mean that masturbation may be inherently guilt-producing for many, if not all, Muslim men. Some Muslim men attribute their own infertility to the "damage" and "punishment" they have brought on themselves for practices of masturbation in childhood, adolescence, and young adulthood. In Middle Eastern societies where masturbation is considered "taboo," to use one informant's term, requests to perform masturbation in IVF clinics, especially in semipublic spaces, are considered inherently shameful, causing great moral and emotional discomfort for some men. Therefore, when asked to masturbate "on demand" as part of the IVF and ICSI regime, some Muslim men bring their anxieties about masturbation with them, and are therefore unable to produce critically important semen samples.

Having said this, most Muslim men in my study were able to "perform" when called upon by clinic staff. Men's masturbation is now a routine part of assisted reproduction. Somehow, against all odds and despite religious guilt, Muslim men are able to masturbate, reach orgasm, and ejaculate into a plastic cup within the cramped spaces and over the toilets in IVF clinics across the Middle Eastern region. Just as ICSI is serving to normalize male infertility through medicalization, ICSI is also normalizing "medical masturbation" in the Muslim Middle East. Although masturbation may be viewed as *zina* in Islam, millions of Muslim men are masturbating out of medical necessity, and some are even embracing the idea of masturbation as a healthy, pleasurable, and guilt-free form of male sexuality. In short, emergent masculinities in the Middle East now include masturbation, especially on the way to becoming ICSI fathers.

CHAPTER 6

Islam and Assisted Reproduction

IBRAHIM AND HIS FIFTEEN FAILED ICSIs

January in Dubai is a lovely time of year. The sun shines, but the winter temperatures are moderate, making it pleasant to be outdoors. It was on such a day in January 2007 when I met Ibrahim and his wife Nura outside the ultrasound scanning suite of an IVF clinic on the outskirts of Dubai. I was packing my bag to leave for the day, when Ibrahim approached me, having read my study advertisement placed on the waiting room tables. We made a tentative appointment to meet later in the month. But as soon as I stepped into the waiting taxi (with Ahmed, my driver), I received a call from Ibrahim on my cell phone, asking if we could meet sooner, ideally at his home. I agreed, and two days later, on Ibrahim's way home from work, he picked me up at the clinic for the short ride to his and Nura's spacious, high-rise flat, overlooking an inland lake. I commented on the beauty of the couple's home and its view, and Ibrahim proceeded to give me a tour, showing me the second bedroom where he hoped there would soon be a child. We then sat down on the ornate, Louis IV–style furniture in the living room to talk about Ibrahim's infertility problem and the couple's ICSI quest.

Married for thirteen years, Ibrahim and Nura were first cousins, the children of two Palestinian sisters. Ibrahim had grown up in a Palestinian family in Kuwait, but when he visited his mother's family in Jineen (now part of Israel), he met his beautiful cousin Nura, falling madly in love with her. They married "for love" in 1993, and by 1994, the questioning began about why Nura was not yet pregnant. "You know our traditions in the Middle East," Ibrahim said to me. "We get married, and after one year, everybody starts asking what's going on. If you go for more than one year [without a pregnancy], this comes to be seen as a problem."

Nura began the treatment quest by visiting a doctor in 1995. When the doctor told her that she was able to become pregnant, Ibrahim did his first "check up," a semen analysis which proved to be "very bad." The physician advised Ibrahim to go to a "specialist." Ibrahim consulted a urologist and, per Middle Eastern medical tradition, Ibrahim ended up undergoing a varicocelectomy in 1995. Not surprisingly, the varicocelectomy did nothing to improve Ibrahim's sperm count. "After that, I did many tests," Ibrahim explained. "And still, the results turned out to be very bad." He then volunteered, "I have a copy of all my medical reports. I could show them to you on Sunday. Always, the semen count was 400,000 to 500,000, very, very weak. And after one-half hour, everything died. There was fragmentation, also."

"Our journey starts here," Ibrahim told me, immediately launching into a story of thirteen failed ICSI attempts between 1995 and 2007, the last one conducted during the sacred month of Ramadan the year before. In the early days of their ICSI quest, Ibrahim and Nura focused on Jordan, a country with a Palestinian majority, Palestinian-run IVF clinics, and a "famous" IVF hospital in Amman, one of the first to perform IVF in the Middle East. Traveling from their home in Kuwait to Jordan was both taxing and expensive. Nonetheless, Ibrahim and Nura attempted ICSI seven times in Jordan at three different IVF centers. At that time, the cost of one ICSI cycle was 1,500 to 2,000 Jordanian *dinars* (approximately $2,100–2,800), but Ibrahim's monthly salary was only 200 Jordanian *dinars*, or one-tenth the amount of one ICSI. In desperation, Nura contemplated selling her bridal gold. Fortunately, however, Ibrahim secured a good job in Dubai as an accountant, and the couple moved there in 1999.

Within their first year in Dubai, Ibrahim and Nura underwent two ICSIs in Emirati government hospitals, where assisted reproductive technologies were partially state-subsidized. However, both ICSIs failed, and the couple became concerned about standards of cleanliness, having seen cockroaches on the hospital walls.

As the new millennium was fast approaching and their nine ICSI cycles had all failed, Ibrahim became convinced to "stop searching in Arab countries." A Palestinian friend in France made an appointment for Ibrahim and Nura at an IVF clinic in Rouen. There, a chromosome test of Ibrahim's sperm showed "fragmentation," an indication of a chromosomal defect. Reviewing Ibrahim's case, the French doctors told him bluntly, "We can't do anything for you. And since you did ICSI more than nine to ten times, we cannot do it again, because the French rules say that we cannot do ICSI after four times." They then suggested adoption, which shocked Ibrahim. "That's fine for you," Ibrahim told the French doctors. "But for us, as Muslims, we have a different tradition."

Demoralized but not destroyed, Ibrahim began his "research," drawing upon his global network of relatives and acquaintances in the Palestinian diaspora. Fortunately, one of Ibrahim's Palestinian friends in Los Angeles told him that he would be willing to help with the ICSI quest. Despite the difficulty of obtaining visas for travel to the post-9/11 United States, Ibrahim and Nura's patience paid off. They were eventually allowed to seek medical care in America. There, they visited IVF centers in both Las Vegas and Los Angeles, agreeing that their best chances for ICSI success were at UCLA, where, in the words of Ibrahim, a "master doctor" was in charge of the IVF clinic.

For the first time in a decade of ICSI-seeking, Ibrahim and Nura were offered preimplantation genetic diagnosis (PGD). In Ibrahim and Nura's case, the UCLA physician wanted to determine whether the couple's ICSI embryos were carrying genetic defects, causing repeated ICSI failures. After verifying that PGD was religiously acceptable, Ibrahim and Nura agreed to PGD, and learned that eight of their twenty embryos were free from obvious genetic disease. As Ibrahim recalled, "He [the IVF doctor] told me something funny then. He said, 'You have seven girls and one boy.' I said, 'I don't give a damn shit for girls or boys, Doctor! All I want is a child!' So he returned back [to Nura's uterus] three girls and one boy."

Ibrahim and Nura were scheduled to return to Dubai a week after the embryo transfer, and Ibrahim carefully changed their tickets from economy to business class, so that Nura and the four ICSI embryos could "recline" in transit. After their return to Dubai, Nura underwent a pregnancy test— again negative. "My God, you cannot imagine how disappointed we were," Ibrahim exclaimed. Calling me by my first name, he continued,

> In the U.S., Marcia, the trip cost me, with the travel, with everything, around $35,000. Maybe I've spent more than $100,000 in total for all of the [ICSI] trials. If somebody else had done this to Nura, I'm sure she couldn't stand it. Sometimes, I come back home, and I find her crying. The environment here in the Arab countries, I mean, her sister is getting pregnant, my brother's wife is getting pregnant, and sometimes they cannot stop it [their fertility]! Our family is not interfering, and it's a love marriage. But sometimes, you know, I told her, "All of the problem is because of me, not you. It's from my side. If you want, we can divorce." But she refused. She told me, "If there is going to be a baby, it has to come from you."

He then asked me, "It's *so* frustrating; I have to do ICSI. But how and where?" At this point, I broached the delicate topic of sperm donation. Ibrahim responded,

> Somebody suggested sperm donation, but we totally refused. For both of us, it's not in consideration. [Why?] Because I refuse it. If the sperm comes from somebody else, you know, inside your heart, you will know it is not yours. Not our color, not our eyes, different things will come out. That's why we refuse. He will not be my son. But maybe I will go for the other one, cloning, or how they did Dolly the sheep. This cloning I have no problem with. [Even if Islam doesn't allow it?] I'm sure they *will* allow it eventually. IVF started in

the 1980s, and at first, the Islamic authorities didn't accept, but now they accept. Maybe after five years, they will accept cloning. But using a donor, no. It's not from your back [where sperm are thought to be made]. It's not from you."

Nura, who had been quietly following the conversation added, "It's like adoption. I wouldn't do it because I don't like the idea."

Given their opposition to adoption and gamete donation, both of which are prohibited in Sunni Islam, Ibrahim and Nura explained that they must use their own gametes. According to Ibrahim, their reproductive fate is ultimately in God's hands,

> I believe in science, but also God. I believe in science, but if God wants to give, He will. We have the same belief, that if God wants to get us something [a baby], he will give. One of my friends, he was having the same problem as me. Every year, he was going on a vacation with his wife to Jordan and doing ICSI, and it was not happening. Then two years ago, I got back in touch with him. He said, "You'll never believe what happened! I got fed up going to clinics here and there and just spending money. So my wife and I went to Saudi Arabia on the *umra* [a form of pilgrimage], and we were staying there and praying to God. And, yes, it happened."

"So you see," Ibrahim said, "This is from God. You have to believe."

According to Ibrahim, he would be satisfied if God granted him one child. "One baby and that's it! Not more. I told Nura, 'If I get one baby, your ovary, I will remove it!' I don't want to think about it anymore! This is the only, and lonely problem in my life. I don't have any other problem."

Ibrahim told me that he had contemplated going to Belgium, where ICSI was invented, but he had decided against it. "One doctor, he advised us to go to Belgium. But after we tried ICSI in America, I feel that what we do here [in the Middle East] is the same." At the time of our meeting, Ibrahim had placed his hopes in the private IVF clinic on the edge of Dubai where I first met him. Although the IVF physician was a Hindu from India, Ibrahim found him "down to earth," a physician who had still "found hope" in Ibrahim's poor sperm profile. Ibrahim continued,

> When I'm alone, I start thinking, "What's wrong with me?" I don't know how to explain it. Sometimes, I think my problem was caused by the fear I faced in Kuwait in 1991. The Kuwaiti people came back to Kuwait [from Iraq], and I was there after the [First Gulf] war finished. They came back and caught all of the Palestinians they could find [whose leader, Yasir Arafat, had supported Saddam Hussein]. They caught me for one night and tortured me, blindfolding my eyes and beating and slapping me. They took me from my house and I

didn't know where I was going because they put a blindfold over my eyes. I was blindfolded, but I felt that there were about eight people there, in a building or a basement, and they tortured me. Then after that, they threw me out, and when the blindfold was removed from my eyes, my eyes opened, but I couldn't see anything for about one-half hour. This happened two years before marriage, and the shock of that, of this happening in the place where I was born and lived for twenty-five years, I don't know, but I think this experience may have caused my problem.

After this sobering conclusion to our interview, Ibrahim and Nura drove me home, chatting amiably about how much they enjoyed the United States and the"friendliness"of Americans. I was able to show them around the pretty, American-affiliated desert campus where I lived with my family. I promised to keep in touch and to make a few inquiries on their behalf. I was heartened by the fact that Ibrahim and Nura still had three female embryos in frozen storage at UCLA. Ibrahim had told me that returning to America to try a so-called "frozen cycle" with these embryos was too difficult, financially and emotionally. "If it is guaranteed that I will 'catch' these three girls [as my children], I will go and put!"he had exclaimed during the interview. But rightly so, Ibrahim realized that there were no such guarantees.

Several weeks after our interview, I inquired with the clinic's "embryo courier" service about whether it was possible to transport three viable embryos all the way from Los Angeles to Dubai. When the courier replied "yes,"I decided to introduce him to Ibrahim, a meeting that took place after Ibrahim and Nura experienced their fourteenth failed ICSI cycle at the Dubai IVF clinic. Ibrahim was very excited about the prospect of transporting their three embryos from the United States to the UAE but was told by the courier that this would cost approximately $2,500. Ibrahim laughed, "What the hell! After all I've paid, this is nothing!"

I left the UAE in July 2007, after six months of fieldwork at the clinic. I learned from the clinic's embryologist—a fellow Palestinian who had taken a special interest in Ibrahim and Nura's case—that the three embryos were flown from Los Angeles in a cryopreservation tank that was hand-carried all the way from LAX through customs at Dubai International Airport. With the help of the Indian doctor, Ibrahim's and Nura's "three girl embryos," made in America and thawed in the UAE, were transferred into Nura's uterus on the Emirati IVF clinic's operating table.

Unfortunately, God decided that the time was still not right for Ibrahim and Nura to become parents. On the fifteenth attempt at ICSI, the three female embryos did not implant in Nura's womb, and Ibrahim's dreams of fathering three little"American-made"Palestinian daughters vanished.

ISLAMIC LOCAL MORAL WORLDS

Ibrahim's story is not only about a tragic ICSI quest. It is a quintessential story about the local moral world of a severely infertile Muslim man and what is at stake for him in trying to become a legitimate father. Neither sperm donation nor adoption of a child can satisfy Ibrahim's parenting desires. Sunni Islamic mandates have prohibited these options for practicing Muslims, and because Ibrahim is pious, he takes these moral injunctions quite seriously. Without these pathways to parenthood, Ibrahim must use his own gametes to conceive a child. However, Ibrahim's sperm are not healthy. PGD, a technology that has been approved by the Islamic authorities,[1] has detected a chromosomal defect that necessitates culling of some of Ibrahim and Nura's embryos. Despite all of Ibrahim's best efforts—including an expensive trip for the couple from Dubai to UCLA, the hand-carried transport of his presumably healthy female embryonic progeny from UCLA to Dubai, and his ongoing faith in both "science and God"—Ibrahim is never able to become the father of his own biological offspring. He dreams of a day when the Islamic authorities will approve of cloning, which could be used to bypass the problem of his infertile sperm. Unfortunately, Ibrahim's own gametes are seriously "fragmented," which he attributes to the shock and fear of wartime torture, rather than to a chromosomal defect, which could be attributed only to God's divine creation. That God makes some people infertile is stated clearly in the Qur'an:

> Unto Allah belongeth the Sovereignty of the heavens and the earth. He createth what He will. He bestoweth female [offspring] upon whom He will, and bestoweth male [offspring] upon whom He will;
> Or He mingleth them, males and females, and He maketh barren whom He will. Lo! He is Knower, Powerful.[2]

Thus, when Ibrahim poses his "why me?" question, he does not blame God for defective creation. To do so would be sacrilegious. Instead, like most infertile Muslim men, he views God as the great "decider"—the one who makes pregnancy and childbirth possible when the time is right, even in cases of recalcitrant infertility. For pious Muslims such as Ibrahim and Nura, these religious theodicies about infertility and its God-given solution are what keep them going, including through multiple painful cycles of ICSI. Only God can grant children to the infertile, as long as the infertile themselves remain faithful, patient, and active seekers of medical remedy.

In the Muslim world, infertile men and women often speak about their deep faith in God, sprinkling their conversations with formulaic remarks, such as "everything is from God," "only God knows," "it's in God's hands," "we're praying to God," "no one stands in the way of God," "God grants children," and "it's our *nasib* [fate]." For example, a Lebanese man with an infertile wife told me, "We believe that everything is in God's hands. You get up in the morning, and then three weeks later, your wife is pregnant. If it's meant to be, it's meant to be." Another Lebanese man, who was himself infertile, had more to say about God's role in earthly life,

> Every problem is from God. If you go to any company and you do not find good work, it's from God. In Islam, when the baby is born, it is God who gives him his life. Everything in his life is from God; it's written before he is born. If the weather is bad, it's from God. In the end, God is responsible for all things. He brings everything. We can't say, "This one is going to be poor, this one is going to be rich, this one a doctor, a professor, a worker." It is all from God.

Science and medicine are also seen as God given. Islam is a religion that is *scientifically agentive*: It encourages the use of science, medicine, and biotechnology in the face of illness and adversity.[3] Assisted reproductive technologies such as IVF and ICSI are seen as being created by human scientists under God's providence. The Muslim IVF physicians who employ these technologies are seen as doing God's handiwork in helping the infertile. Men in my study were adamant that physicians themselves do not have the power to "create life." Or, as one ICSI patient put it succinctly, "The doctors take the eggs and sperm and make embryos and put them back. But who makes the embryo live? It's God, of course." Another man, a highly educated engineer facing "unexplained infertility" with his wife, had this to say about God's role in medicine,

> We've seen four or five doctors, and all the doctors said, "There is no single problem with you, nothing at all." All the doctors said, "It's from God." I told them, "We're talking to scientists!" But they said, "In this case, it's God." Just yesterday, Dr. [name] said, "Pray." I'm a scientist, but I'm a believer, too. The first two months, I went directly and tried science. I did everything I could do, and found no scientific explanation. So now, I will go to God, just like the doctors.

Ibrahim and Nura's dogged pursuit of ICSI must be seen in this light. As religiously faithful Sunni Muslims who have the financial means to pursue ICSI, they are obliged to keep "searching" for a remedy to their childlessness, leaving the ultimate outcome to the realm of the divine. Because IVF and ICSI are seen as God-given solutions to infertility, it is not surprising that a Middle Eastern IVF industry is flourishing. Infertile Muslims who are believers are expected to seek this biotechnological solution to their childlessness. The Muslim demand for these technologies is reflected in growing Middle Eastern supply-side metrics: Turkey now has more than 110

IVF clinics;[4] Iran has more than 70;[5] Egypt has more than 50; and Lebanon, with its tiny population of 4 million, has more than 15 clinics, one of the highest per capita numbers in the world. IVF clinics can be found in virtually every Middle Eastern country, from Morocco in the west to the small, petro-rich Arab Gulf states in the east.[6] This birth of a thriving Middle Eastern IVF sector is also clearly tied to Islam's inherent pronatalism: the Islamic scriptures encourage the growth of an Islamic "multitude."[7] Hence, the use of biotechnologies to assist in the conception of human life has implicit appeal in the Muslim world.

However, the Middle East cannot be called the "Wild East" of assisted reproduction (as the United States is called the "Wild West" of this industry). Although these technologies have been embraced by Islamic authorities, clear limits have also been set for infertile Muslim couples. Specifically, the Sunni Islamic authorities refuse any form of third-party reproductive assistance, including gamete donation, embryo donation, and surrogacy. These technologies have been compared to adoption, which is also illegal in Islam. The Islamic injunctions against sperm donation and adoption underlie Ibrahim's refusal to consider nonbiological fatherhood. To understand the high premium based on biological paternity, it is necessary to examine the contemporary *fatwas* that have ruled on these technologies, effectively banning the use of third parties for Sunni Muslims such as Ibrahim and Nura. It is also important to explore the subsequent bioethical and legal rulings that are being issued to enforce these *fatwa* rulings in some Middle Eastern countries. Furthermore, it is crucial to investigate the convergences and divergences between "official" interpretations of Islam as manifest in *fatwas* issued by renowned Muslim clerics and the "unofficial" discourses and practices of Muslim men and women such as Ibrahim and Nura, who are forced to grapple with infertility in reality.

My goal in this chapter is to explore the moral dimensions of assisted reproduction in the Muslim Middle East, where religion has guided clinical norms and shaped the assisted reproduction experiences of infertile couples.[8] For religiously pious Muslims, both Sunni and Shia, making a test-tube baby within the permissible bounds of the religion is a matter of grave importance. Even today—nearly thirty-five years after the birth of the first IVF baby in Britain, and twenty-five years after the birth of the first Muslim IVF baby in Egypt—infertile Muslim couples considering the use of assisted reproductive technologies turn to religious authorities for guidance. To that end, they tend to seek out the *fatwas* that have been issued on assisted reproduction.

A *fatwa* is a nonlegally binding but authoritative Islamic religious opinion, offered by an Islamic cleric who is considered to be an expert concerning the Islamic scriptures and jurisprudence.[9] *Fatwas* can be issued by a cleric privately, for example, in response to an individual's specific question. *Fatwa*s can also be issued as public statements (e.g., in the media) by individual clerics, or by *fatwa*-issuing councils of clerics within religious universities and special institutions set up specifically for this purpose. For example, in Egypt, the ancient and renowned religious university, Al Azhar, is considered the authoritative source for *fatwa*s. In recent years, many *fatwa*s on a wide variety of reproductive health issues have been issued by Al Azhar and by *fatwa*-granting institutions in other Muslim countries.[10] These *fatwa*s are now disseminated through a variety of means, including religious institutions (e.g., the *fatwa* offices of religious universities or the administrative offices of various religious leaders), books, infertility clinics, and now the Internet, where a great deal of information on Islamic principles and teachings may be found. Today, there are many ways for Muslims to access *fatwa*s on reproduction and other topics, including through media channels, printed collections of clerics' *fatwa*s, and Web sites maintained by clerics' offices. In addition, individuals may place direct queries to those offices, either in person or through telephone, fax, email, or Web sites. In some cases, they may meet directly with a cleric to make a personal inquiry and receive an expert opinion. Once received, the very pathways through which these *fatwa*s are circulated, borrowed, redeployed, and interpreted by followers—particularly in the era of the Internet—are complex and convoluted. In the end, what religious clerics mandate through their *fatwa*s may or may not be realized, understood, accepted, or actualized in daily life.

In general, *fatwa*s issued across the Muslim world have been permissive regarding the practice of IVF and ICSI, considering these technologies to be an acceptable solution to marital infertility and childlessness. But as we shall see in this chapter, major divergences have occurred in the *fatwa*s being issued by Sunni and Shia religious authorities regarding the permissibility of third-party reproductive assistance. In recent years, new *fatwa*s emerging from the Shia world have condoned third-party gamete donation, whereas gamete donation continues to be banned across the Sunni Muslim countries.[11] These divergent Sunni and Shia Islamic approaches toward gamete donation have affected the moral decision making of infertile Muslim couples in ways that are only beginning to be realized.[12]

SUNNI ISLAM AND ASSISTED REPRODUCTION

Sunni Islam is the major branch of the religion. Of the world's 1.6 billion Muslims, 80 to 90 percent are Sunni Muslims. Egypt is a case in point: Of its nearly 80 million people, approximately 90 percent are Sunni Muslims, with a 10 percent Coptic Orthodox Christian minority. Sunni-dominant countries are found across North Africa (Morocco, Algeria, Libya, Tunisia, Egypt, Sudan); through most of the Arab Gulf states, including Saudi Arabia, where a very conservative form of Sunni Islam is practiced; across the Levantine countries of Syria, Jordan, and Palestine; and in the non-Arab country of Turkey. The remaining Middle Eastern countries have a mixture of Sunni and Shia Muslims, as well as Christian minority populations.

IVF was first practiced in the Sunni-majority countries of Egypt, Saudi Arabia, and Jordan, where IVF clinics opened simultaneously in 1986. Egypt's early entrance into assisted reproduction was especially important from a religious standpoint, because the *fatwa* condoning IVF came directly from Egypt's famed religious university, Al Azhar, widely regarded as the seat of Sunni Islamic learning. The Grand Shaykh of Al Azhar issued the first widely authoritative *fatwa* on assisted reproduction, which is reprinted in its entirety in the appendix to this book. The *fatwa* was issued on March 23, 1980—only two years after the birth of the first IVF baby in England but a full six years before the opening of Egypt's first IVF center. More than thirty years later, this original *fatwa* has proved to be enduring. It has subsequently been reendorsed by the Al Azhar clergy and reissued in 1991, 1997, and 2000 during conferences on assisted reproduction organized by Al Azhar's International Islamic Center for Population Studies and Research.[13] In addition, the Egyptian Medical Syndicate has based its bioethical guidelines on the Al Azhar *fatwa*. A variety of other Sunni Muslim Middle Eastern countries have followed suit: *fatwa* institutes in Saudi Arabia, Kuwait, Qatar, and the United Arab Emirates have all issued *fatwas* confirming the basic tenets of the original Al Azhar *fatwa*.[14]

The degree of consensus across the Sunni Muslim countries is quite striking, as are the ways in which these *fatwas* have guided the clinical practices of the Middle Eastern IVF community. The content of the Al Azhar *fatwa* on assisted reproduction has been made known to the Middle Eastern medical community through the writings of Gamal I. Serour, one of three founding members of the first Egyptian IVF center, a professor of obstetrics and gynecology at Al Azhar University, the director of Al Azhar's International Islamic Center for Population Studies and Research, and the president of the International Federation of Gynecology and Obstetrics (FIGO). In a series of major articles published between 1990 and 2008,[15] Serour has spelled out the main points of the Sunni Islamic position on assisted reproduction. Sunni Islamic authorities have agreed that the following ten technologies are *halal*, or religiously permitted:

1. Artificial insemination with the husband's semen is allowed, and the resulting child is the legal offspring of the couple.

2. In vitro fertilization of an egg from the wife with the sperm of her husband, followed by the transfer of the fertilized embryo(s) back to the uterus of the wife, is allowed, provided that the procedure is indicated for a medical reason and is carried out by an expert IVF physician.

3. An excess number of fertilized embryos can be frozen through cryopreservation. The frozen embryos are the property of the couple alone and may be transferred to the same wife in a future frozen cycle but only during the duration of the marriage contract.

4. Sperm or gonads may be cryopreserved before exposure to radiotherapy or chemotherapy and used later in life by the same individual who has survived cancer treatment.

5. Pregnancy in postmenopausal women is allowed using a woman's own cryopreserved embryos, oocytes, or, in the future, ovaries.

6. Multifetal pregnancy reduction (a.k.a. selective reduction) is allowed if the prospect of carrying twins or a high-order multiple pregnancy (HOMP, i.e., triplets or more) to viability is very small. It is also allowed if the health or life of the mother is in jeopardy. As a form of selective abortion, the intention is to preserve the life of the remaining fetuses and minimize complications for the woman.

7. PGD is allowed and even encouraged, where feasible, as a diagnostic option to avoid clinical pregnancy terminations among couples at high risk of genetic disorders in their offspring. PGD may also be used in cases of "family balancing," when couples have children of only one sex.

8. Embryo research, for the advancement of scientific knowledge and the benefit of humanity, is allowed for fourteen days after fertilization on surplus embryos that are donated for research with the informed consent of the couple. These research embryos should not be returned to the woman's uterus.

9. In the future, gene therapy may be approved, not to promote genetic advantage or privilege in offspring but rather to remediate genetically or otherwise physically inherited genetic diseases and pathological conditions.

10. In the future, uterine transplantation will be allowable as a remedy for women who are lacking a competent uterus. The transplanted uterus may be obtained from a postmenopausal donor or a woman of childbearing age who has completed her family. Uterine transplantation has been performed in the Middle East (i.e., Saudi Arabia), but to date, a viable pregnancy in a transplanted uterus has yet to occur.

However, the Sunni Muslim countries of the Middle East cannot be described as an "anything goes" environment. The Sunni religious authorities have not condoned every possible assisted reproduction practice. The list of technologies that are *haram*, or religiously forbidden, is almost as long:

1. No third party should intrude into the marital functions of sex and procreation, because marriage is a contract between the wife and husband. This means that a third-party donor is not allowed, whether he or she is providing sperm, eggs, or embryos. The use of a third party is tantamount to *zina*, or adultery.

2. All forms of surrogacy—both "traditional," using the surrogates own eggs, and "gestational," using embryos transferred to the surrogate's uterus—are forbidden. Although initially allowed by a Saudi Arabian-issued *fatwa* in cases of polygyny (i.e., one wife serves as the surrogate for another), this approval of surrogacy was withdrawn within one year (1984–85), before assisted reproduction was ever carried out in the Middle East.

3. A donor child conceived through any of these illegitimate forms of assisted reproduction cannot be made legitimate through adoption. The child who results from a forbidden method belongs to the mother who delivered him or her. He or she is considered to be a *walad al-zina*, or an illegitimate child.

4. Establishment of sperm banks is strictly forbidden. Sperm donation threatens the existence of the family and the human race and should be prevented.

5. If the marriage contract has come to an end because of divorce or death of the husband, assisted reproduction cannot be performed on the ex-wife or widow using sperm from the former husband (i.e., posthumous assisted reproduction).

6. PGD or sperm sorting techniques for the purposes of sex selection are forbidden, so as to avoid discrimination against either sex, but particularly the female child.

7. Genetic alteration of embryos is forbidden.

8. Reproductive cloning for the creation and birth of a cloned child—who would be the genetic twin of the cloning parent—is forbidden.

Furthermore, it is important to note that physicians are considered the only qualified personnel to practice assisted reproduction in all its permitted varieties. If a Muslim physician were to perform any of the aforementioned forbidden techniques, he or she would be considered guilty of a crime, his or her earnings would be sequestered, and authorities would be required to stop him or her from the morally illicit practice, including through imprisonment and even death.[16]

Clearly, these decisions about which technologies and techniques are *halal* (permitted) and which are *haram* (forbidden) bear considerable weight in Sunni Islam. Most important from a Sunni Islamic perspective, IVF and ICSI are *halal*, as long as the gametes come from a currently married husband and wife. However, third-party donation is *haram*, whether using donor gametes, embryos, or a surrogate womb. As noted by Islamic studies scholar Ebrahim Moosa,

> In terms of ethics, Muslim authorities consider the transmission of reproductive material between persons who are not legally married to be a major violation of Islamic law. This sensitivity stems from the fact that Islamic law has a strict taboo on sexual relations outside wedlock (*zina*). The taboo is designed to protect paternity (i.e., family), which is designated as one of the five goals of Islamic law, the others being the protection of religion, life, property, and reason.[17]

Accordingly, at the ninth Islamic law and medicine conference, held under the auspices of the Kuwait-based Islamic Organization for Medical Sciences (IOMS) in Casablanca, Morocco, in 1997, a landmark five-point declaration included recommendations to prohibit all situations in which a third party invades a marital relationship through donation of reproductive material. Such a ban on third-party reproductive assistance is effectively in place in the Sunni-dominant countries. In the same year as the IOMS declaration was issued, a global survey of sperm donation among IVF clinics in sixty-two countries provided some indication of the strength of this anti-donation stance.[18] In all of the Sunni-dominant Muslim countries surveyed—including the Middle Eastern countries of Egypt, Kuwait, Jordan, Morocco, Qatar, and Turkey, as well as a number of non-Middle Eastern Muslim countries including Indonesia, Malaysia, and Pakistan—sperm donation and all other forms of gamete donation were strictly prohibited. As the authors of this global survey stated, "In many Islamic countries, where the laws of Islam are the laws of the state, donation of sperm was not practiced. AID [artificial insemination by donor] is considered adultery and leads to confusion regarding the lines of genealogy, whose purity is of prime importance in Islam."[19]

The statement "the laws of Islam are the laws of the state" bears further investigation, for it is not, technically, accurate. Islamic law, which is called *shari'a*, governs family law (i.e., personal status law) in most Middle Eastern societies. However, separate civil legal codes, often imposed during periods of French and British colonial rule, govern most other areas of law throughout the region.[20] Assisted reproduction would come under the aegis of Islamic family law, given that assisted reproductive technologies are used to produce families for infertile couples. The association of assisted reproduction with Islamic *shari'a* has given religion outstanding power to dictate the scope and contours of clinical practice in the Muslim world, effectively weakening state intervention or civil law in this area. In fact, state laws on assisted reproduction are relatively rare in the Middle East, found only in Turkey, Iran, and more recently, the Arab Gulf. Furthermore, even though assisted reproduction is subject to Islamic *shari'a*, it is actually the Middle Eastern medical community—not the *shari'a* courts—that must enforce the Islamic *fatwa* rulings on these technologies.

Egypt is a case in point. Over the past twenty-five years, Egypt has supported a thriving assisted reproduction sector, with more than fifty IVF clinics. Five of these clinics are located in government hospitals and receive some state funding to offset expenses for the infertile poor.[21] However, as in most Middle Eastern countries, Egypt's IVF industry is highly privatized and exists beyond the official gaze of the state. Opening an IVF clinic requires licensure by the Egyptian Ministry of Health, based on guidelines set forth by the Egyptian Medical Syndicate. However, no laws of any kind have been passed to control clinical practice. Gamal Serour, for one, laments the relative lack of Egyptian state involvement in this process. "Unfortunately, there have not been any attempts to legislate IVF in Egypt," he writes. "The state controls the practice of IVF through licensing these centers. Centers have to abide by the guidelines laid [out] by the medical syndicate concerning premises, personnel, equipment, facilities, sterilization, etc. Every center must obtain approval of the medical syndicate followed by a license from MOH [Ministry of Health] before they start their programs." However, he adds, the "regulations environment in Egypt is poor. It stops at the phase of issuing a license. There is no regulatory body which supervises or inspects the work done; neither is there an obligatory registry for compiling data. Of course, inspection occurs whenever a catastrophe occurs."[22] Concurring completely with this assessment, Mohamed Yehia, a professor of obstetrics and gynecology at Ain Shams University in Cairo and director of a major IVF clinic there, describes the regulatory environment in Egypt as "very loose and mainly governed by the doctor-patient relationship."[23]

The fact that, in practice, doctors and clinics operate with little government interference does not mean that "anything goes" in either Egypt or other Sunni Muslim countries. In fact, what is quite remarkable is the degree to which the *fatwa* banning third-party donation is actually followed by both practitioners and patients in the Sunni Muslim world. Sunni Muslim physicians in the Middle East appear loath to offer gamete donation to their patients. According to them, clinics in the Sunni-dominant countries simply do not use donor technologies, which violate the *shari'a* guidelines. Instead, if couples with recalcitrant infertility ask about gamete donation, they are either discouraged by their physicians from pursuing it further or are referred out of the country, primarily to Europe. According to Yehia, third-party donation is "not even thought about in Egypt," and a recent discussion of gestational surrogacy ended in another Al Azhar *fatwa* banning it.

In summary, in the Sunni-majority countries of the Middle East and the rest of the Sunni Muslim world, prohibitions against gamete dona- tion are effectively in place. Sometimes these prohibitions are enacted in law (e.g., Turkey, UAE), sometimes in professional codes of medical ethics (e.g., Egypt), but more commonly through broad ministerial decrees that are "heavily influenced by the statements of Sunni religious scholars."[24] As a result, third-party reproductive assistance of all kinds (gamete donation and surrogacy) is not practiced in the Sunni Muslim world, with clinics turning away (or referring to other Euro-American countries) couples who require these services.

Shia Islam and Assisted Reproduction

The situation is changing for Shia Muslims, whose leading clerics have taken a radical step in a new direction. Shia is the minority branch of Islam, constituting slightly more than 10 percent of the world's Muslim popula- tion. Iran is the current demographic epicenter of the Shia world, with one-third of the global Shia population. Shia majorities are found not only in Iran but also in Iraq and Bahrain, and significant Shia minority groups are found in eastern Saudi Arabia, Syria, Turkey, as well as Afghanistan, Pakistan, and India. In Lebanon, Shia Muslims are thought to dominate the Muslim population in this otherwise religiously heterogeneous coun- try. Obviously, Shia Islam has drawn considerable attention because of the U.S.-led war in Iraq and ongoing tensions between the United States and Iran.

Initially, many Shia religious authorities supported the majority Sunni Islamic view: namely, they agreed with Sunni *fatwa*s that prohibit third- party reproductive assistance. However, in 1999, the supreme leader of the Islamic Republic of Iran, Ayatollah Ali Hussein al-Khamene'i (figure 12), the handpicked successor to Iran's Ayatollah Khomeini, issued a *fatwa* ef- fectively permitting donor technologies to be used. (See the appendix for a full transcription of his *fatwa*.)

With regard to egg donation, Ayatollah Khamene'i stated in his *fatwa* that egg donation "is not in and of itself legally forbidden." But he stated that *both* the egg donor and the infertile woman must abide by the reli- gious codes regarding parenting. Thus, the child of the egg donor has the right to inherit from her, as the infertile woman who received the eggs is considered to be like an adoptive mother (through breastfeeding-related "milk kinship").

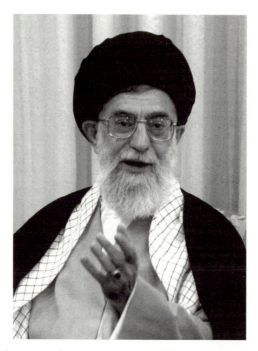

FIGURE 12. Media image of Ayatollah Ali Hussein al-Khamene'i. Atta Kenare/AFP/ Getty Images

With regard to sperm donation, Ayatollah Khamene'i said in his *fatwa* that the baby born of sperm donation will follow the name of the sperm donor and can inherit only from him, since the infertile man is considered to be like an adoptive father.

However, the situation for Shia Muslims is actually much more complicated than this, given two religious practices called *ijtihad* and *mut'a*. Shia religious authorities give considerable precedence to a form of individual religious reasoning known as *ijtihad*, through the use of *'aql*, or intellectual reasoning. There is also a strong tradition of *ijtihad* in Sunni Islam. However, Shia Muslims pride themselves on the greater freedom of their religious authorities to exercise *ijtihad*,[25] often claiming that Sunni Muslims in general—both clerics and laypersons—tend to favor scriptural sources over individual moral reasoning. Through these practices of *ijtihad*, various Shia clerics have come to their own conclusions regarding the rightness or wrongness of gamete donation. Some Shia clerics continue to prohibit gamete donation for their followers, while others have allowed it under certain conditions. As many scholars of Shia Islam have noted, the practice of *ijtihad* has allowed a certain flexibility and pragmatism toward new technological developments, including IVF, ICSI, and a number of other new medical technologies (e.g., contraception, organ transplants, vasectomy, transgender surgery).[26] Furthermore, *ijtihad* has ultimately led to great heterogeneity of opinion and practice *within* the Shia community.

Additionally, Shia Islam allows a form of temporary marriage called *mut'a* (also called *sigheh* in Iran), which is not recognized by Sunni religious authorities.[27] In Shia Islam, *mut'a* is a union between an unmarried Muslim woman and a married or unmarried Muslim man, which is contracted for a fixed time period (e.g., one hour to ninety-nine years) in return for a set amount of money. It is practiced in Iran, as well as in other parts of the Shia world.[28] In the past, middle-aged and older women who were divorced or widowed often engaged in *mut'a* marriages for financial support (and, presumably, sexual pleasure). However, in Iran, following the loss of men during the devastating, eight-year Iran-Iraq war, former Iranian president Rafsanjani recommended *mut'a* as a means of protecting the large numbers of single or widowed women who had no other means of financial support. For Shia men, *mut'a* marriages can be contracted while traveling, or as a means of achieving marital variety and sexual pleasure.[29] Furthermore, young unmarried Shia men and women sometimes contract *mut'a* marriages as a way of gaining sexual experience, or as a way of being together as a "couple" (i.e., boyfriend-girlfriend) without the heavy financial commitment of a formal marriage. In Iran, a kind of legalized prostitution is also made possible through the mechanism of *mut'a*; with *mut'a* marriages enacted privately between prostitutes and their customers, these sexual encounters are made morally licit.

Clearly, *mut'a* marriages have a variety of purposes. However, since the permission of donor technologies by Ayatollah Khamene'i, *mut'a* has also been invoked to make egg donation legal within the parameters of marriage. As shown in anthropologist Morgan Clarke's recent path-breaking book, *Islam and New Kinship: Reproductive Technology and the Shariah in Lebanon*,[30] Ayatollah Khamene'i himself does not stipulate *mut'a* marriage as a requirement for gamete donation, for he believes that *zina* (adultery) requires the physical act of intercourse. However, other Shia clerics disagree. Among Shia authorities, major debates revolve around ten key questions:

1. Should any form of third-party reproductive assistance, including gamete donation, embryo donation, or surrogacy, be allowed at all?
2. Does gamete donation constitute *zina*, if no "touch or gaze" takes place?
3. Should sperm donation be allowed, even if egg donation is made legal?

4. Should the child born of a sperm donor follow the name of the infertile father or the sperm donor?
5. Should such a child inherit from the infertile father or the sperm donor?
6. Are donor children related to the infertile parent who accepted donation, and, if not, could they potentially marry each other, which has implications for proper comportment in domestic life (e.g., bathing, veiling, exposure to each other's nakedness, etc.)?
7. Is donation permissible at all if the donors are anonymous?
8. Should a financial transaction be allowed between gamete donors and recipients?
9. Does the husband of an infertile woman need to do a *mut'a* marriage with the egg donor, then release her from the *mut'a* contract after the embryo transfer (usually two to five days following fertilization of the eggs), in order to avoid *zina*?
10. Can the wife of an infertile husband enact such a *mut'a* marriage?

In order for a married woman with an infertile husband to enact a *mut'a* marriage with a sperm donor, five separate steps would be necessary:

1. "Temporary divorce" of the infertile husband;
2. *Mut'a* marriage to the sperm donor;
3. Establishment of a pregnancy with the sperm donor "husband";
4. Ending of the *mut'a* marriage contract with the sperm donor after the pregnancy is established at three-and-a-half months (i.e., *'idda*, the period required to establish the pregnancy);
5. Remarriage to the infertile husband.[31]

Clearly, the complexities of the Shia religious discourse surrounding third-party donation are rather mind-boggling, given the expansive possibilities presented by both *ijtihad* and *mut'a*. According to Shia religious authorities I interviewed in Lebanon—who accepted the idea of donation, but were strict in their interpretation of how donation should be practiced—a variety of steps should be followed prior to any donation decision:

1. When a donor is needed, a couple should go to a Shia *shari'a* court, where a decision can be made on a case-by-case basis.
2. There should be a determination about which major Shia cleric— or *marja' al-taqlid*, literally, "source of emulation"—the infertile couple follows, to make sure that the particular cleric allows for third-party donation.
3. If so, the decision to donate should be made in the presence of witnesses, the IVF doctor, and with the agreement of both parties (the infertile couple and the donor).
4. Furthermore, strictly speaking, the husband should marry the egg donor for the period of time in which the whole procedure (egg

retrieval to embryo transfer) is taking place, thereby avoiding the implications of *zina*. Polygyny, after all, is legal in all branches of Islam.

However, polyandry—or marriage of a woman to more than one husband simultaneously—is definitely illegal in Islam, in both the Sunni and Shia variants. Therefore, the majority of Shia clerics cannot abide by a married Shia Muslim woman contracting a *mut'a* marriage with a sperm donor. This is true even if she divorces her infertile husband, temporarily marries the sperm donor, and then remarries her infertile husband. In theory, sperm donation might be possible for a widowed or otherwise single woman. However, so far, no Muslim clerics, Shia or Sunni, have accepted this possibility. In the Muslim countries, single motherhood of a donor child is unlikely to be socially acceptable, now or in the future. The child born of a sperm donor to a single woman would be considered a *walad al-zina*, literally, "son of illicit sex," or an out-of-wedlock bastard, without a family name and without a father.

Having said this, divergent gamete donation attitudes and practices have emerged in the Shia Muslim world, as religious authorities come to their own *ijtihad*-driven conclusions about third-party donation in all of its varieties. These divergences of opinion are playing out in interesting ways. For example, Sayyid Muhammad Husayn Fadlallah—Lebanon's most prominent Shia religious authority, up until his untimely death on July 4, 2010—did not agree with Ayatollah Khamene'i's permission of sperm donation and did not condone the use of *mut'a* marriage for women with

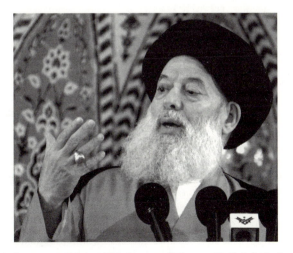

FIGURE 13. Media image of Sayyid Muhammad Husayn Fadlallah, before his death on July 4, 2010. Ramzi Haidar/AFP/Getty Images

infertile husbands to solve the *zina* issue through temporary marriage to a sperm donor (figure 13).[32]

When I arrived in Lebanon to carry out my research, there was a fundamental rift in opinion between those Shia Muslim men who followed the teachings of Sayyid Fadlallah and members of Hizbullah who followed the guidance of Ayatollah Khamene'i in Iran. When I began my study, Sayyid Fadallah agreed with the dominant Sunni Islamic ban on gamete donation and adoption. In a report entitled "IVF in Lebanon: Assessment of Its Current Status," which was sponsored by the American University of Beirut (AUB) medical school, Sayyid Fadlallah and a leading Lebanese Sunni cleric expressed their views on gamete donation in assisted reproduction.[33] Summarizing the two clerics' positions, the AUB report explains:

> To assess the Islamic point of view regarding this issue . . . both agreed that Islam has no objection against any kind of assisted reproduction as long as the parent male and female are the providers of the sperm and egg. . . . Regarding heterologous assisted reproduction, both the Sunnite and the Shiite figures agree that it is *absolutely forbidden* to borrow sperms or eggs from a person other than the involved couple because of the following reasons: 1) The use of sperm from a male other than the husband to inseminate the egg of the wife is seen as an act of adultery because the husband will not be the true biologic father. The same applies in the case of a donor egg. It is of importance to note that polygamy can offer a solution in case of female sterility; 2) The identity of the child will be jeopardized concerning the issues of heritage, life, death and others; 3) This will impose a tremendous social and psychological burden on the infertile male or female partner having to raise a child not of his or her own flesh and blood. Note that in Islam adoption is not allowed and that the adopted child will always be considered a stranger to the (parent) of the opposite sex.[34]

However, Sayyid Fadlallah was one of the only Muslim authorities at that time—either Shia or Sunni—to condone human reproductive cloning as a solution to infertility.[35] Sayyid Fadlallah argued that cloning has great potential in the Muslim world, given that it bypasses sexual reproduction and, hence, concerns about *zina* (or reproduction outside of wedlock). Nonetheless, today, following the death of Sayyid Fadlallah, Muslim religious leaders continue to debate the pros and cons of reproductive cloning, and no authorities except for Ayatollah Khamene'i have come forward to openly encourage human cloning for infertile Muslim couples.[36] Furthermore, worldwide ethical objections to human cloning have put the science "on hold"—although not for other mammals, such as Dolly the sheep.[37]

It is also important to note that Sayyid Fadlallah's position opposing sperm donation squares with the dominant religious discourse in Iran.

Namely, a law on embryo donation passed in 2003 in the Iranian parliament (*majlis*) and approved by the Guardian Council (i.e., a religious "watchdog" body that endorses every bill before it becomes law) has restricted gamete donation to married persons.[38] Even though the law is brief (less than one page), it states clearly and succinctly who can and cannot donate and receive gametes. Egg donation is allowed, as long as the husband marries the egg donor temporarily—thereby ensuring that all three parties are married. Sperm donation, on the other hand, is forbidden, because a sperm donor cannot temporarily marry an already married woman whose husband is infertile. However, quite interestingly, embryo donation—which involves both sperm and egg from another couple—is allowed in order to overcome both male and female infertility. Because an embryo comes from a married couple and is given to another married couple, it is considered *halal*, or religiously permissible.

The social and biological implications of embryo donation are quite interesting. For Iranian couples unable to produce a child because of male infertility, embryo donation allows them to bypass the problem of the husband's weak (or absent) sperm. However, embryo donation does *not* allow a presumably fertile wife of an infertile husband to contribute her own ova, in effect severing her biological ties to the donor child. Furthermore, and most strikingly, embryos donated from another married couple involve *both* egg and sperm donation. In sperm donation, another man's sperm are injected directly into the wife's womb or oocytes. Embryo donation avoids this direct insemination. Nonetheless, embryo donation still disrupts male paternity, because it involves the acceptance by an already married woman of another man's (and woman's) gametes. Furthermore, a woman's acceptance of another woman's egg is effectively like traditional surrogacy, which is strictly prohibited in Sunni Islam. However, gestational surrogacy is now being openly practiced in Iran, despite the lack of firm legislation.[39]

According to Islamic law, a child should inherit only from the biological parents (in this case, the embryo donors). However, under the circumstances of third-party donation in Iran, biological parenthood is not considered sufficient to establish a parental relationship or inheritance duties. In such cases, it is recommended that the recipients of the gametes make a legal commitment to take custody of the child and to specify in their wills that the child will be given the same proportion of the assets as a natural child would inherit.[40] Thus, infertile parents are akin to adoptive parents, with custody over the donor child. The donor child inherits from the infertile parents, as the donors usually remain anonymous throughout the child's lifetime.

Despite the widespread practice of anonymous, commercial, third-party donation in Iran, there are clinical and legal efforts to provide some donor screening. The Iranian law states that the donor should be married, legally and religiously, and should undergo medical testing for physical and mental health, IQ tests for normal intelligence, and screening for drug and alcohol addiction. Because of uncertainties about anonymous donors, donation between kin, especially sisters, remains common and is even preferred by many couples in Iran.[41] The same is true of "sister surrogacy." Iranian anthropologist Shirin Garmaroudi found that gestational surrogacy, in which relatives are sometimes used as surrogates, is becoming increasingly popular in Iran. Among the majority of Shia religious authorities, it is an acceptable form of assisted reproduction.[42]

Whether the future implications of widespread third-party donation and surrogacy have been carefully thought through by the religious and legal authorities in Iran is unclear. Based on her path-breaking research carried out in Iranian IVF clinics, anthropologist Soraya Tremayne notes,

> In reality the lack of clarity in religious rulings has left a wide gap in the ethical, moral and legal aspects of the practice of ARTs [assisted reproductive technologies]. The overall protection that such approvals provide, inadvertently has created a confusing situation for medical practitioners, who, in their everyday practices face complex situations which are not covered by religious rules. . . . But as these gaps emerge, and the medical practitioners, cooperating closely with the "liberal" religious rules, try to close them, the balance of power has gradually shifted in favor of biomedical knowledge as the determining and authoritative source of wisdom as far as ARTs are concerned.[43]

It is important to note that not all Shia clerics are "liberal" when it comes to gamete donation. Some Shia religious leaders both inside and outside of Iran do not agree with the relative Iranian "permissiveness" toward third-party reproductive assistance. Instead, they abide by the dominant Sunni Muslim ban on all forms of third-party donation. For example, in 2006, both Soraya Tremayne and I attended a two-day conference in Tehran on "Embryo and Gamete Donation," sponsored by the Avesina Research Institute in association with the Law and Political Science Faculty of University of Tehran.[44] The conference provided a fascinating example of the kind of rigorous debate that is the norm in Islamic jurisprudence.[45] For example, some clerics, dressed in their stately robes and turbans (black for the *sayyid*s, or descendants of the Prophet Muhammad), argued against the moral permissibility of embryo and gamete donation, while others argued for it. As an example of "*ijtihad* in action," the disagreements generated in public between "pro" and "con" clerics were also debated in the more private recesses of the conference. For example, a Shia *shari'a* judge from Bahrain, who was staying at our guest residence, took great pains to describe to me his opposition to all forms of gamete donation. To prove this point, he provided me with a copy of his book on Islamic personal status law, which had been translated into English and which supported his anti-gamete donation position based on evidence from the traditional Islamic scriptures. According to him, Iranian clergy, who speak Farsi rather than Arabic, are not as familiar with the original Islamic scriptures (in Arabic) that demonstrate the immorality of third-party donation. Thus, in his view, some Iranian clergy are "innovating" in ways that are religiously unacceptable, and which are at odds with the rest of the Muslim world.

Indeed, the degree to which some Shia clergy are "pushing the envelope" in the realm of reproductive science and technology is quite remarkable.[46] At the gamete donation conference in Iran, some Iranian clergy and physicians advocated for future laws permitting all forms of donation (including sperm donation), as well as surrogacy. Meanwhile, despite the existence of a restrictive embryo donation law, many IVF physicians in Iran continue to practice egg donation, sperm donation, and surrogacy without fear of punishment. In Iran, the original "permissive" *fatwa* of Ayatollah Khamene'i—who is, after all, the supreme leader of the Islamic Republic of Iran, even if he is not regarded as the most brilliant intellect and legal thinker[47]—provides adequate moral justification for donor technologies and surrogacy to be practiced quite openly. As of this writing, Ayatollah Khamene'i is the only major Muslim cleric who has allowed all forms of gamete donation, embryo donation, surrogacy, and human cloning. As a result, since the new millennium, third-party reproductive assistance of all kinds (with the exception of human cloning, which is not yet possible) is now widely available in IVF clinics in Iran, with its Shia Muslim majority.

The "Iranian ART Revolution" in Lebanon

This "Iranian ART revolution"[48] has had its most dramatic impact in Lebanon. There, Ayatollah Khamene'i's pro-donation rulings have effectively "opened the door to donation." Thousands of Hizbullah sympathizers in Lebanon follow the spiritual guidance of Ayatollah Khamene'i in Iran. By the year 2000, Lebanon—where the majority of Muslims are thought to be Shia, even though the country's last official census was conducted in 1932[49]—had become the only other country in the greater Muslim world to offer third-party reproductive assistance. As of this writing, Iran and Lebanon are still the only two Muslim-majority countries to offer donation and surrogacy to infertile Muslim couples.

As soon as I arrived in Lebanon in January 2003, it became clear to me that Muslim men's attitudes toward third-party reproductive assistance depended largely on their positionality vis-à-vis Islam. A man's "Islamic masculinity"[50] truly mattered in this regard: namely, whether a man accepted the idea of third-party donation depended upon the Muslim community to which a man belonged by birth, whether a man identified with that community, and what kind of Muslim man each person chose to be as an adult.

Most practicing Muslim men in my study had definite attitudes toward donation. Sunni Muslim men such as Ibrahim, whose story of failed ICSI opened this chapter, tended to reject all forms of third-party donation. Many Shia Muslim men did as well. However, as I was soon to discover in Lebanon, attitudes toward donation among Shia men depended largely on which cleric they followed as their *marja' taqlid*, or source of emulation.

Of the 220 men in my Lebanese study, the largest group (76 men, or 35 percent) identified themselves as Shia. However, many claimed that they were "not that religious," did not "care about religion," did not follow a *marja'*, or were anticlerical (one explicitly and vehemently so). A few of these men described themselves as "Shia by birth" but objected to providing a sectarian label, because they were either nonpious, self-proclaimed Communists or politically opposed to sectarian division in the country. In fact, there was a significant degree of secularism among this population of men. Such secularism in the Muslim countries is largely hidden and underrepresented but is part of the fabric of Middle Eastern religious life.[51]

Of the seventy-six Shia men in my study, thirty-one (40 percent) spoke at some length about their religious convictions, their attitudes toward gamete donation, and whether they followed Ayatollah Khamene'i or Sayyid Fadlallah as *marja'*. It is important to reiterate that these interviews were conducted between January and August 2003, during the initiation of the war in Iraq, and before the rise in the profile of Iraq's Ayatollah Ali al-Sistani as the most senior clerical authority in Shia Islam. At the time, none of the men in my study identified Ayatollah al-Sistani as their *marja'*, although his popularity in Lebanon has grown in the intervening years.[52] Rather, half of the self-identified pious Shia men in my study followed Ayatollah Khamene'i as their *marja'*. The other half followed Sayyid Fadlallah.[53] This division had major ramifications on men's choices about assisted reproduction in the clinic. In an early interview I conducted with a thirty-three-year-old sweet shop worker, Zaher, I asked if IVF was allowed in his religion. He explained assisted reproduction in Shia Islam in this way,

ZAHER: IVF is no problem in Islam if the man's sperm is from the husband and the eggs are her eggs, from his wife. This is *halal*. I want to tell you something about cloning in Islam. If a man has no hope to have a child, it [cloning] is *halal* for Shia. It is not *halal* if the eggs are from outside [a donor], or if the sperm is from outside. I have read extra books from certain *shaykh*s in Lebanon, and this is what they say.

ANTHROPOLOGIST: Is this new? I hadn't heard about that.

ZAHER: Yes, it's new for cloning. For the cloning, as long as there is no hope, and as long as the baby will be born without birth defects, then it's okay, for the service of humanity. It's *halal*.

ANTHROPOLOGIST: That's very interesting. Which *shaykh* allowed this?

ZAHER: As far as I know, there are two Lebanese versions of Shia. And they have different *shaykh*s. But the one I'm following is Lebanese. Another one who is followed is in Iran. I know that the *shaykh* in Iran said that you can take eggs, take sperm from outside. But I don't follow him. He said, in his opinion, in his *fatwa* in Iran, that it was allowed to do sperm and egg donation. This is due to the war in Iran, which left millions of people dead, with lots of widows. In Islam, the *shaykh*s give *fatwa*s to help people. This Iranian *shaykh*, he thinks it is good, it will help these widows to have their own children. But, in Lebanon, it's a different story. In Islam, for every problem, there is a solution. Maybe in Lebanon, it is not allowed today, but they will allow it in years to come. We Shia practice *ijtihad*. This is our difference from the Sunni. We practice *ijtihad* more than the Sunni.

ANTHROPOLOGIST: So who do you follow in Lebanon?

ZAHER: Sayyid Muhammad Husayn Fadlallah. He's the most important in Lebanon. He is so open to *ijtihad*. He is open-minded.

ANTHROPOLOGIST: Is he based in Beirut?

ZAHER: He's in Beirut, but he is not only important in Lebanon. He is followed by others in the Arab world and even in Detroit, Michigan![54] I know people in Detroit, Michigan who follow him. And, in his opinion, donation is *haram*, but cloning is okay. The *Sayyid* had an interview in the newspaper saying if, for a medical reason, there is no other solution [to infertility], then [cloning] is okay. Maybe later on, he will decide this for donation also.

ANTHROPOLOGIST: What do you think about [third-party] donation?

ZAHER: My wife, she was asked by the doctor if she would be willing to donate her eggs. But I asked the Sayyid—I asked him *directly*—and he said, "No." And she didn't have any extra eggs anyway. There will be something wrong if she donates and another person will receive her eggs and the baby will be half from my wife. This is a "relations problem." This is a "mixture of relations" when a baby is half from another person. And another thing he [Fadlallah] said, "If a boy is born from an egg donor, it is *haram* for that boy to be 'shown' [i.e., naked] to the [infertile] wife," because actually, he is not her boy 100%. It is everyone according to his own religion, and so if his religion allows him, he will do it and he will not be punished. But, at the end, God will punish those who will do this and don't have good faith. If you have good faith, you wouldn't do that which is not allowed to you in your religion.

ANTHROPOLOGIST: So you're glad that Shaykh Fadlallah does not allow this?

ZAHER: Yes, he's an expert in everything, medicine, politics. You can talk to him on every subject. All ambassadors go and speak directly to him. Every day, after prayer, you can go and talk to him, and every Tuesday, he holds a meeting where you can write a question and he will answer. He's in a southern suburb, a Shia neighborhood. If you would like to meet him, I can take you there . . .

ANTHROPOLOGIST: Does he meet with women?

ZAHER: Yes, but you would have to cover your hair.

Although Zaher's spontaneous invitation for me to meet with Sayyid Fadlallah never materialized,[55] his comments were an invaluable entreé into the "two versions" of Shia authority operating in Lebanon at that time. According to Zaher, Sayyid Fadlallah was an "open-minded," "expert" cleric, who had approved of cloning as a solution to hopeless infertility. Nonetheless, Sayyid Fadlallah did not agree with Ayatollah Khamene'i's "permissive" position regarding third-party donation of sperm and egg. Ayatollah Khamene'i had introduced a dangerous "mixture of relations" into the Iranian—and potentially the Lebanese—population, according to Zaher.

Given these significant divergences, I began asking other Lebanese Shia men whether they followed the guidance of Sayyid Fadlallah or Ayatollah Khamene'i. Sayyid Fadlallah's followers tended to be ardent in their support for him, explaining that the "majority" of Lebanese Shia Muslims considered him to be their "own Lebanese *marja'*." Sayyid Fadlallah was praised for being a "modernist"—for approaching new issues, technologies, and social phenomena with an "open mind." He was considered a master of *ijtihad*, who could interpret new innovations for the purposes of social advancement. As one supporter of Sayyid Fadlallah explained, "If we look to religion, to Sayyid Fadlallah, he contributes to our advancement, to improving our lives. He uses *ijtihad* because things are changing. We cannot stay at the same point in time. He pushes things for our own advancement."

Assisted reproductive technologies to overcome infertility were considered to be one of these "advancements" and hence subject to *ijtihad*. Karim, a staff member at a Beirut university, explained Sayyid Fadlallah's attitude toward assisted reproduction, before explaining how this Lebanese cleric had diverged from the Iranian-backed Hizbullah, who sought the spiritual guidance of Iran's Ayatollah Khamene'i,

KARIM: In our religion, for Shia, [assisted reproductive technologies] are not a problem, because of Sayyid Fadlallah. I'm not that religious, basically. But Fadlallah said, "This is not a problem." For Shia, it's not a problem to use these technologies. I'm reading only Fadlallah. He's the only religious person I read, because I usually like more open-minded people. Although the media talk a different story, I read many things and I like Fadlallah because he is very open. I'm a man of music, I sing in Arabic, which some say is forbidden in Islam. But I know that Sayyid Fadlallah listens to music, for example, Fayrouz,[56] and he knows a lot of poems. He can talk to an atheist or a non-atheist and both will feel comfortable. He's the least conservative of the ones who understand *fiqh*. But, religiously, he's strict. He's abiding by the Qur'an and hadith and what the Prophet said.

ANTHROPOLOGIST: So most Shia in Lebanon follow him?

KARIM: Well, people here in Lebanon who like Iran don't like Fadlallah, because he said, "Religious leadership should be regional." For example, leaders in Iran won't understand Lebanon, so they cannot make *fatwa*s for Lebanon. The leader needs to live here and know Lebanese society. This made the rift, because Hizbullah are supported by Iran. But we are Lebanese! We are not part of another country.

ANTHROPOLOGIST: And so you prefer to follow Fadlallah?

KARIM: Yes, because Fadlallah is one of those leaders who gives us an opportunity to make a step forward. He is very open in those general things, not just religious ceremonies. And his way of thinking is very good. For example, if he wants to make a *fatwa* for infertile women, he will find doctors at American University Hospital and ask them exactly what happens to women's bodies. People who are not Hizbullah men hold him in high respect because he's a very good thinker.

ANTHROPOLOGIST: And that's really important. . . .

KARIM: Yes, the Shia—this is my opinion, my understanding—the highest thing in Shia is the mind, *al-'aql*, to find out about God, the Qur'an, and anything. In Islam, there are two groups, two main groups. One uses the mind to discover Allah, and when they know Allah, this is it and you should abide by his rules and submit blindly. The other says, no, since Islam started by *al-'aql*, then we must continue to use *al-'aql*. There are certain unchanging principles in Islam, but everything else should be submitted to reason. The Sunnis are in the first group—they start by Allah and [then] they go to the Qur'an and *hadith*. But Sayyid Fadlallah, if he was given a new opportunity, he would have created a new culture where the second group would have flourished.

ANTHROPOLOGIST: But this hasn't happened?

KARIM: I think, no, because of politics. He doesn't have a political group to support him, so he's kind of alone. Hizbullah has Iranian money, while Fadlallah is trying to run his own [charitable] institutions to make money.

As suggested by both Zaher and Karim, Sayyid Fadlallah had, by that point, parted ways with Hizbullah, whose material support and spiritual guidance come from Iran. Shia Muslims in Lebanon who follow Ayatollah Khamene'i are usually members of Hizbullah, whose Lebanese political leader is Hassan Nasrallah. In the IVF clinics, these Hizbullah men stood out; they were usually the only ones to sport beards (a sign of piety), and, out of religious concern, they refused to shake the female anthropologist's hand, sometimes also asking for a male research assistant to be present at the interview.[57] These men's wives were invariably veiled, sometimes wearing full black chadors. In fact, Lebanese IVF clinic waiting areas sometimes looked like "little Iran," with rows of women dressed in black, men with religious beards, and occasionally men wearing clerical robes and turbans. Furthermore, of all the men in the study, these Hizbullah men were among the few to openly advocate for gamete and embryo donation, because Ayatollah Khamene'i had allowed it for his followers. The story of Bassam, a Hizbullah sympathizer from the Shia stronghold of Baalbek, Lebanon, demonstrates the ways in which Ayatollah Khamene'i's decision to allow donor technologies has resonated for Shia Muslims in Lebanon.

BASSAM AND HANNA'S EGG DONATION

On a busy day at a Shia-serving IVF clinic in Beirut, I met Bassam and Hanna, a young couple from Baalbek, which had been a Hizbullah stronghold during the Lebanese civil war. There, Bassam worked as a police officer, although he was studying at night to become a lawyer. Married to his first cousin Hanna, Bassam had assumed the responsibility for their infertility, undergoing repeated sperm tests showing "borderline" results. Highly intelligent and self-taught in English, Bassam attributed his sperm problems to his psychological depression, about which he spoke freely. "I think that there is a main reason for the quantity and quality problems," he said. "It's mainly the quantity of sperm. And it is depression—it affects the number of sperm. I think this is the main reason." When I asked him about the source of his depression, he continued, "It's most kinds of depression—economic, my living situation, in general. It's stress. [The doctor] told me my [variable] sperm counts depend on my mood. And I think my bad mood is permanent!" Laughing, he continued, "After 1996 exactly, the economic situation [in Lebanon] has gotten bad, and also I have a problem in my family. My mother and father got divorced; they split in 1991, but the real divorce was in 1994. And because I'm the only man, the only son, I'm taking care of my mother and my sisters. I have three sisters, and my father doesn't support them. And now he's asking me to support him!"

In addition to these life stresses, Bassam and Hanna had undergone a reproductive rollercoaster. Early in their marriage, Hanna experienced two ectopic pregnancies, the second one of which almost killed her and required an emergency surgery. Since then, Hanna has suffered from tubal infertility and requires IVF in order to become pregnant. Their first cycle of IVF was covered by insurance from the Lebanese Order of Police, but was unsuccessful. In order to finance their second IVF cycle, Bassam took a loan against his future retirement benefits. Because the loan amount was not enough to cover the entire operation and medications, Hanna was in the process of selling her bridal gold at the time I met them.

Fortunately, Hanna produced many eggs during her second IVF attempt, and Bassam was clearly delighted when his sperm count was normal on the day of fertilization. When I saw Bassam and Hanna at the clinic on the day of embryo transfer, they were beaming. A broadly smiling Bassam had his arm around his small, plain wife, who was dressed in a black veil and a pretty blue-flowered jacket. They had been asked to donate their extra eggs to other infertile couples in the clinic, and Bassam explained his and Hanna's decision to donate in this way,

BASSAM: Of course, I asked the *shaykh* first.
ANTHROPOLOGIST: Which *shaykh*?
BASSAM: Sayyid Ali Khamene'i.
ANTHROPOLOGIST: Directly?
BASSAM: I asked at the office. They have an office in Beirut. And they said, "No problem" if you and your wife are agreeing to it. Then there are no other religious problems.
ANTHROPOLOGIST: So you follow Shaykh Khamene'i?
BASSAM: I follow Khamene'i' more than Fadlallah. Actually, we follow Sayyid al-Khu'i, but he's dead. So, in the new things—and we always have new things—we have to go to Sayyid Ali [Khamene'i] for scientific things.
ANTHROPOLOGIST: And I heard that he allows egg donation.
BASSAM: Yes, and so the day before yesterday, my wife was surprised by one of the doctors here. He met her and he told her she has thirty ovules [eggs]! And they asked us if we would give some to people who need them. I said, "No problem."

Hanna's eggs were divided into two groups. Nineteen were kept for Hanna and Bassam's own use, and eleven were donated to other couples.

Unfortunately, only seven of Hanna's nineteen eggs fertilized; five were implanted as embryos in her uterus, and two embryos were frozen for future use. When Hanna left to begin preparations for the embryo transfer, Bassam told me about his feelings for his wife, whom he clearly loved and admired,

> You know, here, most people don't have this kind of information about infertility. Especially in the older generation, when a man and woman get married and there are no children for five years, they always blame the woman, and they tell him to go get married to another. But my mother, she *never* asked or said one word. She said, "Live your life. As long as you are happy with your wife, and everything is good, don't worry yourself about this." And so I take her advice about this. I don't get stressed. And my wife, she is a real good one—a very strong person. She is a believer, and she has hope. She is optimistic, not pessimistic. She is optimistic that she will have children, and I think this attitude will help us to succeed.

Unfortunately, none of Bassam and Hanna's five embryos implanted. Furthermore, all of the eggs that Hanna had donated to other Shia Muslim couples did not to lead to pregnancies. According to the clinic's embryologist, Hanna's eggs were of "poor quality," making the likelihood of an IVF or ICSI pregnancy slim for this couple. But, as religious Shia supporters of Ayatollah Khamene'i, they have another option: namely, to receive another woman's donor eggs in the future.

SHIA DONATION AS MARRIAGE SAVIOR

As seen in Bassam and Hanna's case, some Shia couples are donating and receiving eggs and embryos with little reluctance, although sperm donation is a different matter, as we will see in the next chapter. For infertile Shia couples who accept the idea of third-party donation, they agree with Ayatollah Khamene'i's justification: namely, donor technologies are a "marriage savior," helping to avoid the "marital and psychological disputes" that may arise if the couple's case is otherwise untreatable. Such disputes are clearly dramatized in a popular Iranian movie called *Laila*, which documents the painful separation of an otherwise happily married but infertile couple, and which was released in the mid-1990s before the Khamene'i *fatwa* permitted such marriages to be saved through the use of donor technologies.

In Iran today, donor egg and donor embryo programs have been set up in most IVF clinics.[58] Donor eggs come from three sources: other IVF patients; relatives, and especially egg-donor sisters (even though Islam is

explicitly against the marriage of one man to two living sisters); and unmarried women who agree to participate as egg donors, with or without
short-term *mut'a* marriages for a fee. Such marriages require only a witness and are not officially registered; thus, they take place in confidence in
the back rooms of IVF clinics. Donors who wish to remain anonymous enter these *mut'a* marriages only by written agreement, without ever meeting the female recipients of their eggs or their temporary husbands. They
receive their money following egg harvesting (usually around U.S. $550),
provide no personal information about themselves to the recipient couple,
receive no information about the recipient couple, and generally "go about
their business." In short, egg donation—as well as embryo donation from
other couples—is largely a financial transaction in Iran, with very little
regulation or control over who donates or how donation is enacted. The
same is not true for the receiving of embryos. The 2003 law in Iran specifies clearly that couples requiring an embryo as a result of infertility must
apply in writing to a *shari'a* court in order to receive permission for embryo
transfer. The law specifies that the couple must be morally sound and suit-
able as parents and must be Iranian citizens.[59]

In Lebanon where I have conducted my own research, there is no such
national law governing any aspect of assisted reproduction or third-party
donation, nor is there any government "watchdog" body, as in Iran.[60] Instead, most Lebanese IVF clinics provide donor technologies under the
protective cover of Ayatollah Khamene'i's *fatwa*, which they either post
on clinic walls or keep shelved in clinic libraries for useful reference. For
example, anthropologist Morgan Clarke, who also conducted fieldwork in
Lebanon in 2003, noted, "Doctors keep Khamene'i's *fatwa* collection on
the shelves of their surgeries to demonstrate the permissibility of such procedures to skeptical Muslim patients; and many such patients have prof-
ited from it to undertake donor sperm and egg procedures, even surrogacy
arrangements, with a clear conscience."[61]

As in Iran, some Lebanese donors are other IVF patients such as Hanna;
these Lebanese donors are mostly Shia Muslims who accept the idea of donation because they follow Ayatollah Khamene'i in Iran. Some Lebanese
donors are friends or relatives of infertile women, including egg-donor sisters, who accompany infertile couples to IVF clinics as "designated donors."
However, as we will see in chapter 8, at least a few clinics have developed
true egg-donor programs, where fertile women anonymously donate their
oocytes for a fee. As in Iran, *mut'a* marriages occasionally occur through
written consent forms, but the donors otherwise remain anonymous to
the recipient couple. In at least one Lebanese IVF clinic in which I worked,
some of these anonymous donors were young non-Muslim, American
women, who traveled to Lebanon to donate their eggs for $1,000 of addi-
tional payment. The Lebanese couples most likely to receive these "Ameri-

can eggs" were often Shia Muslims, who accepted the idea of donation because they followed the teachings of Ayatollah Khamene'i in Iran.

In general, in the IVF clinics in Lebanon where I did my research, there were long waiting lists for donor eggs among childless Shia Muslim couples. These waiting lists grew even longer in mid-2003 as a result of a new decision by the local cleric, Sayyid Fadlallah. Through the practice of *ijtihad*, Sayyid Fadlallah eventually decided that the practice of egg donation was morally licit, as long as strict requirements were followed. To wit, the donation should not be anonymous and should be accompanied by a written marriage contract before witnesses. Anonymous *mut'a* marriages behind closed doors were not sufficient, according to Sayyid Fadlallah, because they defied the true spirit of marriage, which is required to make egg donation legal within the Islamic parameters of polygyny.

With Sayyid Fadlallah's April 2003 permission of polygynous egg donation, the door to donation in Lebanon swung open even further. Large numbers of Fadlallah-following Shia Muslim couples began inquiring about egg donation during the time of my study. Shia men, who might otherwise have been pressured by society to divorce their infertile wives, began to reassess their marital options in light of this new *fatwa* from Sayyid Fadallah. In short, choosing egg donation "out of love" for an infertile wife emerged as a new possibility for *all* Shia men in Lebanon by mid-2003. Egg donation—including with American donors—was conceived of as a way for infertile wives to experience the joys of pregnancy and motherhood, while still using their husband's sperm. The permission of egg donation by *both* Ayatollah Khamene'i and Sayyid Fadlallah was a great boon to marital relations, especially for "reproductively elderly" wives and husbands, who were signing up at Lebanese IVF clinics to access the eggs of younger, more fertile donor women.

It is perhaps ironic to consider that the official interpreters of Islam—largely older Shia Muslim male clerics—are leading the faithful in these maritally salubrious directions. In the high-tech world of assisted reproduction, male clerics, particularly in Iran, are using *ijtihad*, or religious reasoning, to interpret and make sense of new technologies that could never have been imagined before the new millennium.[62] The frankly "adventurous" attitude toward third-party gamete donation on the part of otherwise "conservative" Ayatollah Khamene'i has led Shia Muslims to embrace donation as a "marriage savior." Ayatollah Khamene'i's moral justification for allowing donor technologies was included in the text of his *fatwa*: namely, preserving the marriage of the infertile couple by preventing the "marital and psychological disputes" that would inevitably arise from remaining childless indefinitely. In short, preservation of marriage mattered as much to Ayatollah Khamene'i as preservation of lineage—an opinion at odds with the majority Sunni thinking on the subject.

That American donor eggs are being used to save Hizbullah marriages is just one of the outcomes of this brave new world of reproductive "assistance" that could never have been imagined when these technologies were first introduced to Lebanon in the mid-1990s. Furthermore, in multisectarian Lebanon, the recipients of these donor eggs are not necessarily only Shia Muslim couples. Some Sunni Muslim patients from Lebanon and from other Sunni Muslim countries such as Egypt and Syria are quietly crossing international borders to "save their marriages" through the use of donor gametes, thereby secretly going against the dictates of Sunni Muslim orthodoxy. Lebanon and Iran are now the two regional hubs of reproductive tourism. Just as Syrians and Palestinians head to Lebanon, scores of Sunni Muslim Arabs from the Gulf States, such as Saudi Arabia and Kuwait, are traveling to Tehran in pursuit of donor gametes. Their presence in large numbers has necessitated the services of medical translators, who can negotiate clinical encounters in both Arabic and Farsi.

Conclusion

It is fair to state that the Muslim world—generally positioned on the receiving end of global reproductive technology transfers—has nonetheless embraced assisted reproductive technologies with considerable enthusiasm while, at the same time, reconfiguring them in accordance with the local religious moralities so important in this region. Islam is interpreted, debated, and practiced locally. As such, local forms of the religion must be examined and analyzed. This chapter is case in point: Islamic approaches to gamete donation in Egypt are, in fact, very different from Islamic approaches to gamete donation in Iran.

What it means to be a "good" Muslim—and a good Muslim man—takes particular local forms, based on locally grounded and morally imbued interpretations of the Islamic tradition. As we have seen in this chapter—and as we will witness in even greater depth in chapters 7 and 8—Muslim men are doing their best to follow the local religious discourse on assisted reproduction in order to practice these technologies accordingly. Their "Islamic masculinities" are "emergent masculinities." Not only are the technologies themselves rapidly evolving, but so is the Islamic discourse and decision making on issues such as gamete donation. Islamic masculinity thus entails "keeping up with the times," both technologically and religiously. Emergent masculinities in the Muslim Middle East could thus be described as *technoscientifically and morally agentive*: Namely, new scientific technologies and possibilities are being ardently embraced by pious Muslim men such as Ibrahim, whose sad story of ICSI failure opened this chapter. In Ibrahim's case, he dreams of a day when all his reproductive failure will be behind him and he will instead become a father through human reproductive cloning. Although cloning has yet to be approved by Islamic authorities—and has been officially banned by both *fatwas* and bioethical declarations in the Sunni Muslim countries—Lebanon's local Shia cleric, Sayyid Fadlallah, has seen the potential use of human cloning for overcoming infertility in severely infertile men such as Ibrahim. Thus, he has ruled in its favor as a future assisted reproductive technology.

At the beginning of the new millennium, it is important to examine the role of these senior Muslim clerics as "agents of change." Indeed, their own "emergent Islamic masculinities" should be emphasized. Such male religious leaders have often encouraged the acceptance of new reproductive (as well as other life-saving medical) technologies, frequently justifying their decisions based on family welfare.[63] In Egypt, for example, the Al Azhar clergy has issued scores of *fatwas* on reproductive and other medically related issues, including, for example, the support of family planning.[64] In Iran, clerics have paved the way toward an award-winning population program, in which even the controversial practice of permanent sterilization through vasectomy is being recast as "Islamic" and the way to create a healthy, high-quality family.[65]

However, as this chapter has also shown, Islamic clerics are not of one mind in their stances on technoscience. Differences in Islamic attitudes toward assisted reproduction have clearly emerged along sectarian lines. In the Sunni Muslim world, the prohibition on donor gametes has led to an entrenchment of deeply held religious beliefs about the importance of marriage, which no third party should tear asunder. The Sunni proscriptions against third-party donation represent, in some sense, the materialization of conjugal connectivity and the literal embodiment of emotion, in that love of one's partner—including his or her gametes—must prevail over the desire to have children "by any means." In this light, donor technologies represent a betrayal of sorts, a confession that having children is more important than loving one's infertile spouse. For this reason, donor gametes continue to be shunned in the Sunni Muslim world, with donation itself equated to *zina*, or adultery. In short, in the Sunni Muslim countries—which are, by far, the most populous—the use of assisted reproductive technologies has served to reinforce notions of conjugal connectivity, as well as biological kinship, parenthood, and family life. This will become abundantly clear in the following chapter, which examines Muslim men's aversion to "social fatherhood" through either sperm donation or adoption.

Yet, the globalization of these technologies to other parts of the Shia Muslim world has fundamentally altered understandings of the ways in which families *can* be made and the ways in which marriages *can* be saved through the uses of assisted reproductive technologies. In short, the arrival of donor technologies in the Muslim Middle East has led to a brave new world of reproductive possibility never imagined when these technologies were first introduced there more than twenty-five years ago. These technologies have engendered significant medical transnationalism and reproductive tourism; mixing of gametes across ethnic, national, and religious lines; the birth of thousands of egg- and embryo-donor babies to devout infertile Muslim couples; gestational surrogacy arrangements; and in some cases, infertile men's acceptance of donor sperm. Because of the availability of all of these options in Iran and Lebanon, infertile Muslim couples have begun to reconsider traditional notions of biological kinship, even if "social parenthood" of a donor child is still not widely embraced. Moreover, the availability of these forms of third-party reproductive assistance has weakened the Sunni Muslim ban on third-party donation across the region, with some infertile Sunni Muslim couples reconsidering their own anti-donation moral stances. As a result, Shia gametes are finding their ways into Sunni bodies, despite current regional antagonisms between these two branches of Islam.[66]

In my view, these multiple Islamic perspectives on assisted reproductive technologies are powerful indicators of the profound social effects that biotechnology may engender. As the assisted reproductive technologies become further entrenched in the Muslim world, and additional forms of reproductive and repro-genetic technology become available, it will be increasingly important to examine the new local moral worlds that are likely to arise in response to technological globalization. Scholars of Islam must follow these global technologies into the future, anticipating the ways in which PGD, uterine transplantation, human cloning, therapeutic human embryonic stem cells, and the like will make their way into the diverse moral and social imaginaries of numerous Muslim societies around the globe. For, as long as the problem of infertility continues unabated in the Muslim world, the globalization of new assisted reproductive technologies will continue—reaching places such as Egypt, Lebanon, Iran, and beyond.

CHAPTER 7

Sperm Donation and Adoption

HASAN AND HIS RESISTANCE

When I met Hasan in a Beirut IVF clinic, his first words were, "I have suffered a lot in my life." He launched into the harrowing tale of his capture by the Israelis in 1983 and his two-year detention in the notorious Khiam Prison (now a museum) during the Lebanese civil war. He was put in solitary confinement—"where you could not see day from night in some of the cells, and there were no toilets"—and forced to eat the same food, without any meat, for the length of his imprisonment. He was also tortured with electricity to his genitals on three separate interrogations, "and there were many interrogations." As he explained, "I wasn't married then, and I didn't do a sperm test before marriage because I was young then. This was almost twenty-three years ago. But *maybe* this [the torture] is the cause of my sperm problems." In addition, upon his release from Khiam in a prisoner swap with the Israelis, Hasan was involved in a major car accident, breaking twenty-four bones, suffering internal bleeding, and experiencing two months of unconsciousness as a result of a severe head injury that required brain surgery. Unfortunately, such car accidents are common in Lebanon as a result of war-torn roads and general lawlessness. Or, as Hasan put it quite bluntly, "The war was very bad. We lived our life in the war, and we suffered a lot."

Today, Hasan is a forty-two-year-old police officer in southern Lebanon, who describes himself as a member of Hizbullah, or the Lebanese "resistance" (i.e., to Israel). Tall, thin, with jet black hair, a neatly trimmed beard, and a moustache that partly occludes his poor dentition,[1] Hasan has been infertile throughout the nine years of his marriage, suffering from "variable oligospermia," or sperm counts that fluctuate below normal. "I've had *many* sperm tests," he explained. "The number goes up and goes down. It is not fixed. But there is 'weakness,' the doctors said." Although he has impregnated his thirty-five-year-old wife, Khadija, four times, she has gone on to miscarry early in each pregnancy.

In an attempt to overcome his infertility, Hasan has undergone varicocelectomy but believes that this pointless operation helped only the Lebanese physician with his "commerce." In addition, Hasan has taken many hormonal medications, including the brand-name drugs Humegon, Pregnyl, and Clomid, all in unsuccessful attempts to increase his sperm production. Upon learning that his infertile male cousin had visited an IVF clinic and had produced triplets with his wife, Hasan decided to follow suit. As he explained, "We had hoped to get pregnant and make a baby without doing ICSI, since she's been pregnant four times. But she's thirty-five years old now. We've tried, but now I'm forty-two and she's thirty-five, and we're afraid we'll get too old." Hasan continued,

> In our society, when a woman is the cause [of the infertility], the man will leave her and divorce her. So society will not have mercy on a woman who doesn't have a baby. But I'm only afraid that she'll reach an age when she can't have children, and then our society won't have mercy on her. I don't want her to experience this. I won't allow this social pressure. It usually happens, but I don't allow it. In general, I don't allow other people to interfere in my life.

According to Hasan, his wife Khadija has been his only sexual partner, because "I'm committed to my religion, to the *shari'a*. I respect and protect the woman, and I don't just follow my [sexual] desires." As a pious Shia Muslim, Hasan apologetically explained why he could not shake my hand—or any woman's hand—"not because I hate women, but because of my religion" (and its prohibition on "touch" across genders).[2]

Hasan also explained that he and Khadija were committed to each other and deeply in love, despite their unfulfilled desire for a family. He described childlessness as the only major problem in their relationship,

> We *love* children. In my family, we are seven brothers, and some of them have sons who are almost my age. In my family, we do care about having children. I have many nieces and nephews, and I like to treat my nieces and nephews kindly, which makes her jealous. Her psychology is *very, very* affected! We don't have any other problems except this problem of not having children. But she accepts this situation, because if she didn't, she would have asked me for a divorce. She loves me *a lot*! And I would have changed [replaced] her if I didn't love her. It's very easy to divorce. But the husband and wife are one body, one soul.

When asked about whether his infertility had affected his sense of manhood, Hasan said,

> I accept the fact that I'm infertile, but I always seek treatment and medicine to improve my situation. A person doesn't just sit and say,

"This is from God."Of course, in the Qur'an. . . . [he stopped momentarily to explain that in quoting a passage in Arabic from the Qur'an, one must truly understand what the Qur'an is saying, and then he or she will understand"everything"].There's a saying in the Qur'an that scientists are the people most afraid of God, because they get to that point of knowledge to really understand God's wishes.

IVF and ICSI are permitted in Islam, Hasan explained, as long as the gametes come from a married couple,

> IVF is *halal* [permitted], if the sperm is from the man and the egg is from his wife, then there's no problem. But if the sperm is from outside [i.e., a donor], then it is *haram* [forbidden], and the same thing for the eggs, *haram*. But, if the egg is from my wife and the sperm is from me, then it is *halal* for the married couple. But in all Islam, in all religions, donation [of sperm and eggs] is wrong, according to my knowledge. The baby *has* to be from a married couple.

Although Hasan is a member of Hizbullah and follows the spiritual guidance of Ayatollah Khamene'i in Iran, he does not agree with the ayatollah's permissive position regarding sperm and egg donation. He is adamantly resistant when it comes to sperm donation, which has been mentioned by doctors in his case, but which he likens to adoption,

> Sperm donation is like adoption. You can raise an orphan, but he has to stay on his [biological] father's family name. You are only raising him, because if he would be given your family's name, he could grow up and marry his sister without knowing it. This is incest! So you can raise the boy, and this is okay, but *not* change his name.

Although Hasan refuses to consider sperm donation, adoption, or even fostering a child in his home, he and Khadija practice *takafful*, a kind of guardianship in which they support the living expenses of a child in a Hizbullah-run orphanage. According to Hasan, *takafful*—or the care of orphans—is praised as one of the major forms of charity, or *hasanat* (good deeds), to be performed by pious Muslims. According to Hasan, *takafful* "is found in all the Arab countries, and the Islamic countries, including in Iran, Afghanistan, and Pakistan."Members of Hizbullah often pride themselves on providing for orphans in this way.

The fact that Hizbullah is a major provider of charitable services in southern Lebanon is lost on outsiders, according to Hasan."We're known as terrorists,"he explained,"because we don't want our country to be occupied [by Israel]!"Hasan, in fact, prides himself on being a very law-abiding citizen and drug-enforcement officer in the police department, married to

an educated teacher whom he loves and respects, Hasan ended his inter
view by expressing his desire to have a child with his own sperm and the
eggs of his wife, whom he points out "does not have any problems" with
her reproductive body. It is Hasan's love for Khadija—his feeling of being
"one body, one soul"—as well as his Islamic piety, which has kept Hasan
on the "straight path" toward ICSI. According to Hasan, this straight path
to fatherhood does not allow for either sperm donation or adoption, for
such a child "won't be my son."

Assisted Reproduction and New Kinship

Hasan is not alone in his resistance to both sperm donation and adoption
as solutions to his male infertility and childlessness. The vast majority of
Muslims, both Sunni and Shia, reject these options out of hand. As seen
in the preceding chapter, Ayatollah Khamene'i in Iran has allowed sperm
donation for his followers, but it is not a popular option, even in the ayatollah's own country.[3] In the Arab countries, sperm donation is practiced
only in Lebanon, but there, too, it meets with ardent resistance on the
part of most men. As a member of Hizbullah and a follower of Ayatollah
Khamene'i, Hasan is allowed the option of sperm donation. But Hasan
stands firm in his belief that a child should be created within legal marriage, using the gametes of a husband and wife. To take gametes from outside the conjugal unit is *haram*, leading to the birth of a child who "won't
be my son."

Hasan clearly believes that he cannot regard a child conceived through
donor sperm as his legitimate son. Hasan's reaction is not surprising in that
assisted reproductive technologies evoke strong feelings about kinship. Of
all of the anthropological work that has been written about the assisted
reproductive technologies, the most substantial and most foundational, in
some sense, is that which explores the effects of these technologies on
kinship and family life.[4] Marilyn Strathern's book, *Reproducing the Future:
Anthropology, Kinship, and the New Reproductive Technologies,*[5] paved the
way for the new anthropology of kinship[6] and stimulated burgeoning interest among anthropologists of reproduction in how assisted reproduction might redefine and expand notions of "relatedness."[7] Strathern's
major contribution was to question how assisted reproductive technologies might denaturalize and therefore blur the so-called nature-culture in-
tersection: namely, if kinship, as a set of social relations, is rooted in the
"natural facts" of biological reproduction, then the nature of kinship itself
might be called into question by assisted reproductive technologies, which,
in effect, destabilize the "biological" within "parenthood" through the "as-

sistance" of technologies and third parties. As noted by Strathern, assisted reproductive technologies have created "a new convention, the distinction between social and biological parenting, out of an old one, kinship as the social construction of natural facts."[8]

This early insight by Strathern served to spur a wide range of empirical research on assisted reproduction and kinship in Euro-America, leading to a number of major findings.[9] First, given that Euro-American notions of kinship are biogenetically based,[10] many infertile couples now "chase the blood tie"[11] in a relentless quest to produce biogenetically related offspring through the technology-assisted manipulation of their own gametes.[12] The very presence of assisted reproductive technologies has served to marginalize, to some degree, alternate means of family formation through adoption,[13] once regarded in Euro-America as the "natural solution" to infertility.[14]

Second, assisted reproductive technologies have pluralized notions of relatedness and led to a more dynamic notion of "kinning," namely, kinship as a process, as something "under construction," rather than a natural given.[15] In fact, assisted reproductive technologies can be thought of as "deconstructive" in introducing ambiguity and uncertainty into kinship relations, including the fundamental categories of motherhood and fatherhood.[16] With the rapid rise over the past two decades of sperm donation, egg donation, and embryo donation,[17] as well as agencies devoted to surrogacy,[18] the number of potential solutions to infertility has dramatically expanded. As assisted reproductive technologies are applied to an ever-widening range of people and problems, they are unseating core notions of kinship and undermining the traditional family, by introducing a whole range of quasi-, semi-, or pseudobiological forms of parenting.[19] The term "new kinship" has been aptly invoked by anthropologist Morgan Clarke to describe alternative family formation through assisted reproduction.[20] One of these forms of new kinship is exemplified in the Hollywood motion picture *The Kids Are All Right*, which examines "lesbian alternative insemination" among a gay couple (played by Annette Benning and Julianna Moore). The movie is based on the teenaged children's search for their sperm donor "father." Once found, the sperm donor changes all of their lives—with the question "for better" or "for worse" left up to the viewing audience.

Although assisted reproduction has led to a dizzying array of family formations in the West, relatively little is known about assisted reproduction and alternative family formation strategies in the non-Western countries, including Muslim societies, where more than half of the world's population of nearly 80 million infertile people is estimated to live.[21] Furthermore, in most Muslim societies, kinship is central to social organization; thus, the potential impacts of assisted reproduction on kinship and family life could be quite profound.[22]

In light of such realities, it is important to consider how infertile couples living in predominantly Muslim Middle Eastern countries grapple with the new complexities of kinship brought about by assisted reproduction. What do infertile men think about the possibility of their spouse accepting donor sperm and bearing a donor child? Will they consider adopting an orphan? In short, what do Muslim men living in the Middle East think about "social fatherhood"—the very concept that allows so many infertile Western couples to "adopt" others' gametes and embryos, as well as children themselves?

As this chapter demonstrates, the very concept of social fatherhood is culturally contingent and is also deeply embedded in Muslim men's local moral worlds.[23] Local moralities govern ideas about the parenting of non-biological children, including those conceived through biotechnological means. For a number of reasons, the vast majority of Middle Eastern Muslim men do not accept the idea of social fatherhood as a solution to male infertility. As we will see, Hasan is certainly not alone in his resistance.

ISLAM, DONATION, AND DESCENT

In the Muslim world, attitudes toward family formation are closely tied to religious teachings that stress the importance of "purity of lineage."[24] Islam is a religion that privileges—even mandates—biological descent and inheritance. Preserving the "origins" of each child, meaning his or her relationships to a known biological mother and father, is considered not only an ideal in Islam but a moral imperative.[25] In Islamic *fiqh* (jurisprudence), the tie by *nasab* (i.e., filiation, lineage, relations by blood) is considered to be one of God's great gifts to his worshipers. The preservation of *nasab* is emphasized through Qur'anic rules designed to ensure the sanctity of the family and the society; by preserving *nasab*, personal and social immorality are prevented, thus leading to the maintenance of society as a whole.[26]

In the face of such religious edicts, the concept of social parenthood—of either an adopted or a donor child—is considered untenable in most of the Muslim world.[27] The vast majority of Muslim men, both Sunni and Shia, do not accept the idea of third-party gamete donation or adoption as solutions to their childlessness. Sperm donation is seen as particularly abhorrent. Men's moral concerns revolve around four sets of related issues: *zina*, or adultery ("It's like your wife sleeping with another man"); *sifah al-maharim*, or incest ("A brother and sister could accidentally marry each other"); *mahram*, or someone forbidden to you in marriage, thereby affecting gender comportment in family life ("You would have to remain covered in front of this child"); and *nasab*, genealogy or filiation. In addition, two psychological issues are often cited—namely, the feelings of the donor child ("The child won't get the same love as my own child") and men's feelings of fatherhood ("He won't be my son. It would be like raising another man's kid").

With regard to the first issue, Islam is a religion that can be said to privilege—even mandate—heterosexual marital relations. As is made clear in the original Al Azhar *fatwa*, reproduction outside of marriage is considered *zina*, or adultery, which is strictly forbidden in Islam. Although third-party donation does not involve the sexual body contact ("touch or gaze") of adulterous relations, or presumably the desire to engage in an extramarital affair, it is nonetheless considered by most Islamic religious scholars to be a form of adultery, by virtue of introducing a third party into the sacred dyad of husband and wife. It is the very fact that another man's sperm or another woman's eggs enter a place where they do not belong that makes donation of any kind inherently wrong and threatening to the marital bond.

The second aspect of third-party donation that troubles marriage is the potential for incest among the offspring of anonymous donors. If an anonymous sperm donor "fathers" hundreds of children, the children could grow up, unwittingly meet each other, fall in love, and marry. The same could be true for anonymous egg donors. Thus, moral concerns have been raised about the potential for incest to occur among donor children who are biological half siblings. In a small country such as Lebanon, such half-sibling incest is a real possibility in the absence of a donor registry.

A third moral concern has to do with issues of family incest, or how parents and donor children should comport themselves in daily family life. To wit, a donor child is *halal*, or religiously permitted to marry a person who is not related by blood ties. Thus, feelings of attraction might develop between donor parents and their non-biologically-related offspring, especially in the intimate conditions of household life, where individuals are revealed to each other. An infertile parent who is not biologically related to a donor child could, theoretically, marry the child when that child reaches the age of maturity. Thus, in Muslim family life, proper comportment would have to revolve around the diminution of erotic feelings toward a donor child. This would complicate matters such as bathing, praying, veiling, and all matters pertaining to "touch and gaze."

The final moral concern voiced by Muslim men is that third-party donation confuses issues of kinship, descent, and inheritance. As with marriage, Islam is a religion that can be said to privilege—even mandate—biological inheritance. The problem with third-party donation, therefore, is that it destroys a child's *nasab* and violates the child's legal rights to known parentage, which is considered immoral, cruel, and unjust.

Men use the term "mixture of relations" (*ikhtilat al-ansab*) to describe this untoward outcome. Such a mixture of relations, or the literal confusion of lines of descent introduced by third-party donation, is described as being very "dangerous," "forbidden," "against nature," "against God"—in a word, *haram*, or morally unacceptable. It is argued that donation, by allowing a "stranger to enter the family," confuses lines of descent in Islamic societies. For men in particular, ensuring paternity and the "purity" of lineage through "known fathers" is of paramount concern. This is because most Muslim societies are organized patrilineally—that is, descent and inheritance are traced through fathers and the "fathers of fathers" through many generations. Thus, knowing paternity is critical.[28]

Mothers, too, share kinship relations with their children through gestation and especially the sharing of milk through breastfeeding (often called "milk kinship"). However, descent itself is traced through the patriline, flowing through males to successive generations.[29] Thus, sperm donation in particular threatens not only a child's *nasab* but a man's patrilineage. Not surprisingly, then, Muslim men feel strongly about the importance of patriliny and paternity, claiming that a sperm donor child "won't be my son." Coupled with men's feelings that such children are created through *zina*, or adultery—"It's as if my wife slept with another man!"—the child conceived through sperm donation is considered to be of questionable moral character. Together, questions of *nasab* and *zina* lead to strong rejection of sperm donation. Or, as many men explained it, "the child would not be *from me*—it would be like raising some other man's child."

Bringing such donor children into the world is considered unfair to the children themselves, who would never be treated with the love and concern parents feel for their "real" children. Such a child could be viewed only as a bastard—a *walad al-zina*, "a child of illicit sex," or an *ibn haram*, literally "son of the forbidden." Thus, a child of third-party donation starts its life off as an "illegal" child. It is deemed illegitimate and stigmatized even in the eyes of its own parents, who will therefore lack the appropriate parental sentiments.

ISLAM, ADOPTION, AND FOSTERING

This firm conviction that parenthood of a donor child is impossible is clearly linked to the legal and cultural prohibitions against adoption throughout the Muslim world. In the Middle East, most orphans who are abandoned in hospitals or on the streets are *laqits*, or "foundlings," who are considered to be the illegitimate offspring of unmarried persons. Thus, an abandoned orphan, too, is a *walad al-zina*, or *ibn haram*, who is considered morally tainted. As noted by Egyptian historian Amira Sonbol,"Illegitimate children themselves are regarded as a real stigma, almost a threat, a source of evil."[30] This view is upheld in the original Al Azhar *fatwa* on medically assisted reproduction, which states:

> A legitimate child will grow and be raised by his parents in the best manner they can afford, while an illegitimate one is a shame for the mother and her people, neglected in the community and will then turn into a disease. Islamic scholars discussed illegitimate children in the books of Islamic law, [and] explained that they are human beings who deserve to be brought up properly and taken care of so as to stimulate what is best in them and avoid their evilness.[31]

The *fatwa* goes on to state that adoption of such children is explicitly forbidden in the Qur'an,"for the purposes of origin protection and family rights' preservation."

Nonetheless, the Islamic scriptures, including the Qur'an, encourage the kind fostering of orphans—whether these children are orphaned through the death of parents, parental poverty, or out-of-wedlock conceptions. The Prophet Muhammad himself was orphaned when his father died during his mother's pregnancy, and then his mother died when he was age six. He was fostered first by his grandparents and then his uncle. He, in turn, fostered an orphan child named Zaid. Eventually, he advised against the practice of adoption, or *tabanni*, involving change of a child's birth name to an adoptive surname, although he continued to encourage the kind upbringing of orphans.[32]

The Prophet Muhammad's ruling against adoption has continued to be followed throughout the centuries in the Islamic world. Today, Islamic *shari'a* does not allow legal adoption as it is practiced in the West, whereby an orphan takes the legal name of the adoptive parents (usually the father's surname) and is treated as if it is a biological child through the mutually reinforcing mechanisms of co-residence, inheritance rights, and ongoing affective relations including unconditional love. This sort of "fictive kinship" is explicitly forbidden in Islam. Instead, numerous Islamic scriptures emphasize *nasab*, or blood relationship, as the only basis for paternity, making adoption, or *tabanni*, a sin equal to *kufr*, or apostasy.[33]

The only three Muslim Middle Eastern countries where legal adoption is practiced are Tunisia and Turkey (Sunni-dominant but also "secular") and Iran (Shia-dominant and an "Islamic" republic). Iran's permission of adoption is not surprising, given its unique acceptance of gamete donation as well. In 1975 an adoption law was ratified, giving Iranian couples the right to legally adopt orphaned children, including the transfer of surname, birth certificate, and inheritance rights.[34] The law has not been modified since that time; thus, infertile Iranian couples have the option to adopt as a way of overcoming their childlessness. After a six-month period of "adjustment"—where social workers from government child welfare agencies follow the interactions between the adoptive parents and child—the child receives a birth certificate in the adoptive couple's name.

Having said that, strong cultural resistance to adoption has been reported for Iran. Infertile couples there describe their "fear of people's words," concerns about the child being "illegitimate," and worry about the problems that might arise if "the child's parents turn up and want the child back."[35] Thus, even in "permissive" Iran, legal adoption is viewed as a "last resort" among infertile couples.[36] In short, in the Muslim Middle East, few infertile couples, either Sunni or Shia, will contemplate *tabanni*, or legal adoption, stating with conviction that it is "against the religion."

Child fostering is legally permitted and even encouraged in most Middle Eastern Muslim societies.[37] Nonetheless, fostering an orphan in the home is relatively rare and may be shrouded in secrecy. Infertile couples who do foster an orphan may attempt to pass the child off as their own biological offspring in order to avoid the severe stigma of such a fostering arrangement.[38] Anthropologist Jamila Bargach, in her book *Orphans of Islam*, calls this scenario "secret adoption," and describes how legal fostering in Sunni-dominant Morocco is shrouded in secrecy, falsification of birth records, and dissimulation.[39] In Lebanon, a Sunni Muslim family court judge I interviewed explained secret adoption in this way,

> Adoption? In Islam, there is no adoption. In Christianity, yes, there is. But not in Islam. And given that my wife is very religious—she prays and fasts a lot—I don't think that *she* would agree to taking in an orphan. It would be a burden on us, because if the child wouldn't be registered in court by Islamic law, there are later problems at the time of marriage. Usually, when orphans are born, they manage to register them only by "cheating"—by false birth certificates—and they bring other liars as witnesses. It becomes a game for supposedly bearing children!

SUNNI MUSLIM MEN'S RESISTANCE

Given these attitudes, I was curious to know whether men in my Lebanese study would ever consider sperm donation or adoption as routes to social fatherhood. I was especially interested to know whether Sunni and Shia Muslim men might feel differently about sperm donation and adoption, given the permission of these practices in Shia-dominant Iran. Not surprisingly, anti-donation and anti-adoption stances were expressed more vehemently by Sunni Muslim men in my Lebanese study. For example, of the forty-four Sunni Muslim men I interviewed about adoption, thirty-four of them (77%) absolutely refused the idea. Opposition to gamete donation was even stronger. Of the forty-eight Sunni Muslim men I interviewed about gamete donation, forty (83%) refused the idea completely, with nearly 100 percent opposition to sperm donation. Of all the Sunni Muslim men interviewed in Lebanon, only one man admitted to even contemplating sperm donation. He was an infertile Syrian physician, who had come to Lebanon with his Palestinian wife to try ICSI using his own sperm. At the end of his interview, he admitted to recently checking some anonymous sperm donation Web sites,

> I did this secretly, because I know sperm donation is not allowed, and I don't like "mixing." It will create problems if it's not controlled by law. For example, it's a problem if, after one to two years, I have this [donor] son, and the donor knows to whom he gave the sperm, and he comes and says, "Okay, it's *my* son." It's not enough to control [donation] by religion; it needs to be controlled *by the law.*

This man's ambivalence about sperm donation is not surprising. In more than twenty years of studying assisted reproduction across the Middle East and Arab America, I have *never* met a Sunni Muslim man who ultimately agreed to using donor sperm. In general, Sunni Muslim men have a rather clear set of responses on various paths to social parenthood: absolute no to sperm donation, no to egg donation, no to embryo donation, no to adoption, no to in-home child fostering, and a qualified maybe to financial guardianship of a child living in an orphanage. When I broached these subjects further in some of my interviews, Sunni Muslim men often went well beyond the expected "It's against the religion" response to explain in a more nuanced fashion why they could not accept these various practices. As one infertile carpenter explained,

> Egg and sperm should be from the couple themselves, not from an egg or sperm donor. If I didn't have sperm and took it from another man, for example, this would be *haram,* considered to be adultery. Other people may do it, but they don't abide by Islamic law. They just want to have a child. Personally, I wouldn't consider it, because it is *haram,* and I wouldn't really feel the effect of this thing that's forbidden until many years later. It's the same with adoption. I have a concern that when the child grows up, he won't regard us as his own parents. If we adopt, we wouldn't really feel comfortable looking at this child, given that

he's not our biological child. When he grows up, we would have to tell
him honestly that he's not our child. Then his psychology would be affected. He wouldn't feel that hopeful. There would be a "gap" because
he's not our child. If you have your own biological child, you will feel
differently. He *is* your own child, so you feel attached.

Similarly, an infertile physician who had already been successful on two
previous ICSI attempts explained that his wife still worried about whether
excess embryos created in the IVF laboratory were donated to other couples,

> My wife has her worries about fertilized embryos. Do they give them
> to other people? So, we asked the doctor, "What do you do with the
> embryos? "They said, "We will not kill them, but we let them out-
> grow their nutrients." He probably knows our religious background,
> because in our religion, it is not allowed to share genes. So he didn't
> offer donation for that reason. Neither egg nor sperm donation are
> allowed. Donation is not accepted in Sunni Islam. I've never seen a
> specific *fatwa*, but it's just a feeling that I have based on my knowl-
> edge of the religion. In Sunni Islam, if you breastfeed someone else's
> baby, it becomes a brother or sister to your child.[40] Egg donation is
> much stronger than that. It's like bringing a stranger into your family.
> So this is my assumption that donation is not accepted.

As suggested by this man's statement, Sunni opposition to gamete and
embryo donation leads to abiding concerns about the disposition of excess
embryos (i.e., will they be frozen, discarded, or donated to other couples?).
In addition, Sunni Muslim IVF patients are often extremely concerned
about the proper handling of sperm and eggs in IVF laboratories. With the
routinization of assisted reproduction in Lebanon and other Middle Eastern countries, fears about laboratory "mix-ups" have clearly diminished
over time, given that none have ever been reported for the Middle Eastern
region.[41] Nonetheless, embryologists described to me the great care taken
in sperm processing and egg and embryo handling—especially in the absence of government regulation or laboratory monitoring of any kind. One
Lebanese embryologist described the "paranoia of the lab—not to mix, not
to lose embryos." Having said that, Sunni Muslim men in my Lebanese
study still occasionally conveyed their concerns about intentional or un-
intentional "sperm mixing," especially with "black *bizri*" (black "seeds," or
sperm), which would lead to the birth of a clearly non-Lebanese, multiracial, nonbiologically related child. These fears of "laboratory miscegenation" were clearly fueled by the media, as one Lebanese man explained,

> Doing IVF is not a problem for me, because it has become more com-
> mon. But I read that a lot of mistakes are made. Recently, in London,

a woman brought black twins, even though she was white! I read this in the newspaper just last week, and it made me *very* worried. But, here, I see them always writing the names on the sperm containers. So I didn't question them about this.

Most men said that they trusted the IVF clinics where they were undergoing their ICSI procedures, as they had watched the careful labeling of semen containers. Men sometimes made funny quips about their fears of sperm mixing, joking that they would turn to DNA testing to confirm their paternity. Some typical remarks, made in jest, spoke to men's underlying fears: "They can't escape from me! If I have a son, the first thing I will do is a DNA test! I would sue them and get many millions!" Another man stated, "Not all people understand IVF, what it means. Perhaps they will think bad things about sperm donation or egg donation, and I'm worried about that. I'm paying a lot, and not for a black baby!" Or, as one man laughed, "Someone will get shot for that!"

Men who were timid about conveying their concerns to laboratory staff nonetheless openly worried about sperm mixing in interviews. As one man lamented, "Oh yeah—I'm worried! I didn't ask, but I made sure that she [the embryologist] labeled that cup!" Another man explained, "It occurred to me that they could make a mistake with my sperm. But I have no choice! I cannot follow them around with my sperm! And I'm not that kind of a person to ask the doctor about the precautions they take." When I asked another man whether he was concerned about laboratory mix-ups, he told me how he was forced to confront this issue in the clinic,

> Oh, yes! Because there were two Fadias in the clinic that day. Another doctor came out and asked me, "Is your wife Fadia?" I said, "Yes." "Fadia Muhammad?" "No!" There were two women named Fadia that day, and thank God, they figured that out. So I told [the embryologist] to write *my* name on the [sperm collection] cup, because I'm white and maybe a black child would come from this!

Men's fears of sperm mixing, questionable paternity, and racial miscegenation were repeating themes, especially among men who had already experienced untrustworthy medicine in Lebanon. For example, one infertile man, who had undergone a botched varicocelectomy and whose wife had undergone three unnecessary pelvic surgeries for ovarian cysts, was very, very angry at Lebanese doctors, calling them *haramis*, or "thieves." Although this Sunni Muslim infertile couple had no option but to undergo ICSI using their own gametes, the husband was very concerned about sperm mixing, claiming that at least one Lebanese IVF physician was performing sperm donation without the consent of his patients. Although I never heard this story repeated during my stay in Lebanon, the man I interviewed claimed the following,

> First of all, after three years of marriage, some doctors told me to do [intrauterine] insemination. However, I was afraid of that—that they would take another man's sperm, to put it in my wife. And of course, right now, I'm afraid, honestly. They told me that I have sperm, so there is no need for sperm donation. But if a baby comes, I will see if he looks like me! I would do DNA testing! Maybe if it's *very black*, like a black person, I will ask for that! [Really? Do you think that could happen?] It's impossible that they would take sperm from a black man, I think, but I do have some fear. Some doctors told me that there is a doctor [in Lebanon] who does this, but the patient doesn't know this. It is a crime, but this has happened in Lebanon. Some man who had no sperm, the doctor told him, "Don't worry! The next time, come to the lab and everything will be okay." And so the doctor just picked up any sperm, and it wasn't from the [azo-ospermic] man. Now there is a criminal investigation about this.

Lebanese men's anxieties about "black babies" are perhaps less an indicator of underlying racism—although color-based racism is certainly present in the Middle East—than about fears of phenotypic dissimilarity. Namely, men want their children to resemble them, for strong father-child resemblance is "proof" of paternity, including to the outside world. Children who do not resemble their fathers may elicit curiosity, even taunting by others, especially if their test-tube origins become known. The desire for father-child phenotypic similarity reflects men's desires for clear biological paternity (i.e., without the need for DNA paternity testing), clear patrilineal descent (i.e., without concerns about the child's *nasab*), and the prevention of social ridicule (i.e., without concerns about the child's future social well-being).

In my study, concerns for a child's social welfare were often found in Sunni Muslim men's narratives about adoption, and why they could not tolerate the possibility of adoptive fatherhood. One Sunni man who had briefly toyed with the idea of fostering a child in his home explained his reluctance in this way,

> Here in Lebanon, not everything you believe you can do. For me, it's no problem to raise an orphan child. Maybe I could take this child home and not be embarrassed to raise him. But I can't do it because of the social environment. For me, personally, there would be too much embarrassment, for me and for the child. In Lebanon, maybe one in a million people would do this. There are cases, but they are very rare.

There is a program, an Islamic program called *takafful*, where you support an orphan and pay a certain amount every year, and you know the kid you support. I said to my wife, "There is no affection. You are just supporting a child. It's only financial." So I don't want to do this. And [gamete] donation, I would *never* do! If my wife ever mentioned this, I would say to her, "Shut up! I'm already convinced [not to do it]."

As suggested in this man's comments on *takafful*, Islam encourages the kind upbringing of orphans as a form of *zakat*, or charity to the less fortunate. Of the Sunni Muslim men I interviewed in Lebanon, fifteen men said that they would consider caring for an orphan, primarily through financial contributions to an orphanage. However, these were primarily Muslim men with adequate financial means. The thought of actually raising an orphan child in the home—either as a legal foster child or as an actual legal adoptee—was rejected out of hand by virtually all of the Sunni Muslim men in the study. One infertile man, an affluent physician, explained why adoption was equivalent to gamete donation, and why his wife was resistant to fostering,

Similarly, adoption is prohibited, and you're not allowed to take a baby and pretend like it's a "natural" baby, as if the name is your name and it's your child. Eventually you *must* tell the child that he is adopted. There is a *fatwa* about this. You have to tell them they're adoptees, and we can't give them our name. Many people here do "adopt" children, but not what you would call adoption in the States. It crossed my mind for a while, but my wife is against it. I considered it because I worked in a hospital [in the United States] where there are many children of teenaged mothers. I told my wife, "There are plenty we could raise," but she refused.

Another financially well-to-do Sunni Muslim lawyer explained why he considered legal fostering to be a better option than either gamete donation or adoption,

Donation is not allowed. From the religious point of view, he will not be your child, or he will be a "half-child." And even for those who want a child *very* much—they can't live without a child—this is still a problem. In my opinion, it's not good. It's better to take a child from an orphanage. This child will not take our name, but we can help this child, on a humanitarian and religious level. We haven't considered this yet, because we want to have a child [of our own]. But I *can* help another child. I like to help another family, another neighbor, another man who needs services. But I don't like to take a child by adoption. I can only be a *kafil* [guardian], and offer this child help.

Despite these affluent men's professed desires to help orphans, neither was practicing *takafful*. Financial guardianship was quite rare among the Sunni Muslim men in my study.

Of all the 220 men in my Lebanese study, there was only one man, a Sunni Muslim Palestinian, who was raising an orphan child in his home. But this was not *any* orphan; it was his niece, the daughter of his dead brother, who shared the same family surname. Yet, this depressed, infertile, impotent man did not mention the child until the very end of an otherwise long interview, which focused on the suffering of the Palestinians and on his own depression, or his feelings of being "down." When I asked him how many children he would eventually like to have, he mentioned, almost as an afterthought, "Actually, we have one girl, my brother's girl. He died in a car accident, and so did his wife. The girl was with them, but she survived. She was two months old at the time, so I'm taking care of her." At this point, the man's pretty young wife, who was his first cousin (once removed) and also biologically related to the child, entered into the interview room dressed in her Betadine-stained hospital gown. She immediately launched into the following story,

> We have a daughter. She will be five years old in July. She needs a brother. This is why we're doing this [ICSI]. She needs two to three boys to protect her. Because of her, we are trying this. This is the third time. [Do you consider her your daughter?] She *is* our daughter. She doesn't know [about her parents' death]. I am her mother, and she has the same family name as my husband. We wish we could adopt her, but we can't because we're Muslim and they don't allow this. We both have green cards to the States, and we thought about moving there, but she needs adoption papers. But we can't get them, because Islamic courts won't allow this. They just give papers saying that this is our equivalent of adoption. But, she doesn't have the official adoption papers like the ones needed for the States. Because of this, we will not go to live in the States, because Deena, our daughter, can't. This is our problem. In the States, they require legal adoption papers. We did some papers in the *shari'a* courts, and I have papers which say the Islamic law is like adoption in the States, but the U.S. Embassy didn't accept this. In the Arab countries, there is no adoption. It is "custody" only.

Clearly, this couple differed in their attitudes toward adoption. The husband could not consider his biological niece (his dead brother's daughter) to be his adopted daughter, whereas his wife could. She was clearly interested in adopting the child legally and had pursued this issue in the Sunni Islamic *shari'a* court and with the U.S. Embassy in Lebanon. However, because adoption is not legal in Sunni Islam, her pursuit to adopt the child ultimately failed.

SHIA MEN'S AMBIVALENCE

So where does this leave Shia Muslim men in Lebanon, who, one might argue, have been the beneficiaries of the permissive attitudes toward both sperm donation and adoption in Iran? How do Lebanese Shia Muslim men feel about sperm donation to overcome male infertility? Similarly, how do they feel about adoption, which is legally practiced in Iran?

Interestingly, given the marginal economic status of most of the Shia Muslim men in my study, one of my most striking findings was the degree of *takafful* in the Shia population. Most Shia Muslim men in my study hoped to become economic guardians of orphans when their own financial situations improved in the future. Furthermore, seven of the Shia men in my study were already serving as guardians through regular monthly contributions to an orphanage. This included one man who worked as a physical education teacher in one of Sayyid Fadlallah's orphanages and earned only $400 a month. Nonetheless, he was following Sayyid Fadlallah's encouragement of *takafful* (a.k.a. *kafalat il-yatim*, or guardianship of orphans) through a regular monthly donation to one of the orphanages run by Sayyid Fadlallah's charitable organization, Jama'iat il-Mabarrat.

The significant practice of *takafful* among Shia men in my study clearly reflected the ravages of the civil war and the subsequent Israeli occupation of southern Lebanon, as found in Hasan's opening story in this chapter. Whereas Hasan lived to tell his story, many Shia civilians and male fighters were killed, leaving children without parents or at least a father who could support them. In some cases, war-related poverty had forced desperate Shia parents to place their children in orphanages, where at least they would be clothed, fed, and educated.

Although the Shia men in my study were acting generously and humanely toward the war orphans in their midst, few of them supported the idea of actually adopting and raising an orphan as a son or daughter. The overall opposition to *tabanni*, or legal adoption, was almost as pronounced among Shia Muslim men as among Sunni Muslim men in the study. Of thirty-seven Shia men I interviewed about adoption, thirty-two (86%)

were firmly opposed, with only five men saying that they would consider this possibility. As explained by the Fadlallah orphanage teacher, "Adoption is *haram* in Islam. I *can* be a guardian to a child, but I can't let him live with me, because if he lived at my home, he would be like an adoptee, and this is forbidden."

Just as most Shia Muslim men opposed *tabanni*, they adamantly opposed sperm donation. One Shia businessman, who had spent many years outside of the country, had this to say,

> I don't think any Muslim can accept that idea [of sperm donation]. Even in Europe, the majority of the people don't like it. It's very complicated to find yourself with another person's child. "Look at me, look at you." It will complicate your life. And there could be medical matters where the child needs assistance. If it becomes public and widespread, it could be problematic. If ten people can be the same looking from the same donor, an anonymous donor, and you're looking for that one guy, you may never find him. So you would have to think about this, because it will affect your life.

Quite interestingly, half of those men who identified Ayatollah Khamene'i as their *marja'* disagreed with his permissive position on sperm donation. This was true even among those men who were azoospermic (i.e., no sperm found in their ejaculate or testicles), for whom sperm donation was their only viable procreative option. One of these men, Kamal, a Hizbullah electrician whose five semen analyses had failed to identify a single spermatozoon, had asked at Khamene'i's office in Beirut about what he should do to become a father. Kamal and I had the following conversation about what he was told, and what he ultimately decided,

KAMAL: They told me that if the [IVF] doctor is a woman, it is better.[42] But if it is a man, you must know that he's honest. In the Islamic *shari'a*, it *is* allowed for a woman to have a male doctor, and it *is* allowed to bring another sperm from another man [for donation]. But if you do it, the wife has to make a *katb al-kitab* [marriage contract], because the child will go to her other husband [the sperm donor] for inheritance. Sayyid Khamene'i said this.

ANTHROPOLOGIST: Would you do this?

KAMAL: No! I don't feel it's logical. There's not even a one percent chance that I will do this. Religiously, it's okay in the *shari'a*, but I thought about it, and I said, "No, absolutely not."

ANTHROPOLOGIST: Does your wife agree with you?

KAMAL: My wife, she didn't accept this either, even though she knows it's in the *shari'a*. It is difficult. For the woman, it is not difficult to take another one's egg like it is for the man [to take another man's sperm]. If you get a child and it's a girl, when she's fifteen, sixteen, or seventeen, she's not like your daughter. How will you behave with her? In the religion, you could marry her.

ANTHROPOLOGIST: So it's too difficult.

KAMAL: It's *very* difficult. I'd prefer not to have a child than to have a child and always think about this.

ANTHROPOLOGIST: So you wouldn't consider adoption then?

KAMAL: It's the same problem. It's not my child, and if I bring home a girl, she could be my wife.

In Kamal's discussion of sperm donation, he criticizes his avowed *marja'*, Ayatollah Khamene'i, for allowing a procedure that is, in his words, "illogical." Notably, Kamal uses his own intellectual powers of reason and interpretation—*'aql* and *ijtihad*—to arrive at this conclusion. And Kamal is not alone in this regard. Of the 220 men I interviewed in Lebanon, only one man had actually undertaken sperm donation. Moustafa, a poor, weathered carpenter from southern Lebanon, had suffered from persistent nonobstructive azoospermia throughout his ten-year marriage. When a Christian doctor had broached the subject of sperm donation with him, he and his wife had gone directly to their local *shaykh*, a follower of Ayatollah Khamene'i. The *shaykh* indicated Ayatollah Khamene'i's approval of the practice and showed them the actual *fatwa*. This had "encouraged" the couple, who saw it as their only way to make a baby. They returned to the clinic, where Moustafa's wife was prepared for the donor-ICSI procedure. The doctors would not let the couple meet the medical-student donor, who consented to sperm donation only on the basis of strict anonymity. However, the doctors did allow the couple to visualize the semen sample, taken directly from the medical student on the morning of the ICSI procedure. Moustafa's wife said a little prayer over the semen in the plastic cup.

On this very day, I happened to meet Moustafa in the clinic, and he agreed to be interviewed, perhaps as a form of guilt-reducing catharsis. Upon reading and signing the human subjects consent form, the first words out of Moustafa's mouth were literally, "The sperm are not from me." He then became taciturn, answering most questions with the briefest of responses. Nonetheless, he made it clear that he had sold his land to go through with the $2,000 donor-ICSI cycle; he had no idea who the sperm donor was; and he and his wife had vowed to keep this a secret, including from their families, for the rest of their lives. Indeed, the interview was more like a confessional than a conversation, with Moustafa ending by saying "I just want to have a child." The anthropologist, privileged recipient of Mouctafa'c revelation, replied "*insha' Allah khayr*" the formulaic expression of divine intervention said as an expression of good luck within Lebanese clinics.

SPERM DONATION IN PRACTICE

Because of the widespread disapproval of sperm donation in Lebanon among both Sunni and Shia Muslim men, it is rarely practiced. Despite reports of a mysterious "sperm bank" in southern Lebanon, I was told by IVF physicians and embryologists that a Lebanese sperm bank does not exist. Rather, donor sperm are generally procured in one of three ways: from European or U.S. sperm banks, through direct mail order; from family members (e.g., brothers, cousins) who are brought to the clinic for semen collection; or from anonymous Lebanese donors, who are usually medical students or hospital employees and who are paid between $100 and $500 for their services.

Physicians whom I interviewed about Lebanese sperm donation were mixed in their attitudes toward this practice. Proponents of sperm dona-tion saw it as a "solution to social problems" in the absence of adoption or any other known medical solution for men with absolute azoospermia. Because sperm donors are generally medical students—at purportedly "low risk" for infectious diseases—they are seen as a "safe" and "intelligent" population of sperm donors. Physician opponents of sperm donation, on the other hand, have multiple reasons for rejecting the practice. First, there is no local donor registry of any sort, or a reliable regulatory system in the country. As a result, sperm donation is being carried out behind closed doors, in the unregulated, sometimes secretive environment of private IVF clinics.[43] As a result of this lack of regulatory oversight, practices that would never occur in Euro-American settings do, in fact, take place in Lebanese IVF clinics. For example, "fresh" semen samples are used in sperm dona-tion, without any kind of mandatory screening for HIV virus, hepatitis vi-ruses, and other sexually transmitted infections. Similarly, no mandatory genetic testing is performed with either donors or recipients. Hence, seri-ous genetic diseases, such as cystic fibrosis, may be perpetuated within the Lebanese population. Finally, the very legality of sperm donation in Leba-non is a matter of concern for the Lebanese IVF community. The Lebanese Maronite Order of Physicians has developed ethical guidelines which for-bid donor insemination. Some physicians and embryologists I interviewed said that sperm donation may eventually be made illegal in the country if a law is ever passed.

Meanwhile, in the absence of a national law, sperm donation does occa-sionally take place. Religiously pious Lebanese Shia men such as Moustafa are the most likely to accept donor sperm, and even some Shia clerical opinions toward sperm donation have transitioned over time. According to one Lebanese Shia physician—who offers sperm donation in his clinic and has repeatedly sought the advice of Shia clerics on this subject—sperm donation has moved from being a practice that is *haram* (i.e., totally forbidden and for which a person will go to hell) to being *makruh* (i.e., a practice that is reprehensible and should be avoided, but is not absolutely prohibited, or *haram*). According to his interpretation of the clerical debates, sperm donation now falls into this category of *makruh*—namely, a practice that should not be done if it can be avoided, but if it cannot be avoided, then it is acceptable. Or, put another way, even though sperm donation is "disliked" in Shia Islam, it is not entirely forbidden and therefore will not send a person who practices it to hell. According to this physician,

> [The Shia position] has *evolved* over the years, especially on sperm donation. Depending on the question and the way it is asked, and whether they think the person asking is "liberal" or not, they [clerics] give differing answers. And this is a gray zone—sperm donation is not automatically seen as "guilty." With sperm donation, the rationale is that sperm which is banked is the same as medicine in a pharmacy. With sperm donation, you're prescribing medication for the wife, which is given to her. As long as there is no physical intercourse, and the husband knows, then the practice is *makruh.* But the child cannot inherit from the infertile father, only the sperm donor. He can give him everything, but he can't bequeath his inheritance.

When I told this physician that I had never before heard about this "gray area," he explained that it is a "Shia thing," allowing a great deal of flexibility, even beyond the practice of *ijtihad.* This was the only time I ever heard mention of this—or of donor sperm being like a "prescription medicine." In other words, this may have been the Shia-but-secular physician's own rationale for performing sperm donation in his clinic—a kind of individual *ijtihad*, or interpretive strategy, which is invoked by some Shia Muslims in their moral decision making.

Nonetheless, it is fair to say that between Ayatollah Khamene'i's permissive *fatwa* and other Shia clerics' constantly evolving positions on gamete donation, sperm donation has definitely entered the lexicon and practice of Lebanese reproductive medicine. This is largely due to the high numbers of Middle Eastern azoospermia cases—men who have no spermatozoa whatsoever in their semen. Why is there so much Middle Eastern azoospermia? According to the physicians and embryologists I interviewed, many of whom had trained in reproductive medicine in both Lebanon and the United States, so-called nonobstructive azoospermia cases are much more common among Arabs, including Arab American men with male infertility. These nonobstructive azoospermia cases may be due to three major causes: undescended testicles that are not surgically corrected early in a male infant's life; genetic causes, which may be linked to high rates of consanguineous marriage; and cancer treatment in which male fertility preservation through semen collection before chemotherapy or radiation therapy is not offered. Some Middle Eastern men also have "obstructive azoospermia," in which sperm are present in the testicles, but are obstructed from exiting the body during ejaculation. Such obstructions may be due to three major causes: prior infections (e.g., sexually transmitted, adult mumps orchitis, chronic prostatitis, genital tuberculosis); trauma (e.g., being hit or tortured in the testicles); or genetic factors, such as men who are born without the vas deferens (a marker of cystic fibrosis carrier status). In these cases, sperm may be found inside the testicles upon testicular aspirations or biopsies. However, in some azoospermia cases, no sperm whatsoever is discovered, in which case men may be offered sperm donation as an alternative.

In my studies in Lebanon and Arab Detroit, I came across thirty-one azoospermia cases (table 14). Six of nineteen men in Lebanon and four of twelve men in Arab Detroit were offered sperm donation as a solution to their problem. In addition, while in Lebanon, I met the wives of two azoospermic Lebanese men who were currently living in the United States and had been offered sperm donation there. But they decided to return to Lebanon for sperm donation because they wanted a Lebanese donor. I interviewed all ten men in Beirut and Detroit who had been offered sperm donation and who were thus forced to seriously consider this possibility. Only one of them, Moustafa, confessed to going through with it. One other religious Shia man was considering using his brother as a donor but had yet to ask his sibling. Kamal, the Hizbullah electrician who disagreed with Ayatollah Khamene'i's opinion, refused sperm donation altogether. Shaykh Ibrahim, whose story opened chapter 5, knew about Ayatollah Khamene'i's permissive opinion but found it very "difficult" to accept sperm donation, as did his Iraqi wife, who eventually divorced him. One Lebanese Shia man, who had migrated with his family during the Lebanese civil war to Arab Detroit, had been living in the States since age fourteen but was appalled to be offered sperm donation at age thirty-one upon discovery of his azoospermia. He was clearly troubled by this possibility, beginning his interview in this way,

> The doctor kept encouraging me to do donor sperm. Never! I know they do it in America, but in Arabic men, no, because I don't know who's the father. A lot of problems are going to happen in the house.

TABLE 14. Azoospermia cases and responses to sperm donation

Country	Religion	Cause of Azoospermia	Sperm Donation Offered	Response
Lebanese	Shia Muslim	Congenital absence of vas	No	
Lebanese	Shia Muslim	Undescended testicles	No	
Lebanese	Shia Muslim	Undescended testicles	No	
Lebanese	Shia Muslim	Mumps orchitis	No	
Lebanese	Shia Muslim	Obstructive, unknown cause	No	Thinks about asking his brother to donate sperm
Lebanese	Shia Muslim	Nonobstructive, unknown cause	Yes	Refuses the idea, although he follows Ayatollah Khamene'i
Lebanese, living in Netherlands	Shia Muslim	Obstructive, unknown cause	No; has ICSI son	
Lebanese, living in Cote d'Ivoire	Shia Muslim	Genital tuberculosis	No; has son from early in marriage	
Lebanese	Shia Muslim	Nonobstructive, unknown cause	Yes	Accepted anonymous sperm donation, because he follows Ayatollah Khamene'i
Lebanese	Sunni Muslim	Nonobstructive, familial (genetic)	No	
Lebanese	Shia Muslim	Mumps orchitis	No	
Lebanese	Maronite Catholic	Unknown cause	Yes	Accepts the idea, but is trying ICSI with testicular aspiration first
Lebanese, living in Saudi Arabia	Sunni Muslim	Nonobstructive, unknown cause	No	
Lebanese	Maronite Catholic	Post-chemotherapy	Yes	Accepts the idea of sperm donation, since no sperm were found with testicular biopsy
Lebanese	Sunni Muslim	Nonobstructive, familial (genetic)	No	Refuses the idea of sperm donation, but no sperm were found with testicular biopsy
Lebanese	Sunni Muslim	Nonobstructive, unknown cause	No; has ICSI son	
Lebanese	Sunni Muslim	Nonobstructive, unknown cause	No	

TABLE 14 Azoospermia cases and responses to sperm donation (continued)

Country	Religion	Cause of Azoospermia	Sperm Donation Offered	Response
Lebanese	Shia Muslim	Nonobstructive, unknown cause	No	
Lebanese	Druze Muslim	Post-chemotherapy	Yes	Refuses the idea of sperm donation, because child is "not part of me"
Lebanese	Maronite Catholic	Nonobstructive, unknown cause	Yes	Refuses the idea of sperm donation, although his wife accepts after ten failed ICSIs without a single embryo
Lebanese, living in USA	Shia Muslim	Klinefelter's syndrome (XXY)	Yes	Refuses the idea of sperm donation; "Never!"
Lebanese, living in USA	Shia Muslim	Undescended testicles	No	
Iraqi, living in USA	Shia Muslim	Nonobstructive, familial (genetic)	No	
Syrian, living in USA	Refused to identify	Mumps orchitis	No; married a woman with four children	
Yemeni, living in USA	Sunni Muslim	Adolescent testicular infection (maybe mumps)	No	
Lebanese, living in USA	Shia Muslim	Congenital absence of vas	Yes	Agreed to sperm donation, but his wife did not; "I gave her the divorce"
Yemeni, living in USA	Sunni Muslim	Mumps orchitis	No	
Lebanese, living in USA	Shia Muslim	Undescended testicles	No; underwent six testicular aspirations	
Lebanese, living in USA	Maronite Catholic	Obstructive, probably from STIs	Yes; has two adopted sons	Agrees to sperm donation with second wife; "I'm open. Children are children."
Palestinian, living in USA	Sunni Muslim	Hirschprung's syndrome (genetic)	No	
Iraqi, living in USA	Shia Muslim	Undescended testicles	Yes	Refused the idea of sperm donation, as did his wife, who divorced him

Like, I can't say, "Swear to your father." It's easier to remarry someone who has kids, you know what I mean? That way, I see the child, and I can feel something for the child. But, if it's not "my blood" [by sperm donation], especially his looks, I'll never feel that he's my child. Here [in America], you can pick the way you want him to look. What is it—a factory? I can't do that.

In short, even Shia Muslim patients who were religiously allowed to use donor sperm, and who were living in the donor-tolerant United States, were resistant to this practice. None of the Shia men I interviewed in Arab Detroit had gone through with anonymous sperm donation. They either refused sperm donation altogether, were deeply ambivalent, or had never seriously considered the possibility.

In religiously heterogeneous Lebanon, I interviewed five other men, including three Christians, one Druze, and one Sunni Muslim man, who had been offered sperm donation. Only two—both Maronite Catholics—consented to sperm donation, but *only* if sperm could not be found in their testicles. In one of these cases, one thousand sperm were found on the day of the testicular biopsy; the other case was "negative." The negative case was especially poignant, as this handsome man, Bernard, had survived Hodgkin's disease and was now healthy and happily married. However, Bernard's oncologist had never asked him to bank his own sperm before chemotherapy, which destroyed his testicular function. Bernard was thus forced to resort to sperm donation. On the day of Bernard's testicular biopsy, before he knew the outcome of the procedure, we discussed his attitudes toward sperm donation at length:

ANTHROPOLOGIST: Would you consider using a sperm donor?

BERNARD: Sperm donation? It's one of the different options we've been given. If we have "zero" [sperm] today, then we agreed that rather than go for adoption, we would go for sperm donation, so this way, my wife would feel the sense of motherhood.

ANTHROPOLOGIST: Do you know where the sperm come from?

BERNARD: I know nothing about the sperm donors. We didn't talk about this yet. Perhaps they come from China! Japan! Honestly, I'm not interested in knowing from where. But, instead of adopting a child, why not adopt a sperm?

ANTHROPOLOGIST: So you feel comfortable with this . . .

BERNARD: We have had this problem now for two years, and in the end, if it's not going to work, one should adapt to the situation and get convinced [about sperm donation].

ANTHROPOLOGIST: Does your family know?

BERNARD: Yes, my family knows about ICSI, but not about the donor, be
cause, until now, it's our secret between me and my wife. They only
know about ICSI. The sperm donation—it's our secret.

ANTHROPOLOGIST: Do you think you would tell the child some day?

BERNARD: Yes, maybe we will tell the child. If at the end of the day, when
the child reaches a certain age and is able to comprehend and accept,
then why not tell? But, if you tell too early, it may complicate things.

ANTHROPOLOGIST: Have you inquired about the religious aspects?

BERNARD: Now, I'm not thinking about the Maronite opinion or my religion. I'm thinking about my life. It's between me and my wife, and
not me and my priest. As long as a child is born and the church allows us to baptize him, it would be okay. The most important point
is to solve our problem, and this is between me and my wife. We
are a family, me and my wife, and if everything inside our home is
okay, then everything outside must be okay. Because we have some
limits, we have our privacy. And that's why we have a good marriage.
[Laughing] And she is beautiful and she cooks very well!

Although Maronite Catholics are allowed to adopt children from Catholic orphanages, Bernard chose to pursue sperm donation as a way for his
beloved wife to experience pregnancy and motherhood. He equated sperm
donation to "sperm adoption," perhaps making sperm donation seem less
morally problematic in this way.

But, not all Christian men I interviewed were as sanguine about sperm
donation as Bernard. Joseph, another Maronite Catholic, had been offered
sperm donation but adamantly refused—despite the fact that his wife was
willing to consider sperm donation after enduring ten failed ICSIs without a single viable embryo formed. As a religious Catholic, Joseph had
asked his priest about both ICSI and sperm donation and had come to
this conclusion,

There is no problem in the religion with ICSI. But sperm donation, I
don't like. I don't want to bring a "stranger," even though [my wife]
would consider it. From the first time ICSI didn't work, from the very
first year, Dr. [name] said he could bring sperm from someone other
than me to get my wife pregnant, and I refused. [The doctor] said, "I
can take sperm from another man and do the operation, and then
you can adopt the child." But I refused, even though he said it would
be much easier to take sperm from "outside" to make the ICSI succeed. My wife also prefers ICSI over sperm donation, but she would
do sperm donation. And here in Lebanon, they do do sperm donation, but they don't tell who the donor is.

The two other men in my study who were offered sperm donation—one a Sunni Muslim and the other a Druze—absolutely refused to consider this option, even though their cases were fairly hopeless. As noted in earlier chapters, the Druze are a Muslim subsect who are generally considered to be an offshoot of the Shia. Although the Druze have accepted IVF and ICSI—or as one Druze man put it, "even the *shaykhs* and *shaykhas* are doing this!"—all forms of donation are strictly forbidden, unlike the "donor-permissive" Shia. The story of a Druze banker named Marwan bespeaks the heartbreak of surviving cancer only to be diagnosed as azoospermic and then experiencing the emotional rollercoaster that was to follow.

MARWAN, TESTICULAR CANCER, AND AZOOSPERMIC MANHOOD

When I met Marwan, his first words to me were, "I want to do the study," but he cautioned me that he was pressed for time, as he had to return to a banking job he hated. A forty-one-year-old Druze man, Marwan described how he had been unable to "enjoy" his American University of Beirut college days because of the civil war, and how his family's home was leveled by bombs, although no one was seriously injured. Fortunately for Marwan, he was able to migrate to the United Arab Emirates, but, soon after his arrival, he began experiencing testicular pain. Seeking medical care, he underwent repeated semen analyses, as well as a testicular biopsy. This was in 1991, and it was then that Marwan learned he was infertile, suffering from a very low sperm count. What the physician failed to diagnose was the testicular cancer, which was causing Marwan's testicular pain. It took a full six years for the cancer to be properly diagnosed, and Marwan underwent an urgent removal of his left testicle, along with chemotherapy. Marwan's Lebanese physicians had caught his cancer in time; repeated pelvic scans and blood tests showed that the testicular cancer was gone and had not spread to other parts of his body.

In the joyous aftermath of a cancer cure, Marwan began a new relationship with a woman he wanted to marry. Given his medical history, he decided to undergo premarital semen analysis. The results, he recalled, were "shocking," a term he used over and over to describe what he learned,

> I went to check and I was surprised that it was a zero count, and it was very big shock—shocking! It was shocking, and it caused a failure of this new relationship with a girl, because she didn't accept thinking of marrying me. It was a shock for me. It was *very, very* shocking, especially when it resulted in that failure of that relation-

ship. Maybe at that time, when I knew about it [the azoospermia], I didn't feel the difficulty of this issue. But when this case happened, I felt that this *is* a big problem, a big deal.

Marwan continued,

When I discovered, when you hear about cancer the first time, you will imagine nothing but death. But when you have the treatment, and I was cured, then everything will not be that difficult compared to the cancer case. So when I discovered that I had no sperm, it was not that difficult for me. But after this case [of relationship failure], I felt the manhood problem for the first time. I felt a little deficient. But *only* at that time. Before this, I considered it God's will. What can I do? I will do my best.

Without stopping the narrative, Marwan then began to explain how his self-esteem had been affected by his "weight problem." In fact, Marwan was obese—which was very unusual, given that Lebanon can only be described as a weight-, beauty-, and fashion-conscious nation. Although some of the men in my study could be described as "stocky," "pudgy," or slightly overweight, the majority were trim, even thin, often because of excessive smoking. Marwan himself was a regular pipe smoker, sometimes also smoking cigars or cigarettes. But, this did not seem to control what he called his "obesity problem," describing it to me as follows,

I have the problem of fatness, which I've been following since 1984. I've reached as high as 131 kilograms, and in 1991, as low as 78 kilograms, because I'm always dieting, "yo-yo dieting." This is one of the major problems in my life. I want to be able to maintain one weight. But I'm sedentary, and now I'm 109 kilograms.

According to Marwan, many people have counseled him about his weight over the years,

In our society, you will find a lot of people talk about a lot of subjects, whether or not they know about it. "Go for the operation [to staple the stomach]!" "No, no, no, don't go for the operation!" This weight problem is what makes everything for me even more difficult.

Fortunately for Marwan, at the age of forty, he finally found a wife, Sherine, who accepted him for who he was—in spite of his history of cancer, azoospermia, and obesity. At the time of our interview, Marwan and Sherine had been married for less than a year.

Of course, Sherine knew before our marriage about the cancer. I was not trying to deceive her by not telling her. Maybe it's her faith. It will be our pleasure if God is willing to give us. And if not, we won't have children. This is the way she is, and she has no problem dealing with it. And, also, if there is any scientific way to deal with this problem, she's ready. And, by the way, she is *very* afraid; she's afraid of everything. She's afraid of injections. She hates medicine, drugs.

Given Marwan's azoospermia and Sherine's fear of medicine, I asked whether they would consider sperm donation via simple intrauterine insemination (i.e., the "turkey baster" method, but with injection into the uterus). I learned then that Marwan's family physician, as well as his IVF physician, had both advised him to consider sperm donation. Marwan had a great deal to say on this issue,

> The thing I would like to emphasize is that I do *not* prefer any sperm donation. If I have sperm, I will go ahead with ICSI. If not, up until now, I'm not convinced about that sperm donation. My family physician said, "You can go for that." And Dr. [name] said, "If you are willing, you can have a baby through sperm donation." In fact, I'm still afraid that nothing, ultimately, will be found [i.e., absolute azoospermia]. And let's be frank, I have no other choice. Any person in my shoes will not have any other options. But, you're either confident in doing these things [i.e., sperm donation] or you're not.

I asked Marwan what made him uncomfortable about sperm donation. He replied,

> The sperm, it's from other people. Still, I can't accept this. I don't know, maybe it's our culture, you name it, our environment. Still, to me, as a person, still maybe there are so many people who have a problem with that. I don't feel that this child is our child. In our culture, I don't feel that this child is part of me and my wife. I will not be feeling this is part of *me* and my wife. Maybe this is seen as selfishness in some other cultures, or a lack of understanding. Everyone has his own opinion about sperm donation. And I'm telling you as of this day, I don't accept it. And adoption, it is the same for me as sperm donation. My attitude toward it up till now, just to be clear with you, is the same. It's not a problem in the religion [i.e., adoption]. It's a matter of personal acceptance. This is how I feel today, but no one knows what will happen in the future.

Fortunately for Marwan, approximately 1,000 spermatozoa were found in his testicular biopsy sample on the day of Sherine's oocyte retrieval. Unfortunately, in the ensuing days, embryos formed, but did not divide. Marwan's ICSI cycle was therefore canceled.

Lineal Masculinity, Genealogy, and Fatherhood

Marwan's rejection of both sperm donation and adoption is telling in several ways. On the face of it, Marwan is a most likely candidate for sperm donation. He is educated, he is a cancer survivor, he faces intractable azoospermia, and he is secular in his outlook. Both his family doctor and his IVF doctor have recommended sperm donation as his most likely path to parenthood. Yet, Marwan speaks at some length in his interview about his feelings of diminished masculinity and his inability to "personally accept" the thought of fathering either an adopted or sperm donor child. He is one of the few men to use the gender-neutral term "child." In most cases, men use the expression, "He won't be my *son*," to explain their rejection of both adoption and sperm donation.

Clues to this overarching rejection can be found in what anthropologists Diane King and Linda Stone have termed *lineal masculinity*.[44] As they note, the Middle Eastern region is exceptionally patrilineal. Kinship, inheritance, and a person's very sense of identity are seen as flowing "to and through men over the generations."[45] According to King and Stone, "a patriline is not only a line of fathers and sons through time but it is also a 'mascu-line' that enhances and gives form to masculinity."[46] Lineal masculinity, in their view, involves perceived social ontology; manliness is socially enacted through a man's ability to pass along his name, his lineage, and his achievements to future generations. To do so requires actual biological reproduction, or the passage of "seed" (*semen* in Latin), which is the very essence of kinship substance. As King and Stone explain it,

> Neither kinship nor lineage membership nor lineal masculinity can be transmitted any other way. . . . A man, but not a woman, lives on through reproduction, through the transmission of his semen. . . . Living on, passing on one's semen and transmitting one's collective and individual lineal masculinity are considerable inducements for men to reproduce, especially to reproduce sons, indeed, many of them. Having many children, especially sons, itself counts as a plus in a man's enhancement of the lineal masculinity he receives from his ancestors.[47]

According to King and Stone, lineal masculinity underlies Middle Eastern pronatalism, as well as son preference.[48] It is also the basis for men's concerns about women's "honor," given that sexual transgressions may threaten the "purity" of the patriline. In addition, among the Iraqi Kurds studied by King, lineal masculinity is manifest in men's desires to found their own lineages, and to be remembered as powerful heads of clans and tribes. In short, lineal masculinity provides a powerful conceptual heuristic for understanding men's investments in patriliny. Although it does not and cannot explain all male behavior in the Middle East or in other regions where it is said to operate, it nonetheless provides clues concerning why men may reject sperm donation and adoption.

Furthermore, men's feelings about patrilineal genealogy, or *nasab*, are critical. As Morgan Clarke has noted for Lebanon, *nasab* is "a key term, although difficult to translate and not common in everyday speech."[49] Variously glossed as kinship, genealogy, consanguinity, or filiation, *nasab* is viewed in much Islamic discourse as "the primordial relationship upon which the wider set of relationships of rights and obligations which form human society is built."[50] Men in my Lebanese study clearly saw both sperm donation and adoption as disruptive of *nasab*, or of what they considered to be the primordial relationship between father and child. As they explained this in genealogical terms, "He won't be my son. It would be like raising another man's child." Men in my study argued that sperm donation and adoption "confuse," "destroy," or "mix" *nasab*, which is both morally illicit and devastating to the child. Just as a child has the "right to know" his or her true *nasab*, so does a man. In other words, a father wants a true patrilineal descendant, ideally a son, created from his own sperm.

Men spoke to this genealogical desire when I asked them why having children was so important. Although men had many reasons for wanting children—often telling me how they "loved," "adored," and "needed kids"—issues of patrilineal continuity and personal immortality were prominent in some men's statements. For example, men told me: "Children help their father and continue his family." "I want children to continue my name, so that people will say, 'This is the son of so-and-so.'" "Children will continue our family heritage." "The child will carry my name to future generations." "Having children creates a memory; you will leave someone, a son to take your name." "Boys carry the name, for the continuity of generations." Some men were slightly more expansive, enumerating several reasons they wanted children. For instance, one man told me, "First, marriage is *for* children. Why else would we marry? Second is name continuity. Third is work. Children take over the family business. Fourth is the inheritance which you leave to your children. That's *why* men work." Another infertile man enumerated his need for children in this way, "First is normality, to be a normal family. Second is continuity, to continue the family into the future. Third is old-age security, to have someone to take care of you when you're old. But honestly, all I want is to have a child who's healthy; that's all."

Naming, and more specifically "carrying the family name" into the future, emerged as a major theme in these comments. Middle Eastern naming practices can differ from country to country, according to both local custom and national law. Generally, however, all children, both boys and girls, share their father's patrilineal surname. In most Middle Eastern countries, women retain their maiden names (i.e., the father's patrilineal surname) after marriage and on all official identity documents, although in Lebanon and Syria, it has become common for women to be called by their husbands' surnames (i.e.,"Mrs. So-and-so") at the time of marriage. In Lebanon, sons are often given the first name of paternal grandfathers. In Egypt, most people adopt their own father's first name as their"every-day" last names, leaving familial surnames for official records. Furthermore, as soon as a man marries and bears a child, he is no longer called by his first name. Instead, he is given the teknonym,"Father of So-and-So."If a man's first child is a girl, he will keep her name in his teknonym until he bears a son, at which point the teknonym will be changed to signal a male heir.

Given the intimacy and interconnection of these naming practices, it is not surprising that naming is one of the problems mentioned in reference to both adoption and sperm donation. Changing a child's surname to match an adoptive father's is considered to be a form of legal evasion that is immoral, a legal fiction that confuses *nasab*. Similarly, with a child of sperm donation, questions and debates center on naming practices; namely, does the child take the surname of the sperm donor, or of the fictive infertile father? The Shia authorities who have allowed the practice of sperm donation have suggested that naming, inheritance, and biological descent rest with the sperm donor and not with the infertile man.

These complexities of naming and *nasab* are thus critical in understanding men's aversions. Marwan is like most Middle Eastern men in this regard. In Marwan's own words, a sperm donor or adopted child will not be "a part of *me*."For Marwan, social fatherhood of a child who is not a direct genealogical descendant and who, on a legal level, should not carry his own family name, is clearly out of the question. In fact, these feelings of estranged fatherhood have also been reported for Iran, the Middle Eastern Muslim country where sperm donation is most widely accepted in practice. As shown by Soraya Tremayne in a poignant essay, men who have chosen to use donor sperm may later regret their decisions, taking out their angst and anger on hapless wives and donor children.[51] Increasingly, these Iranian women and their donor offspring are fleeing to the West, seeking political asylum from abusive spouses/fathers. Furthermore, the Royan Institute, one of the major assisted reproduction and stem cell research centers in Tehran, has conducted survey research on attitudes toward sperm donation among infertile men.[52] Despite Ayatollah Khamene'i's approval of sperm donation, Iranian men continue to be morally ambivalent about the practice, finding it much less acceptable than either egg or embryo donation. It is important to note here that donated embryos, too, are created from other men's sperm; yet, Iranian men seem to accept this practice with greater enthusiasm. At the time of this writing, Iran is the only Middle Eastern country to encourage embryo donation, and the reasons why infertile men there prefer it over sperm donation have yet to be fully investigated.

Given everything I know about Middle Eastern third-party donation, I would surmise that Iranian men find "donated embryos" akin to "adopted children" in a country that also allows for the latter practice. Furthermore, transferring donor embryos into a wife's uterus is symbolically quite different than injecting her uterus with another man's sperm. For men, sperm donation implies extramarital intercourse. In my own study, men clearly equated sperm donation with *zina*, or adultery, and could not bear the thought of "strangers' sperm" impregnating their beloved wives, to whom they were sexually faithful.

Such aversions to sperm donation are not unique to the Middle East, nor are they indicative of a uniquely Middle Eastern lineal masculinity. Perhaps lineal masculinity underlies most men's desires to father biological offspring and to rest assured about their paternity. This is true even in the purportedly "progressive" West. Even though donor insemination is the "oldest" assisted reproductive technology—having been practiced in the United States and Europe for nearly a century[53]—anthropologists have revealed the stigma and secrecy incumbent in this practice.[54] In the West, men seem to have less trouble donating sperm—usually for a nominal fee—than accepting it from another man. In order to abide by sperm donation, infertile men must find ways to reframe their sense of fatherhood, convincing themselves that they are able to feel deep love for individuals who are not biologically related to them. Moreover, infertile men and their spouses must make difficult decisions regarding donor disclosure. For example, should friends and family be notified that a child is the product of sperm donation? Should parents disclose this information to a donor child, and at what point in the child's life? Do a child's rights to medical knowledge trump parental desires for secrecy? As shown in anthropologist Gay Becker's fascinating work on sperm donation in the United States, "to tell or not to tell" becomes a major ethical dilemma in the local moral worlds of infertile American men and their wives.[55] Some couples choose absolute secrecy, while others deem disclosure necessary to prevent dishonesty and deception. In some cases, couples choose the path of least resistance by delaying the decision indefinitely. In short, sperm donation troubles American men, too, even though they may not reject the practice out of hand.

CONCLUSION

Moustafa, the only man in my Lebanese study who secretly "chose" sperm donation, was not alone in his moral angst. In the new millennium, sperm donation continues to be one of the most stigmatizing reproductive technologies, even though, before ICSI, it was widely practiced in the West in cases of male infertility. The introduction of ICSI around the world has dramatically reduced the demand for sperm donation.[56] However, as seen in this chapter, ICSI has not erased the practice of sperm donation altogether. For numerous reasons, genetic and otherwise, there will always be men without sperm. Furthermore, there will always be recalcitrant sperm that resist the fertilizing power of ICSI.

When ICSI fails, sperm donation is now offered in two Middle Eastern countries, Iran and Lebanon. Along with "secular" Tunisia and Turkey, Iran is also the only Muslim Middle Eastern country to offer legal adoption to infertile couples. Nonetheless, as shown in this chapter, both sperm donation and adoption are widely resisted as routes to social fatherhood in the Middle East, including among men who are otherwise allowed these avenues by law, religion, or both. Men's reasons for feeling this way are complex but lie in deeply entrenched Islamic and local moral concepts of *nasab*, *zina*, and patriliny. Or as Middle Eastern Muslim men themselves put it, quite simply, "He won't be my son."

CHAPTER 8

Egg Donation and Emergence

Eyad is the only Middle Eastern man I have ever met whose specific dia-sporic dream was to emigrate to the American state of Wisconsin. Perhaps because of his unusual longing for the great dairy state, Eyad and I imme-diately bonded in the Beirut IVF clinic where I met him. Although I have not lived in Wisconsin for more than thirty years, I was born there, leaving only after I graduated from college. When Eyad told me that he hoped to one day reunite with an emigrant brother in a rural town outside of Mil-waukee, I was touched. And, if it weren't for the fact that we were meeting in a crowded Beirut IVF clinic, I might have taken Eyad for a bratwurst-eating, beer-drinking, "cheesehead." This is because Eyad had very "white" skin, upon which he would later comment at length. Furthermore, he was a large, corpulent man, who had shaved his head to hide his baldness. In short, Eyad did not fit the American stereotype of a Middle Eastern Arab man. But, as I would soon discover, he had spent his entire, tortured life in the Middle East, where he had moved from country to country in an at-tempt to find peace and happiness.

Eyad was a Sunni Muslim Palestinian man who had lived for many years in the Arab Gulf as a worker in the petroleum industry. As a Pales-tinian refugee, the whole of Eyad's life had been extremely difficult and stressful. With the formation of the state of Israel in 1948, his parents were impelled to flee their home in Haifa. They ended up in a Palestinian refu-gee camp in Saida, Lebanon, where they eventually bore ten children. Be-cause of the appalling living conditions in the camp, and then the outbreak of the Lebanese civil war in 1975, nine of the ten children, including Eyad, fled the country. (The only remaining sibling died in the war.) When Eyad emigrated at the tender age of fifteen, he left behind his childhood sweet-heart, Lubna, who was also his *bint 'amma*, or paternal first cousin (i.e., his father's sister's daughter). He had promised to marry her when the war ended. But, the bloody conflict raged on for a full fifteen years, and this was followed by ten years of the Israeli occupation of southern Lebanon. Thus, Eyad was effectively barred from returning to southern Lebanon to retrieve his waiting fiancée.

Eventually, at age thirty, Eyad married a Palestinian woman from the West Bank of Jordan, who bore him two daughters and a son. As stateless Palestinians, they chose to migrate to Kuwait, where Eyad could make a better living as a crane operator in the oilfields. Despite a decent standard of living and company benefits, Eyad's marriage and family life were unhappy. His feelings for his first love Lubna had never waned, and this contributed to a marriage fraught with tension and fighting. Furthermore, when Iraq invaded Kuwait in 1990, the Palestinian residents of Kuwait were caught in the middle. PLO leader Yasir Arafat supported Saddam Hussein instead of the Kuwaiti monarchy and its allied forces; therefore, most Palestinians were ostracized and then ousted from the country. In Eyad's case, he and his two brothers were kidnapped and brutally beaten, before being turned over by their Kuwaiti captors to the American forces in Desert Storm. (Although the American forces imprisoned Eyad and his brothers for several days, they fed and treated them well before releasing them, according to Eyad.)

At this point, Eyad fled with his family to Damascus, Syria, where he found a safe haven for his family and schools for his three children. But Eyad could not find work in Syria, a relatively poor and isolated Middle Eastern country without major oilfields. Given few options, he returned by himself to the Arab Gulf, this time to Dubai in the United Arab Emirates, where he renewed his work in the petroleum industry. Living by himself for nearly ten years (1992–2002), Eyad experienced deep loneliness and sexual frustration. As he explained to me, "I can't sleep with my wife [in Syria], so I feel pain, pain in the testicles. Any man who sees some beautiful girl and can't have sex will feel this way."

Given his ongoing marital problems and his sense of isolation, Eyad decided to take a lover, even though he realized that adultery is a form of *zina*, a major sin in Islam. In Eyad's case, his lover was his Filipina housemaid, whom he had hired to cook and clean for him. "I got one girlfriend [in the UAE] because I haven't a wife [to have sex with]," Eyad said. But he then added, "She loves me *too* much, that girlfriend. She was a Filipino [*sic*]. She wanted to get one baby to look like me, but I said no."

In fact, Eyad had no intention of either marrying or impregnating his Filipina maid-cum-mistress, although she lived in his apartment—first as a maid, then sharing his bed—for nearly a decade. Instead, when political conditions in Lebanon improved with the retreat of Israeli forces from southern Lebanon in May 2000, Eyad decided to ask his first love, Lubna, to become his second wife. Lubna had never married during the war years and thus remained a forty-year-old virgin, with few if any marital prospects. Eyad proposed, and Lubna agreed, although Eyad's first wife vociferously objected. (Eyad never described to me the reaction of his Filipina maid-mistress, or whether he continued to have sexual relations with her.)

Eyad married Lubna in the summer of 2000, although she continued to live with her mother in Lebanon, and Eyad continued to work in the Gulf. Because Lubna lived in a United Nations–supported refugee camp, her rights to exit Lebanon as a refugee were severely restricted. Moreover, the UAE does not grant political asylum or citizenship rights to foreigners living in the country.

As newlyweds already in their forties, Eyad and Lubna faced infertility problems from the beginning of their marriage. Eyad's semen was tested at a laboratory in the UAE, where he was deemed to be fertile. When semen analysis was repeated on the day of our interview in Beirut, Eyad described his positive semen test results with me, joking, "Very good! Should I marry a third one?"

Lubna, however, had entered perimenopause, and doctors told her that her chances of conceiving were less than 5 percent, even with a cycle of IVF. If Eyad had been able to marry Lubna when she was still a teenager, they might have had children together quite easily. But now, at age forty-one, Lubna needed an egg donor, according to the IVF physicians in the Beirut clinic.

"She needs eggs," Eyad explained. "He told me to do this [IVF] with donor eggs. He didn't tell me I must do this, but he said that she *needs* this operation [to become pregnant]. If he sends me to any other hospital or doctor, they will say the same thing." In fact, Eyad had already inquired about Lubna's case at an IVF clinic in an Islamic hospital in Sunni-dominant Jordan, but he was told that Lubna was too old to conceive and that egg donation was not allowed in the religion.

Given his bad experiences with war-related violence and ongoing discrimination against Palestinian refugees in Lebanon, Eyad would have preferred to undertake IVF in the UAE. But, he knew that accessing IVF for Lubna in the UAE would be virtually impossible for two reasons: first, Lubna would have great difficulty traveling to the UAE as a stateless Palestinian refugee without an official passport; and, second, he learned that third-party gamete donation was not allowed in the Sunni-dominant UAE, even though "global" Dubai was known for its cosmopolitanism. As Eyad soon determined, the only option for him and Lubna was to attempt IVF with egg donation in Lebanon.

However, since Eyad did not reside in Lebanon, he began his career as a reproductive tourist—namely, a person who travels between countries for so-called cross-border reproductive care.[1] Flying back and forth from Dubai to Beirut on several occasions to deposit his semen in the IVF clinic, Eyad was a man on a mission—namely, to get his beloved second wife Lubna pregnant through assisted conception. When I met Eyad and Lubna, they were in the midst of a donor-egg cycle. He explained his decision to use donor eggs in this way,

In Islam, donation is *haram*. I mean, in Islam you should try to get the eggs from the wife and the *bizri* ["seeds," sperm] from the husband if you want to make IVF. The eggs from the wife and the *bizri* from the man, not from outside. Since we're using an egg donor, if I get a baby, it's *my* son, because it's my *bizri*. But it's not *her* son, because the eggs came from another girl. The other girl—that's her mother.

He continued,

But my wife, she *really* needs a child. It's more important to her to be a mother than following the religion. So I don't mind. I'm not too much a Muslim. I pray, but sometimes you should "move" a little. For her psychology, she *needs* that baby. I could go to take a baby already born from outside and bring it to our house [i.e., fostering]. But when she puts it in here [he points to the belly], day by day, she's feeling it growing inside her. It's born *from* her. She's feeling that it's *really her baby*. But if I get [an orphan] from outside, she won't feel it's *her* baby. And my wife *should* be its mother. Because she will care for him in the future, and she feels the pains from today and *forever*!

My wife loves babies *so* much, because she cared for the children of her sister, and they love her too much. All the time, by telephone, they're calling and saying, "Auntie. Where is she?" She loves them, because they are the children of her sister. And she'll make a great mother, because she hasn't any children, and she loves children.

She wants a baby. She needs a baby. So I'm doing this IVF for *her*, yes, for *her*. We're doing it very secretly, because maybe it's not a baby who looks like me or his mother, and people will ask, "From where did you get that baby?" People will talk. In America, it's normal [to use a donor], and in Europe. But with us here, it's difficult to do—*very* difficult. If we are in America, or outside the Middle East, it would be normal. But in the Middle East, we'll have to tell people that we did this operation [IVF] from her eggs and my *bizri*, so people will believe this is our child.

Interestingly, despite Eyad's desire to convince the world of a biological conception with his dark-haired, olive-skinned wife, he had become fairly obsessed with a "white" American egg donor, whom he happened to spot in the Lebanese IVF clinic. In fact, this particular Beirut-based clinic employed both Lebanese and American egg donors; the latter were paid an additional $1,000 to travel to the Middle East for egg harvesting. When Eyad spotted the pale-skinned, bleached-blonde donor in her khaki shorts and tank top, he became immediately smitten with her beauty and manner. He extolled her virtues to me in this way,

Yesterday, I saw a very beautiful girl outside [in the hallway]. She's American, I'm sure. So I told the doctor, "Take $1,000 more! And give me the eggs from that girl!" She was fat a little bit, and really, really very beautiful. There was something quiet about her, and something about her face. Directly, my eyes went to her. She was really beautiful and my heart opened to her.

He continued, half joking and half serious, "I hope my wife gets some eggs from that girl, because my child, she'll be coming white—already American!—and not black like my wife. My child, when he comes, he will take the American passport in the future!"

At that point in the interview, I asked Eyad how he had spied the donor, given that egg donation in the clinic was intended to be anonymous. He explained, "Yesterday, at one o'clock, maybe twelve thirty, when I was about to give my *bizri*, I went up, and I see her going inside [the operating room]. I told my wife about it. 'I've seen a girl who is too much beautiful! I hope we get eggs from her.' I also told the doctor then, 'I'll give you $1,000 more!' "

He explained further, "I want a child who looks like an American. My father looked like an American. His face was white. My sisters, they are white, and their hair is very blonde, and me and two of my brothers. The others look like my mother [i.e. dark hair, olive skin]. My wife [Lubna] is too dark, and my first [wife] even more. I'm the only one who is white. So I hope that the baby will be coming white like me." He laughed, "If she gets a white baby, I'll give them $1,000!"

I asked Eyad what the doctors thought about his request, and if they were willing to grant his wish. "No," he responded sadly. But he added, "I told them, 'Please, if you give me eggs, *not* from a Sri Lankan, *not* from an Indian, but white like me.' My sons and daughter are *asmar shway* [slightly brown], like their mother. I want a white baby to look like me. But [the doctor] just laughed. He said that none [of the egg donors] are Sri Lankan or Indian or from the Philippines. From *America* they're coming."

I then asked Eyad why he preferred an American donor. "Why not?" he exclaimed. "American girls are giving their eggs all over the world. In the future, all people will look like they are Americans!"

When I asked Eyad whether people would believe that a very white baby had been conceived with his darker-skinned wife's eggs, he replied, "People here will say it's okay. Nothing's wrong, because I am white. Also, if my wife does not get a white child, it's okay. I'm white, but she's brown, so if the baby is brown, it's no problem. But if the baby is coming Filipino, then that's a problem, and I will refuse it! That means that one man who is Filipino slept with my wife! Or that's what people will say if my wife uses eggs from a Filipino."

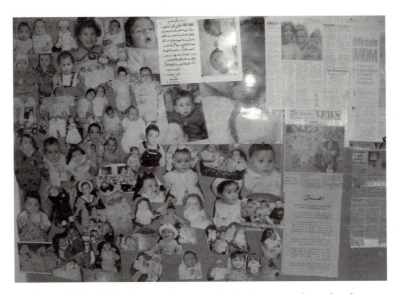

FIGURE 14. Bulletin board of Lebanese IVF baby photos, with study advertisement (*on lower right*)

Whether Eyad and Lubna went on to produce a donor child is unknown, as I never encountered them again at the clinic. I did discover, however, that the eggs of the "beautiful" American donor were, indeed, used in Eyad's and Lubna's IVF cycle. According to one of the clinic's embryologists, this fact was a coincidence based on the donor's egg quality, rather than acquiescence on the part of the clinic to Eyad's request, or any attempt by Eyad to bribe the clinic for a particular donor's "white" eggs.

The egg donor, for her part, was entirely unaware of Eyad's longing. She was a working-class, twenty-four-year-old from the Upper Midwest, who waited tables and tended bar in a chain restaurant. She had been "recruited" into egg donation by a friend, and she was hoping to eventually pay off all of her credit-card bills through repeated egg donation in Lebanon (for which she was paid $3,000 per cycle). Additionally, as an American Christian, she had no moral qualms about donating her eggs to Middle Eastern Muslim couples. She believed that she was performing an altruistic act, by allowing couples who desperately wanted a child to become parents. As we passed by the clinic's bulletin board—which was crowded with photos of Lebanese IVF babies (figure 14)—she pointed out to me, "This one is mine," based on what she perceived to be the phenotypical similarities that Eyad had so admired, namely, the baby's light skin and large "Caucasian" eyes.

EGG DONATION AND DOUBLE FORMS OF EMERGENCE

Eyad's story is morally complex and open to multiple readings and interpretations. From a critical feminist perspective, Eyad could be viewed as
a callous polygynous adulterer, who cares little for the feelings of his first
wife and his long-term mistress. Furthermore, Eyad seems racist, main-
taining a hierarchical preference for "whiteness" that is manifest in his
yearning for a "white" American egg donor. Moreover, Eyad could be accused of being a postcolonial "cultural dupe," who has become convinced
of the superiority of America, a country that has done almost nothing to
help the Palestinians as a people. Finally, from a Sunni Islamic perspective,
Eyad has committed a kind of "triple *zina*"—the grave *zina* of extramarital
sex with a Filipina lover, the *zina* of fertilizing another woman's eggs with
his sperm, and the "fantasy *zina*" of a white American egg donor "mother-
ing" his child. In this reading of Eyad's life, he appears as both a bad man
and a bad Muslim.

A different and more sympathetic reading of Eyad's story casts him in
another light. He is a man who has maintained one true love throughout his lifetime but who has been thwarted from consummating this love
by the circumstances of war and political oppression. In exile, Eyad made
"second best" choices for marital and sexual fulfillment. However, as soon
as the political situation reversed in May 2000, Eyad married Lubna, the
love of his life. In so doing, he did not abandon his first wife, which would
have left her and their three children economically and socially vulnerable.
Polygyny on the part of Eyad signifies his feelings of responsibility toward
two women—a first wife whom he never loved but who is the mother
of his children, and a first cousin with whom dreams of marriage were
crushed by twenty-five years of civil war and occupation. Under normal
circumstances, Eyad and Lubna would probably have married in their early
twenties and would have gone on to become parents of several children.
Eyad's lonely isolation and his resort to sex with his maid—his only other
lifetime sexual partner—would never have happened.

Even though their best reproductive years are already behind them,
Eyad clearly loves his new bride, Lubna, who works as a schoolteacher
in a Palestinian refugee camp. She is neither white nor beautiful like the
American egg donor, but Eyad has adored her since childhood, and he
feels great sympathy toward her as a maritally and reproductively frustrated woman who waited for him for nearly thirty years. Lubna has been
emotionally hurt in the process, as Eyad took another wife and raised a
family. But Lubna's patience has been rewarded. Eyad not only loves her
enough to marry her but also chooses to pursue costly IVF cycles with her.
Already the father of three and in his late forties, Eyad does not desire

more children. But he is willing to pursue IVF "for her," because he appreciates Lubna's ardent desires for motherhood.

Eyad's decision to overcome Lubna's infertility takes moral courage, because in order for Lubna to become a mother, a religiously forbidden technology, egg donation, is required. Eyad justifies this by pointing to Lubna's right to motherhood, his own relaxed approach to religion, and his belief that Islam must "move" to take advantage of emerging technologies that are widely accepted in Euro-America.

In order to access egg donation, Eyad is forced to leave the Sunni-dominant UAE and to help underwrite the costly importation of an American egg donor to Lebanon. Once the process is set in motion, he does not look back, nor does he question the fact that the American egg donor is undoubtedly not a Muslim. Rather, he cares about her skin color and phenotype, because he wants a white (and beautiful) baby to resemble him. He is also concerned that the birth of a racially or phenotypically mixed child would cast doubt on Lubna's morality, or how she has produced the baby. Questions about *zina* and *nasab* would be sure to arise. Against such moral aspersions, Eyad seeks to protect her.

In the end, Eyad's story is about *double forms of emergence*—both technological and masculine. On the one hand, new forms of reproductive technology are continuously emerging, and once they reach the reproductive marketplace, they are being rapidly discussed, debated, and, in most cases, deployed in Middle Eastern IVF settings. Egg donation is a case in point: after entering Iran in 1999, it spread within a year to Lebanon, where Shia Muslim couples were the first to access this reproductive technology. By 2003, when Eyad and Lubna married and decided to try egg donation, Middle Eastern couples from all religions, Sunni, Shia, Druze, and Christian, were beginning to employ this technology in hopes of overcoming age-related and other forms of female infertility.

The willingness of Middle Eastern husbands such as Eyad to accommodate egg donation is a powerful marker of their emerging masculinities. These men have effectively prioritized their wives' own motherhood desires and their conjugal happiness over religious orthodoxies and various practical obstacles and apprehensions. For example, in Eyad's case, he has become a male reproductive tourist; he has engaged in a sophisticated transnational process of commercial foreign egg donation; he has demonstrated his marital love and commitment through costly purchase of IVF and donor eggs "for her"; and he has displayed a form of religious resistance by refusing to abide by Sunni Islamic imperatives. As seen in Eyad's story, the emergence of new forms of assisted reproductive technology has gone hand in hand with emerging masculinities in the region.

Egg Donation Enters Multisectarian Lebanon

As of this writing, Lebanon is the only Middle Eastern country outside of Iran to offer egg donation to infertile couples. Although Lebanon has a large Shia Muslim population, other Middle Eastern countries with large Shia populations, such as Bahrain and Iraq, have not followed suit. This then brings us to the question: Why Lebanon? The answer, I believe, has to do with three interrelated factors: Lebanon's unusual level of multisectarianism, or religious diversity; its entrepreneurial culture, including in the field of medicine, which is largely privatized, as we have seen; and its weak legislature, which has been unable to formulate an assisted reproduction law.

With regard to the first factor, Lebanon is the most heterogeneous Middle Eastern society, and perhaps the most religiously heterodox of all societies in the larger Muslim world. Demographers agree that Muslims constitute a solid majority in Lebanon—almost 60 percent, with Shia outstripping the Sunni population by several percentage points (approximately 27% versus 24%, with Druze at 5% of the total population). Christians constitute the remaining 40%, with the largest group being Maronite Catholics, followed by Greek Orthodox.[2] It is widely believed that the Christian population of Lebanon, once the largest single group, has declined significantly during the past thirty-five years of civil war and ongoing political violence. Meanwhile, the Shia population has increased disproportionately, not only because of higher fertility rates but also because relatively fewer of the poor Shia Muslims of southern Lebanon were able to emigrate from the country. Until the Lebanese civil war, Sunni Muslims dominated the coastal cities of Lebanon, such as Tripoli in the North. Although they are not counted as Lebanese, nearly half a million Sunni Muslim Palestinians live in twelve registered refugee camps in the country.[3] Other significant refugee populations include Armenians (who fled the Turks), Iraqis (fleeing recent wars), and Syrians (fleeing poverty). Given this multisectarian, diverse composition of Lebanese society, it is important to understand how the local IVF industry has developed there, and how exactly egg donor programs came into being to help infertile couples such as Eyad and Lubna.

Lebanon is a relative latecomer to assisted reproduction, compared to Sunni-dominant countries such as Egypt, Jordan, and Saudi Arabia. The first IVF clinics did not open in Beirut until the mid-1990s, nearly a decade later than in Egypt, for example.[4] This "Lebanese delay" has everything to do with the fifteen-year civil war. It was not until the early 1990s, after the fighting stopped, that Lebanon was able to start rebuilding its medical infrastructure, which had been severely damaged during the period of prolonged battle.

Before the civil war, Lebanon was well known in the Middle Eastern region for the medical "3 Es": education, entrepreneurship, and excellence. By the mid-1990s, these aspects of Lebanese medical society had begun to return. Local gynecologists began opening their own small hospitals and private IVF clinics. Expatriate Lebanese physicians, trained in the West, returned to the country to start IVF clinics staffed by local doctors. Eventually, several of Lebanon's major private hospitals opened their own IVF centers. By 2003, when Eyad and Lubna began seeking assisted conception, the country boasted between fifteen and twenty clinics, depending upon how clinic was being defined.

Before the year 2000, it appears that all Lebanese IVF clinics abided by the Middle Eastern regional ban on third-party reproductive assistance. Lebanese IVF physicians, circulating through regional medical conferences, were clearly aware that the Islamic religious authorities did not approve of any form of donation or surrogacy. They knew that third-party donation was not being practiced in any Muslim country at that time, and thus they felt obliged, even if they were Christian, to follow the local religious norms. To do otherwise would be to incite potential anger and resistance among Muslim clients of Lebanese IVF centers.

Nonetheless, the year 2000 was a watershed in Lebanon. At a Middle East Fertility Society (MEFS) meeting held in Beirut, an Iranian female IVF physician—dressed in her black chador—was giving a lecture on problems of ovulation in women. A Shia Muslim physician, who had heard that Iranians were performing egg donation, asked, "If patients don't respond to medication, what do you do?" The female physician answered, "We use donor eggs." The assembled audience of Middle Eastern IVF practitioners literally gasped in shock and awe—or, perhaps, horror—at this big news. However, the Iranian physician calmly explained that egg donation was *halal* in Iran, because Ayatollah Khamene'i had issued a *fatwa* the year before effectively permitting both egg and sperm donor technologies to be used.

This "millennial moment" in Iran had an almost immediate impact in Lebanon. Shia IVF physicians were the first to respond, developing informal egg donation arrangements within their clinics. In general, they used only "designated donors," usually female family members or close female friends chosen by the infertile patient. Occasionally, married Shia women who had produced excess eggs, but did not want to pay extra for embryo freezing and storage, were asked by clinics to donate their excess oocytes to other infertile couples, mostly other married Shia couples. However, by 2003, when Eyad traveled to Lebanon, he was able to find a majority Shia-serving IVF clinic, which had developed a full-fledged egg donation program, complete with anonymous donors flown in from America. This is the clinic in which I met him and Lubna in early June 2003.

In addition, Christian IVF practitioners soon joined the pro-egg-donation bandwagon in Lebanon, setting up informal programs within their clinics. Many Western-leaning Lebanese Christian IVF practitioners had been frustrated by the MEFS's pressure to conform to the Sunni-inspired regional ban on third-party assistance and, hence, were happy

and relieved that Iran had opened a path to donation. Being able to provide gamete donation—and even surrogacy—allowed them to offer the
full spectrum of possible assisted reproductive technology services to their
IVF patients. It is fair to state that Lebanese Christians—both physicians
and patients—were as eager as Lebanese Shia Muslims to introduce third-
party reproductive assistance to Lebanon, even if their own inspiration
was European, rather than Iranian. Third-party reproductive assistance in
Lebanon could showcase Lebanon's European-style modernity, while also
providing a tremendous source of profit to the local IVF industry. Furthermore, many Lebanese Christians did not have any moral qualms about
using donor technologies. Rather, they considered donation to be an act
of altruism, similar to child adoption, which most of them condoned on
Christian religious grounds.

For example, in the second IVF clinic in which I worked in Lebanon, all
three physicians were Maronite Catholics. Although the Catholic Church
bans all forms of assisted reproductive technology, including gamete donation,[5] at least two of these three Catholic physicians were solidly supportive of egg donation. The physicians reported performing three to four
egg-donor cycles each month, using designated donors brought by infertile couples to the clinic. Without a full-fledged egg donation program of
their own, these physicians sometimes referred their patients to four other
IVF centers, where egg donation was regularly being offered. As one of
the Catholic physicians in this clinic told me, "There's no egg donor program here because of hospital restrictions. But we would if we could. And
we would attract *many* Middle Eastern patients!" He added, "When you're
in this situation, what are you going to do to solve your problem? The
Catholic Church, when you get married preaches to you not to do 'artificial'
things like IVF. But I've seen Catholic priests using such 'artificial' methods
for other medical conditions. It's easy to say this when it's not your problem. But when it's your problem, you do what you have to do."

In short, the "door to egg donation" was opened even for Catholic IVF
practitioners in Lebanon as an indirect result of the Iranian *fatwa* allowing donor technologies. Generally speaking, these Christian clinicians followed their Shia Muslim colleagues' lead. Starting with entrepreneurial
Shia IVF physicians who cited the new Iranian guidelines, the local Lebanese Shia clergy soon followed, issuing formal *fatwa*s on egg donation,
which most agreed was now *halal*, or religiously permitted.[6] Not surprisingly, the Lebanese clerics of Hizbullah, loyal to Ayatollah Khamene'i,
were the first to agree to egg donation, inciting significant demand for
donor eggs among the most conservative Hizbullah faction of Lebanese
Shia Muslims. As noted in chapter 6, the local Lebanese cleric, Sayyid Fadlallah, was a relative holdout regarding egg donation, deciding that it was
halal only in mid-2003. Nonetheless, in April of that year, a *fatwa* was issued from Sayyid Fadlallah's Beirut office announcing that he would now

permit egg donation for his followers, as long as each infertile couple was "sure prior to taking the eggs that the woman is without husband and without sexual partner and that there must be an 'agreement' [marital], even if temporary, with the donor; otherwise, it is not acceptable."

Ironically, Sayyid Fadlallah's stipulation of a written marriage contract served only to increase the demand for *American* egg donors. Why? "Egg harvesting" requires ultrasound-guided penetration of the ovary, with the insertion of the speculum and retrieval devices through the vagina. Such egg harvesting essentially "deflowers" an egg donor who is a virgin; hence, it is unacceptable for the vast majority of unmarried Shia Muslim women who care about their premarital virginity. As a result, recruiting unmarried Shia Muslim women to donate their eggs is very difficult, even though it occasionally happens. For example, in my own study, one older Syrian Armenian Orthodox couple recruited their own designated donor, who happened to be a strikingly beautiful, twenty-two-year-old Shia Muslim woman. Although she was unmarried, she agreed to the egg donation out of love for this couple, who had supported her successful medical treatment for a congenital heart defect. Using the donor's healthy eggs, the forty-five-year-old wife conceived triplets. This case, however, was highly atypical and was mostly conveyed to me by the niece of the husband, who accompanied this couple to the clinic.

Given the difficulty of finding unmarried Lebanese egg donors who were willing to go through the vaginal egg-harvesting procedures, a demand for American, unmarried, but nonvirgin women was created in Lebanon. Not only would they be willing to undergo vaginally penetrative gynecological procedures, but they might even be willing to undergo temporary marriage contracts by simply signing a written document (in Arabic) "as a formality" in front of clinic staff. Quite interestingly, the greatest demand for such American female egg donors came initially from infertile Shia Muslim *wives*, who pushed their husbands to formally enact these marriage contracts. By doing so, they could abide by Sayyid Fadlallah's demand for written, temporary, polygynous marriage, thereby ensuring that no unlawful *zina* was taking place. As a Shia Muslim IVF physician explained this rather surreal situation to me, "I had four Shia Muslim women patients coming to see me, all in premature ovarian failure. They all wanted their husbands to do a temporary marriage with the donor. And so they want an *American* donor, because the husband can *marry* her!" Then he added, "And we have Sunni couples coming to Lebanon from Egypt, Kuwait, all over the Middle East. They have searched the Internet, and they are calling me about coming here for egg donation."

At any given time, this clinic maintained an egg donor waiting list with ten to twenty Middle Eastern couples, most of them hoping to receive American donor eggs. Middle Eastern Muslim women's desires to find *unmarried* donors and Middle Eastern men's desires to find *white* donors

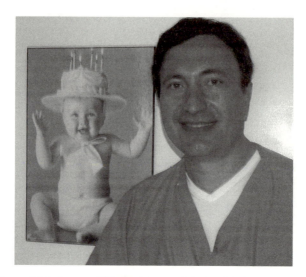

FIGURE 15. Lebanese IVF physician and "white" baby photo

appeared to trump any concerns about the donor's own religious back-ground. This says a great deal about racial preferences for "white" babies and the perceived transmissibility of race—rather than nationality or religion—vis-à-vis donor gametes (figure 15). As egg donation becomes more firmly ensconced in Lebanon, such issues of "difference" surround-ing race, religion, and nationality require further investigation. Suffice it to say here that egg donation in Lebanon—and some men's willingness to pay extra for the eggs of attractive, white, unmarried American women—is a fascinating subject for study in the dramatically emergent assisted reproduction sector.

Also quite interestingly, this demand for American donor eggs never ceased, even in the immediate aftermath of the 2006 sixty-day war in Leb-anon. The supply of American donors rebounded almost immediately as soon as the war ended. Who were these American "foreign traveling egg donors"?[7] As we will see, problems of social class featured quite promi-nently in these donors' lives, trumping for them other concerns about donating their eggs across racial, religious, or national lines, or about the embodied risks of further political violence.

AMERICAN DONOR DAYS IN LEBANON

In general, American women restrict their egg donation to the United States. So why would American women be willing to travel to war-torn Lebanon? During the course of my study in Lebanon, I was fortunate to be present at two "American donor days" in the Shia-serving clinic in my study. I was therefore able to meet and interview three young American women donors, who had come to Lebanon from the "motor state" of Michigan, where I was living at that time as a professor at the University of Michigan. My being a fellow "Michigander" came as a pleasant surprise, as well as a source of comfort to these young women, who had traveled so far from home. I tried to help them navigate their way through Beirut, and two of them took me into their confidences.

As it turns out, American egg donation in Lebanon began with one of their acquaintances from Michigan. She was both a college student and an avid golfer, and she used her egg donation earnings to pursue her love of the sport. She had already undertaken five egg donation cycles in the United States when a Lebanese-American IVF physician asked her if she would be willing to consider an expense-paid trip to Lebanon to donate her eggs to Lebanese couples. Eager for more money, she readily agreed. Between 2000 and 2002, she made five trips to Lebanon to donate her eggs, playing golf on the newly emerging Lebanese courses. According to the IVF physician who initially recruited her, "She made a few friends in the process, and then she retired after she made all of these babies." Although I never learned the total number of IVF children conceived from this woman's eggs, the number was considerable. According to a Lebanese Shia Muslim IVF physician who worked with the Lebanese recipients of her eggs,

> In December, the American woman came to donate her eggs. There were about twenty patients in need of eggs. About thirteen patients received her eggs, which is problematic in a small country. This donor has done it ten times—five in the U.S. and five in Lebanon. This is crazy, because the research suggests that one should never donate more than five times. There are long-term risks of breast and ovarian cancer. But she is young, a college student, and she now loves Lebanon. At first, her family was worried about her, and she had to call home when she arrived, so that they know what she is doing. But she makes money each time and all of her expenses are paid. So she pleads with [the clinical director] to come, even though he tries to tell her to wait.

Although I never met this initial donor who underwent so many cycles of egg donation, it was through her friendship circle that American egg donation in Lebanon blossomed. The donor convinced some of her skeptical girlfriends that Lebanon was now a safe country. And because these young, working-class women desperately needed money, they agreed to check out the clinic's Web site. There, they discovered that an egg donor in Michigan is reimbursed $2,000 per cycle for egg harvesting—one of the lowest rates of reimbursement in the country.[8] But, by agreeing to travel to Lebanon, they could make an additional $500 to $1,000 per cycle, plus receive an expense-paid vacation in a foreign land. Few of these young women had ventured beyond the state of Michigan, with the farthest journeys being taken across the borders to Canada and Mexico.

In Michigan's crumbling economy, foreign egg donation thus represented a financial opportunity for young, working-class American women. All were white, and two of them were working their way through community colleges. Eyad's "dream girl," Becky, was a twenty-four-year-old bartender and four-time repeat donor, who was using the $12,000 she had made so far to, as she put it, "pay for my past mistakes" in the form of significant credit card debt. Having been kicked out of the house by her divorced mother, she had lived on her own since her late teens, making only $450 a week as a bartending waitress. Becky was blunt about needing the extra income egg donation could provide. When I asked her if she was receiving "several thousand" to donate her eggs in Lebanon, she explained to me,

> Well, not *several*, but $3,000. If we only stayed in Michigan, it would be $2,000. But if we agreed to travel, it would be $3,000. Other states pay more, for example, $5,000 in Indiana and California. I don't know why, except that California has a higher cost of living. But even $3,000 is something, and I figure that if someone is willing to pay that much money for someone's eggs, then they must really want a child, and they'll be good parents.

At that point, I mentioned that they would be helping many couples who would love to have children. Becky responded, rather wistfully, "The families seem closer here. . . . I wish it was more like that in the States." When I joked that the resulting babies would be "half-American," Becky replied, "Yeah, we were surprised they'd want Americans." Becky herself had blue eyes and brown hair with bleached blonde highlights. She was overweight, though not obese, showing off her voluptuous figure in khaki shorts, a short-sleeved top, fashionable sunglasses, and sandals. Having been to Beirut four times, she volunteered that the Lebanese seemed concerned about their weight; thus, she was surprised that they would want "a donor like me, as I do *not* have a skinny body—never did, never will!" Nonetheless, she had noticed that Lebanese men, both on the street and in the clinic, stared at her. I described to Becky the traditional Middle Eastern male preference for "full-figured" women, which seemed to please her. Eyad was one such man. As he had told me, he considered Becky's being "fat a little" to be very beautiful and arresting.

Jill, whom I would meet on Becky's second trip to Beirut that summer, had been described by the physicians as "Middle Eastern" in appearance, because of her dark hair and olive skin. However, Jill was also nearly six feet tall, which would be rare for a Middle Eastern woman. Similar to Becky, Jill was twenty-three years old and the child of divorced parents. She had lived most of her life with her father, a construction worker who had been unemployed throughout much of the 1980s. "We were poor," Jill told me, "but not all the time, just for a while." During this period, she made extra money on a paper route, taking her first salaried job at age fourteen. She had been working as a personal trainer at a woman's gym in order to pay for college on a "semester by semester" basis. Jill's hope was to become a mortician—not the dream of every young Midwestern woman, but a way to bring some financial stability into her life.

Still living at home with her father, whom she called to reassure that she had arrived safely, Jill mentioned her thirty-one-year-old musician boyfriend, whom she described as "very talented with anything that involves strings." When I asked what he thought about her coming to Lebanon for egg donation, Jill said matter-of-factly, "It's not his decision. I don't let him dictate any aspect of my life." He, too, was underemployed and rarely had any money. Although Jill described him as "so kind, generous, and very loving," she admitted that he would probably never have enough money to support a family, which was one of the reasons she believed she would never have her own children. Selling her eggs, therefore, made sense to Jill. She could give her eggs to infertile women who needed them, while at the same time making money to go to college. Although Jill described her fear of flying as significantly worse than her fear of the "political stuff in the Middle East," she nonetheless took the sixteen-hour flight from Detroit to Beirut in order to anonymously donate fifty fertile eggs to infertile Middle Eastern couples.

"Anonymity," in this case, deserves some further explication. Unlike in the United States, where basic egg donor information and usually photographs are shown to recipient couples, such practices are not common in Lebanon. As mentioned in the last chapter, there is no Lebanese donor registry of any sort, and so infertile recipients have little if any information about physical features or the health of donor women. In this particular clinic, all egg donors were screened for hepatitis, HIV, and syphilis. However, the results of these tests were not conveyed to recipient couples. They were told only that the donors hailed from America. Neither background information nor photographs were provided.

This does not mean, however, that total anonymity prevailed. Because of the clinic's relatively cramped quarters and narrow entryway leading directly into the waiting area and front desk, the American donors ended up passing by a waiting room filled with "recipients." A passage from my field notes captures the somewhat surreal clinic scene on "American donor day" in Lebanon:

> I went downstairs [after an interview], and it is all of a sudden *packed* with people—standing room only. I just asked [a clinic staff member] what had happened, and he said, "Most of these people are recipients."

Apparently, they have all been called in this afternoon, so that the husbands can provide their sperm. Many of the women look old, and the men haggard. Most are veiled Muslims. I only see one young couple with a very pretty wife; I notice they are linking arms as they wait. The place is "hopping." The waiting room is full, the corridors have many men, husbands, most of them smoking, and the upstairs hallway is also full of people. It is so crowded and somewhat chaotic. Very interesting—the arrival of the American egg donors, and the clinic is abuzz!

Shia Muslim Marital Imaginaries

So, who were these mostly older, weather-beaten Muslim men who were embarking on egg donation with their middle-aged, veiled wives? Through my study, I came to realize that these were mostly working-class, Shia Muslim men from southern Lebanon and Beirut's southern suburbs, who had decided to move forward with egg donation because it was religiously allowed by Ayatollah Khamene'i and then by Lebanon's Sayyid Fadlallah. However, as suggested by the presence of the young, arm-in-arm couple in the preceding vignette, not all of those receiving donor eggs in Lebanon are Shia Muslims.

In general, how men reacted to egg donation was, to a large extent, shaped by their religious affiliation in this multisectarian setting. Overall, Lebanese clinics practicing egg donation report low rates of patient acceptance—much less than the 20 percent of all IVF cycles undertaken in the United States—because many infertile couples are simply reluctant to try IVF of ICSI with another woman's eggs. For example, in the major Shia-serving clinic in my study, the clinical director estimated that only two of the fifty IVF cycles undertaken each month, or 4 percent, involved egg donation. Rates of sperm donation were significantly lower, and surrogacy was truly rare, having occurred only twice in the history of this clinic.[9] Embryo donation—quite common in Iran, because of its sanction by law—was not practiced at all in Lebanon, with most couples hoping to use their embryos in future "frozen cycles." As the clinic director explained, third-party reproductive assistance in general was not widespread,

> Sperm donation, in our clinic, occurs once in a blue moon, and only when the husband accepts. But men don't like it. It *does* happen, but *very* infrequently, maybe once every three to four months. Egg donation occurs about two times a month. But it's very hard for women to agree to be recipients. It takes forever for them to be convinced. They will not willingly do it without asking questions.

However, this physician explained why he himself believed in the importance and permissibility of egg donation,

When I first started [IVF] in Lebanon, there was a couple sitting in my office. The wife's ovaries were failing and they wanted my help, but I could not help them [without donor eggs]. Two months later, he returned to my office. He had married another woman. If told that they had another option, this might not have happened.

He continued,

And what's wrong with it [egg donation]? The reason *to* allow it is this: in Islam, a man can marry so many wives. But rather than marry another, he can get eggs and stay with one. This is "to save marriage." I've read the *fatwa* [from Khamene'i], and that's what they say. In the U.S., about 20 percent of cases use egg donors. If it is allowed in the U.S., why is it not okay here?

Even if egg donation is viewed as a last resort in Lebanon, it is important to point to its growing acceptance. By the time of my study, some of the Shia Muslim couples I interviewed were beginning to receive donor eggs, as well as donating their eggs to other infertile couples in IVF clinics. When I asked Shia Muslim men themselves about their attitudes toward egg donation, they were the least likely of all the men in my study to oppose this practice. Whereas 83 percent of Sunni Muslim men in my study opposed all forms of gamete donation, just 64 percent of the Shia Muslim men did. The other 36 percent of Shia men agreed with the idea of egg donation, and some had already tried this with their wives. Among these men, egg donation was clearly seen as less *haram* than sperm donation, because it did not affect a child's *nasab*, or patrilineal genealogy, in the same way as using donor sperm. Furthermore, the introduction of donor technologies was clearly viewed as a "marriage savior," helping to avoid the possibility of divorce over infertility. These men clearly valued their marriages and often spoke lovingly of their aging wives. Their main desire was to have children by them. As one Shia airport mechanic, whose wife was two months pregnant following a donor egg cycle, explained to me,

She's pregnant now, with an egg from another female, but sperm from me. I don't know from whom the egg came. Dr. [name] is doing the treatment, and offered us the donor eggs. I accepted the fact because of my wife—because she's loving and she wants a baby. She wanted to take the eggs from outside; she accepted this. And they told me it's okay in Shia Islam. But, for me, it's not because of the religion that I accept this. I accept the fact that the sperm is *from me*, so it's okay. I asked, and they told me it is okay, according to the religion. But I accept it not because of the religion, but because of my wife.

To understand why this Shia Muslim man views egg donation as being for his wife, it is important to reiterate what can happen to an infertile marriage in the absence of egg donation. Both IVF and ICSI require healthy, fertile eggs in order to be successful. However, egg quality begins to decline by age thirty-five, and then precipitously after age forty.[10] A middle-aged woman, who may have been fertile earlier in her life, may no longer be able to produce viable oocytes for the IVF or ICSI procedures. When a man is informed that his wife's age may be a major limiting factor to success, one option is for him to divorce her and then remarry a younger, potentially more fertile woman, as suggested by the Shia Muslim clinic director. In my earlier study in Egypt, undertaken shortly after the emergence of ICSI, such cases were beginning to occur.[11] Because Sunni Islam does not allow egg donation, once-fertile Egyptian women, who had "stood by" their infertile husbands for years, even decades in some cases, were at risk of being divorced by their husbands. Had egg donation been an option in Egypt, such marriages would likely have been preserved.

By contrast, in Lebanon, Shia Muslim men's growing acceptance of egg donation has brought with it the possibility of new marital imaginaries still unthinkable in the "anti-donation" Sunni Muslim countries of the Middle East. Egg donation is now saving marriages among older Shia Muslim couples in Lebanon, allowing them to stay together out of love and still create a happy family. For older Shia Muslim women, egg donation has truly emerged as a kind of salvation, allowing them to bear children from their bodies, using the sperm of the husbands they love.

SUNNI MUSLIM MEN AS MORAL PIONEERS

Clearly, such new marital scenarios speak to the importance of understanding the local cultural context, particularly the local moral worlds in which new reproductive technologies such as egg donation are being rapidly deployed. In Lebanon, Shia Muslim couples have not been the only beneficiaries of egg donation. The emergence of egg donation seems to be giving infertile couples of *all* religious backgrounds new hope that their infertility problems can be overcome. Some Sunni Muslim men such as Eyad—as well as Druze and Christian men of all sects—are also quietly "saving their marriages" through the use of donor eggs, thereby secretly going against the dictates of Sunni Muslim and Christian orthodoxy. This transformative possibility of egg donation as a Middle Eastern marriage savior was probably never imagined when this technology first arrived in the Middle East at the beginning of the new millennium.

In my own study, a small number of Sunni Muslim men stood out as "moral pioneers"—a term I borrow from medical anthropologist Rayna

Rapp to signal the personal challenges to religious orthodoxies that arise in the face of new reproductive technologies.[12] These pioneering men clearly "broke the mold" and decided to "go against the religion" in order to achieve fatherhood and happiness in their marriages. Of the seventy Sunni Muslim men in my study, four men had already accepted donor eggs, four other men were considering this option, and most of these men were also considering legal adoption of a child, if the egg donation did not succeed in producing offspring. In addition, one Sunni Muslim man was considering surrogacy to overcome his wife's bicornate (divided) uterus. In almost every case, there were unique features of these men's personal histories that might have made them less compliant with the prevailing religious norms. For example, several men had spent considerable time outside of the country, including in the United States, where two men were currently residing. Two were educated Palestinian men, who were aware of the plight of orphans and children in refugee camps. One man, born Sunni Muslim, now considered himself "nonpracticing" and said that he had deep respect for the "good" in all religions.

An abiding theme of the interviews with these non-conforming men was the deep love and respect they felt for their wives. Most of these men said that they would undertake egg donation or adoption "out of love" or "for her." Several had been the first to offer these possibilities to their wives, even though some of their wives did not accept these options at the outset. Each man revealed a personal story of marriage and love that was often quite touching. Excerpts from three of these interviews will help to capture such sentiments. These excerpts also reveal the complex moral decision making undertaken by men who have decided, usually on their own, to defy the Sunni ban on all forms of gamete donation.

RAFIQ: A Lebanese man who had lived for several years in the United States but had recently married a woman living in Lebanon, Rafiq had decided to use an egg donor to overcome his wife's premature ovarian failure. Rafiq described their situation as follows,

The doctor told me, "There is no way you can get her pregnant, because her FSH [follicle-stimulating hormone] level is 50 and an FSH level at 27 is considered impossible. Her ovary does not respond." [The doctor] said, "There is nothing we can do to get her pregnant except with an egg donor." But we said, "No." Actually, I said "no" at the beginning. Basically, I said, "Thank you." But then I started to think . . . and I started searching the net, asking for advice. I started asking from the religious point of view, if doing it was right or wrong. I called everybody here in Lebanon, and I asked a *shaykh*. Actually, no one gave me the right answer. So I sent her to talk with the doctor, and because he is a Muslim, it made my wife feel better.

By that point, I was going to do it anyway, but she's the religious one. It didn't bother me, but it bothered her. None of the explanations from the religious point of view made sense to me. But I needed to support my wife and make a family with her—to make it easier for her—even though no one yet has made it easier for me.

At this point, I have no problem with it [egg donation], other than that she get pregnant. We went through lots of discussion and research. To me, over here [in Lebanon], the culture still has not accepted [egg donation]. There's no social discussion over here yet. I told my colleagues in the U.S., and they didn't have a problem with it. Everybody wished me luck. Everybody over here thinks I'm "playing God" by using eggs. I'm not God, I'm just using God.

I had to search on my own, and I didn't find any *clear* indication about why this would be wrong. Islamic legislators are still behind in serving the Muslim community according to new scientific findings. According to me, as a Muslim, they are behind in science. Religion is a common sense thing. I use my common sense, because all of the [Islamic] legislators are behind the times. So I had to make my own assessment. My relationship with God is personal. I take care of what I can, and if not, fine with me! All the *shaykh*s haven't faced this situation, but I have. So I follow my own religion, which is being a good person and doing the best you can.

KHALED: A Bahraini man who worked in an Arab Gulf oil refinery, Khaled traveled to Lebanon with his infertile wife in order to undertake IVF with donor eggs. He had also encouraged her to consider adopting an orphan, but, to date, she had refused. Khaled's acceptance of both egg donation and adoption was clearly out of sync with local moralities in Bahrain, as he explained to me,

[Egg donation] is not allowed, not in Islam. You know why? The mixing of blood, of inheritance, and everything. It's like *zina*, like sleeping with a woman you don't know. And afterward, for inheritance, you don't know your roots. It's like mixing families and tribes.

Orphans, however, you can take them and feel you have a family. You can raise [them] in the family. Islam is always encouraging this, but no one follows it. In Bahrain, there are *so* many conditions to adopt. You have to have a house, your salary has to be okay, and they come on sudden visits, to see how you treat the child. I told her I'd do this, but she doesn't want. She said, "I want something from my body." I said to her, "There are two benefits: one, you raise a poor orphan, and two, a girl will get you to heaven, because the *yatim* [orphans] have no relatives." I told her, "This is no problem for me." But she rejects the idea. She wears the *hijab* [veil], and if she takes a boy, she can't go without *hijab*—unless her sister or relative breastfeeds the baby and he becomes a family member.[13] And if it is a girl, when she gets older, I can't touch her.

My wife doesn't want to take an orphan, because they are illegitimate [children] and maybe they are bad. And there are too many conditions and very complicated rules. But this is my idea, and she rejects it.

MAZEN: A Palestinian man who had been born and raised in Beirut, Mazen had married late in life to a Palestinian woman also in her forties. Both were teachers for Palestinian children living in Lebanese refugee camps. They were trying IVF, but were unlikely to succeed because of the wife's advanced age. When I asked Mazen about egg donation and adoption, this is what he said to me,

I heard about egg donation, but I didn't think about it. Until now, I didn't consider it, but in the end, I think my wife is much more religious than I am so she wouldn't consider it. According to me, I am scientific more than religious. Depending upon the problem—if the source is from me or from her—for example, if the problem is from me, she would refuse [sperm donation], but if the problem is from her, maybe we would do [egg donation]. We don't have a clear position yet, because we didn't discuss it.

As for adoption, yes, why not? I thought about this. So even though you raise a kid who is not originally your kid, with time, he'll get used to you and you to him, and he will be like your kid. But she's not supporting this idea. She prefers to have her own kid. But I think, in the long run, if I had to adopt, eventually we would get used to it and we would treat the child as our own. She would feel the motherly affection, and I think it's a good idea, a humanitarian act. A human being is a human being. And I love children—*any* child. I can, I think, feel pleasure to have any child. Sometimes I feel myself a father of any child. I can play with him, talk with him; most of the children love me.

From the beginning of marriage, I made it clear to my wife—before marriage—that we could adopt a child, because we married at an older age, and this shouldn't affect our marriage or our life. I think in the long run, my wife will ultimately be affected if we don't find a solution, because, by nature, the wife is much more emotional than the husband. I mean, it's affecting her personhood. She feels inferiority, that something's lacking, and she feels down, depressed. Despite the fact that I *told* her that having our own children doesn't matter, I'm sure, ultimately, that it will affect her. Two times when the operation [IVF] failed, she felt depressed and cried. I tried to ease her pain and tell her that it doesn't succeed from the first operation. We're both old, and because of our age, our chances are less. So now, we're both trying to sort it out.

Indeed, all of these Sunni Muslim men were in the process of "sorting out" their feelings and intellectual responses to egg donation and adoption, given their awareness that neither option is accepted in the Sunni Islamic religion. Some men tried to distance themselves from religious orthodoxy; they explained that they valued science over religion, found Sunni authorities to be scientifically outdated, and thus were forced to form their own moral responses to new biotechnological developments in assisted conception. Furthermore, all of these men considered themselves less religious than their more pious wives, who, despite their husbands' willingness, sometimes refused to go forward with alternatives, especially adoption. All the men professed great concern for their wives' feelings, including their feelings of lost personhood and suffering. They also valued their wives' strong desires to experience the feelings of pregnancy and become mothers. When they realized that their wives' chances of becoming biological mothers with their own eggs were slim (often because of advancing age), they offered either adoption or egg donation as acceptable solutions.

It is important to reiterate features of these men's biographies that might have led them to nonconforming moral stances. These men were mostly educated professionals, who had spent considerable time outside of the country. Furthermore, reflecting the disruptions of the civil war and a postwar trend of delayed marriage,[14] these men had married late in life to women they knew were reproductively "elderly." In the case of the Palestinian-Lebanese men, their own experiences of exile and discrimination made them perhaps more open to the possibility of alternative family formation. As one of them put it in a way that was uncharacteristic of most men in my study, "I feel myself the father of any child."

In summary, all of these men were in the process of reconsidering the religiously guided rules of family formation that have been authorized within Sunni Islam and to which most Sunni Muslims strictly adhere.[15] That other Sunni Muslim men might be renegotiating religious norms was apparent in the Beirut IVF clinics in which I worked. There, I saw Sunni Muslim couples from a variety of economic classes, social backgrounds, and Middle Eastern nations. These included some young couples, who were clearly in love with each other despite the wives' premature ovarian failure. They were secretively signing up for donor eggs, thereby "going against" the mandates of Sunni religious orthodoxy.

CHRISTIANS AMID MUSLIM MORAL WORLDS

These Sunni Muslim men were not alone in taking pioneering moral stances. In my study, more than one-quarter of the men (26%) were Christians, including 17 percent who were either Maronite or Roman Catholic. As noted earlier, the Catholic Church bans all forms of reproductive technology (including contraception and abortion), even though IVF is practiced widely in the Catholic countries of Europe and Latin America.[16] With regard to assisted conception, the Catholic Church disapproves of IVF because it disassociates procreation from sex, both of which are intended to occur only within the holy covenant of matrimony. According to the Catholic doctrine of "natural law," no artificial barriers or aids to conception are to be used during the procreative act. Replacing loving intercourse with the masturbation and surgical procedures required in IVF will necessarily erode marital unity.[17] A life that is created by medical practitioners—rather than through an act of conjugal love between two married people—"establishes the domination of technology over the origin and destiny of the human person."[18] The technology of IVF, therefore, threatens the unity of marriage; IVF physicians themselves become "third parties" to a marriage, intruding into the marital functions of sex and procreation. Similarly, all forms of third-party donation—of eggs, sperm, embryos, or uteruses, as in surrogacy—are seen as "offenses" to the conjugal unity of the couple, introducing an "emotional and spiritual wedge between husband and wife both symbolized by and enacted in sexual infidelity."[19] In this regard, the association of infidelity with third-party donation is similar to one of the moral justifications undergirding the Sunni ban on this practice.

In addition, the Catholic Church considers life to begin at the moment of conception; hence, all human embryos created through assisted reproduction are considered to be sacrosanct. As a form of human life, embryos must never be forsaken. Yet, according to the church, the processes of assisted reproduction "destroy" embryos—and hence, human life—in multiple ways. For one, multiple embryos are often transferred to a woman's uterus in a single IVF cycle, without all of the embryos implanting. The high failure rates following embryo transfer are considered to be a loss of potential human life, to which the Catholic Church objects.[20] Furthermore, the Catholic Church is concerned with the overproduction of embryos in assisted reproduction, leading to problems of "embryo disposition."[21] Excess or unused embryos that are produced through ART may be cryopreserved (i.e., frozen), but their "quality," clinically speaking, declines considerably during long-term storage. After five years of cryopreservation, some IVF clinics routinely dispose of all excess embryos from cold storage. Furthermore, some unused embryos—especially those of poor clinical quality (and, hence, less likely to implant)—are routinely disposed of in IVF laboratories, while others are destined for human research. The Catholic Church's view is that the destruction of *any* embryo is inherently wrong; such a view underlies the church's ban on embryonic stem cell research as well.

This view of the embryo as a human life from the moment of conception is not shared by any of the schools of Islamic jurisprudence. Embryo disposition is a problem in Islam only if an embryo is donated to a third party. Embryo disposal and even multifetal pregnancy reduction (i.e., a form of selective abortion) are allowed by the Sunni Islamic authorities, particularly if the prospect of carrying the pregnancy to viability is markedly reduced or the health of the mother is in serious jeopardy.[22] Embryo research is similarly allowed, if the latter occurs within fourteen days of initial fertilization. This consensus on embryo research—and hence stem cell research—was reached at a conference on the "Dilemma of Stem Cell Research" held in Cairo in November 2007.[23]

In short, in Islam, the human embryo simply is not sacrosanct as it is in Catholicism. As a result, Islam has been significantly more permissive than Catholicism in allowing assisted reproduction, including various procedures that involve manipulation, removal, and disposal of the embryo and fetus (e.g., cryopreservation, preimplantation genetic diagnosis, fetal reduction).[24] Because these forms of embryo and fetal demise do occur in assisted reproduction, Catholics who follow the teachings of the Vatican closely cannot participate in assisted reproduction of any kind. Not surprisingly, the Vatican officially criticized the awarding of the 2010 Nobel Prize to Robert Edwards for his invention of IVF.[25]

In Lebanon, with its significant percentage of Catholics, assisted reproduction has its Christian detractors, including many priests, who condemn the practices of IVF, ICSI, and third-party gamete donation, but especially multifetal pregnancy reduction and embryo disposition (i.e., donation or disposal). However, one-half of the IVF physicians I worked with in Lebanon were Catholics, and nearly one-fifth of the men I interviewed in IVF clinics were Catholic as well. Despite the Catholic Church's condemnation of all forms of assisted reproduction, Catholics in Lebanon are using these technologies, including gamete donation. In fact, some of the Catholic men in my study condemned the Catholic Church for its condemnation! One Catholic man described his evolving attitude toward IVF and the church in this way,

> In terms of the religion, it is not bothering me, but it *is* bothering me in a way. Before getting married, they told us that these kinds of things shouldn't happen, anything not "natural," but specifically IVF. We undergo premarital counseling as Catholics. So at the beginning,

yes, I *was* uncomfortable. But, at the end, it was just logical thinking at the end. It's either that way [without IVF] or that way [with IVF]. We have to choose, and we will not be the first or the last to choose IVF.

He continued,

Actually, the religion needs to think logically as well. We have the religion, but if you're desperate, you have to take all measures in a logical way. The Catholic Church is *not* with these kind of things, but how many people have done it? If I'd asked a priest, he was going to say, "No, this is totally immoral." But, in the end, you come to the age of forty, and your wife is also forty, so what is it going to be? No family? You do what you have to do, and in the end, if God wants, it will happen, and if not, it won't happen. These days, medicine has evolved, and is it feasible for the Catholic Church to say to people not to have an IVF and then to get the couple divorced?

Another Catholic IVF patient put it more succinctly, "Science is advancing faster than the priests!"

Just as with some of the Sunni Muslim men in my study, four of the Catholic men I interviewed (two Maronite Catholic, two Roman Catholic) told me that they supported the practice of egg donation, even though it is prohibited by Catholicism. In addition, seven Christian men in my study (mostly Catholic, but also Greek and Armenian Orthodox) were also considering adoption as an alternative route to parenthood. This latter number is actually small, given that most Middle Eastern Christian denominations run their own orphanages and encourage Christian couples to adopt. Nonetheless, it reflects the social taboos on adoption described in the preceding chapter. Furthermore, many of the children put up for adoption in Lebanese Christian orphanages are of "mixed" heritage, usually the illegitimate offspring of housemaids who are from Ethiopia, the Philippines, Sri Lanka, and other resource-poor countries. One Catholic man, who lost his "lovely" ICSI son one week after birth (as a result of a birth injury and probable malpractice), had this to say about adoption,

This is our fifth or sixth IVF. The first one went very well; she got pregnant, then we lost our baby. Then we did IVF three to four times with no success. Our psychological state is bad following the death of our child. My wife's psychological state is *very* bad. But this is the last time we'll do IVF, and my wife is saying this, too. And if there is no success, we'll adopt a black boy. That's what I'd like to do. [Really?] It's not easy to be black in Lebanon, but that's what I want, because if I want to do something good, I have to do it for the person who needs it most. Nobody here will adopt a black boy. So, if I'm going to do something good, I will do it for someone good.

Then he added,

I'd like to be a father. When I see a man who is walking with his wife and child in the street, I'd like to be holding a baby, too. I'd like to be a *good* father.

Like the Sunni Muslim moral pioneers in my study, this Christian man saw adopting a black child as a way to do something good and to be a good father to a child in need. I met several of these Christian moral pioneers during my time in Lebanon. Another man, for example, had found an abandoned newborn in a Muslim section of Tripoli, a Northern Sunni-dominant Lebanese city. He had made every effort to adopt the male child but was prevented from doing so by the Lebanese police, who turned the infant over to a Muslim orphanage.

Other Christian men saw egg donation as the most viable way to build their families. They were all married to infertile women but pointed out that their marriages were "for life." The vows of marriage among Christian Middle Eastern couples are considered sacrosanct; divorce is not an option, and annulments can be obtained only with great difficulty. In this regard, pursuing egg donation was not about saving marriage, as it was for Shia and Sunni Muslim couples. Rather, positive attitudes toward egg donation among Christian men were generally couched in terms of lifelong love and respect for an infertile wife. The experiences of three Catholic men are revealing in this regard.

JOHNNY: A Lebanese Maronite Catholic man, Johnny was facing problems of both male and female infertility and had decided to consider all forms of gamete donation, as well as adoption. He knew that IVF—along with gamete donation—was not allowed by the Catholic Church. But he had this to say about the subject,

In the Maronite Church, the priests, they don't like this work [IVF]. But like us, if I ask the priest, "What can we do? I want a baby. Give me the solution," then I think it *is* our solution. I never asked a priest about this problem. But we don't have a problem with doing this, even if I ask a priest. If you see this is your solution, then it's okay. I know that Christians take donors in Europe and America. I know everything about the Christians there, and they even take donor sperm, which I would do, but wouldn't tell anyone.

And adoption, yes, we don't have a problem with it. Maybe we will do this. But if someone can give me a baby with my own sperm [through ICSI], it's perfect. And if I don't, then I would adopt. I would do it for her, and she would accept.

If you ask me about our problem—if this [infertility] is a problem—I would say we have no problems. If I married another time, I'd take my wife. She's my baby.

ROLAND: A Lebanese Roman Catholic man, Roland had undertaken multiple failed IVF cycles with his pretty wife, with whom he had been married for fifteen years. He emphasized how much he loved her, and how little he cared about the religious rulings on IVF and egg donation,

I have no religious concerns. I really don't put myself into all the trouble of that. I'm a Catholic. I'm a Christian, but I don't go into all the details of what the Church has to say. When you're desperate for a child, you don't go for the details.

I'm not intending to kill a human being, an embryo. But it's part of the process. If embryos are going to be lost during IVF, they can also be lost during a natural pregnancy. The Church calls this "killing," yes?

It took a little time for us, from my part, I don't know. But you have to be realistic—not emotional, not religious—if you want to go for this subject. Dr. [name], three or four years ago, he mentioned egg donation, and my wife told him, "No, no, no. Don't mention it!" But now, with time, we've come to accept the idea.

MOUSSA: A Syrian Roman Catholic man, Moussa had come to Lebanon seeking donor eggs for his wife's premature ovarian failure. Moussa emphasized that having children was "not important for him." His pursuit of cross-border egg donation in Lebanon was "just to satisfy my wife." Interestingly, Moussa and his wife were accompanied by their Syrian Catholic gynecologist, who was now regularly bringing his infertile couples to Lebanon in order to seek donor gametes. Moussa had a great deal to say about this reproductive tourism from Syria to Lebanon,

IVF is allowed in Syria, if the sperm and eggs are from husband and wife. That's why we came to Lebanon. In Syria, there is no sperm donation or egg donation. There are only two IVF centers, and our government is an Islamic government. What's not allowed in the Islamic religion is not allowed in our country, because the government is an Islamic government.

But we Christians, we don't care about [gamete] donation. We consider it normal. This is not the religious point of view, but it is some point of view. I have a friend, and he has the problem [of infertility]. He's ready, okay, with taking sperm donation. He's Christian, and he's the only son, and he's very rich.

The important thing is raising your children. It doesn't matter if you have sperm or eggs from outside. It's how you raise your kids. I'm also not against adopting. I'm ready to adopt, but since we found this way, she will have the embryo in her body, and we thought it would be better.

We don't know where the egg comes from, but I insisted on two things. First, she shouldn't be from Africa; she should be white. And second, she should be free from AIDS and hepatitis. I insisted that they [the clinic] should do hepatitis and AIDS tests, her features should be white and a little close to my wife—a little Arab looking.

As for the number of children, I'd like two children, and if she gets pregnant with more, we'll have to do a fetal reduction. My generation prefers one or two, not three, because the economic situation is not so good. And I'd prefer girls. The girl is better than the boy. She takes care of her parents more than the boy.

Moussa's response is demonstrative of many aspects of emergent masculinities in the Middle East today. Moussa is a willing reproductive tourist, who defies the Syrian government's Islamically inspired ban on gamete donation by traveling with his wife and physician to Lebanon. He chooses to ignore his own church's anti-egg donation stance, pointing also to a wealthy Christian friend who is accepting sperm donation to become a father. Moussa also defies his church's antiabortion position; he agrees in principle to multifetal pregnancy reduction, in case his wife becomes pregnant with triplets or more. Furthermore, Moussa argues that fatherhood is not about biological connection but rather how well a man raises his children. Moussa's only desire for his donor offspring is that they be "white" and a little "Arab looking" like his wife. Because he is doing donor egg "for her," he is concerned about his wife bearing a resemblance to the children, and he also wants to keep her free from life-threatening infectious diseases. Finally and most notably, he wants only one or two children, ideally girls. Moussa points to girls' superior caretaking of their parents in old age. Moussa is not alone in these convictions. Table 15 shows the wide range of men in my study who went through egg donation, their reasons for doing so, and their emerging preferences for small families with daughters.

Fathers, Daughters, and Child Desire

As seen in table 15, most men using egg donors wanted a small number of children. Furthermore, they told the (female) anthropologist that the sex of the child did not matter to them. A few of these men stated a clear gender preference for female offspring. A similar pattern of child desire—

two or three children of either sex[26]—was widespread among the men in my study. Of the 220 men interviewed, I asked 136 of them what they were hoping for in terms of family size and gender of offspring. The vast majority of these men (93%) replied that they wanted families of one to four children, with the ideal being two or three. Few men wanted to have a"lonely" only child; thus, several of the men in my study were undertaking repeated ICSIs in an attempt to provide existing children with siblings. Furthermore, most men were clear in wanting children of both sexes, with two boys and one girl being commonly stated as the "perfect" or "ideal" family by some Lebanese men.

Men clearly had reasons for wanting sons, mostly having to do with patrilineal continuity and the perpetuation of the family name. The few men who told me that they wanted only sons justified their desire by citing the "responsibility" and "worry" they would feel if they were to have daughters in a society which they saw as still being oppressive to women. For example, an educated Sunni Muslim family court judge told me,"I love girls a lot, but not for them to be my own."When I asked him why, he said that he had seen too many difficult gender cases in his work as a judge."In traditional village society, they tell the woman,'God willing, may you bring a boy!'This, by itself, creates pressure on her. So if we have a chance to have kids, I want a boy. It's not that I don't like girls, but it's for their sake. Just in case she is not lucky in her life, because the female is weak in Arab society, and maybe she has no rights."

Despite this judge's pessimistic view of gender relations, many other men in my study were more hopeful. In fact, if there was an emerging gender preference in my study, it was for daughters. Bearing in mind that men were talking to a female anthropologist, it was nonetheless notable that many men provided detailed explanations of why they loved girl children more than boys. Such men repeatedly cited girls' superior compassion and affection, including the love they give in return to their parents (table 16). Although sons continue to be valorized over daughters on a societal level, many men are now investing in their own daughters as much as—or even more so—than in their sons. Furthermore, they can articulate strong feelings of emotional connection to their female offspring. In short, as other Middle Eastern scholars have suggested,[27] so-called"son preference" may be fading away over time, thereby representing another dimension of emergent masculinities in the region.

In general, when men spoke to me about their fatherhood desires, they couched their fatherhood dreams in the language of *hubb*, or love. Just as most Middle Eastern men love their wives, they also profess a deep love for children—of knowing that they always wanted to have children, of loving to play with their nieces and nephews as the"kind uncle," of experiencing great joy in the presence of youngsters. In fact, men's stated child desires

TABLE 15. Men whose wives received donor eggs

Nationality	Religion	Infertility Status	Need for Donor Eggs	Desired Outcome
Lebanese	Shia Muslim	Fertile	Wife is 43 and has two uteruses; used donor egg and produced triplets in one uterus; multifetal pregnancy reduction to twins was performed.	"I will be satisfied with only one girl. I like the girls. I love the babies. The best number is four; it is a complete family with four children, some boys, and some girls."
Lebanese	Shia Muslim	Fertile	Wife is 44 and used donor eggs; she is pregnant with a singleton.	He was married to his cousin for 29 years and has seven daughters and one son. They divorced because of intractable marriage problems. He married his second wife "for love" when she was 42. He would like one more son, and is doing IVF "for her."
Syrian reproductive tourist	Roman Catholic	Fertile	Wife is 40 and has been in premature ovarian failure since her early 30s.	They are cousins, married for twelve years. They want one or two children, and will undergo multifetal pregnancy reduction if necessary. "I'd prefer girls. The girl is better than the boy. She takes care of her parents more than the boy."
Palestinian reproductive tourist	Sunni Muslim	Fertile	His second wife is 44 and is using American donor eggs.	They are cousins and childhood sweethearts, prevented from marrying because of the war. He has two daughters and one son with his first wife. He is doing IVF "for her," and would like two or three children, but "one is enough, praise God!"
Lebanese, living in USA, reproductive tourist	Sunni Muslim	Both infertile	Wife is 40 and is using donor eggs.	He was married to an American woman. His new wife is Lebanese. He is trying "to support my wife, to make it easier for her." He wants only one child, "as a project, to keep me occupied for the next twenty years, to raise it, for the joy of being a parent."

Table 15. Men whose wives received donor eggs *(continued)*

Nationality	Religion	Infertility Status	Need for Donor Eggs	Desired Outcome
Lebanese, living in Kuwait, reproductive tourist	Sunni Muslim	Both infertile	Wife is 42 and has done ooplasm transfer from a donor "to enrich the egg." Considering a donor egg cycle now. "Why not? There's no other solution. It is like eyes or a heart or a kidney transplant."	They are second cousins married 22 years. He would like one or two children. "If I get one, I will stop! A girl or a boy."
Lebanese	Druze	Both infertile	Wife is 42; did one unsuccessful anonymous donor cycle; she is currently on her twelfth ICSI using her 30-year-old married sister's eggs. She asked permission from her sister's husband, and he agreed. Her sister donated "out of love."	He is 62 and delayed marriage because of the war (he lost ten relatives and attempted suicide). This is their last trial, because they have run out of money. He wants only one or two donor children. "Anything, whether a boy or a girl, it doesn't matter."
Lebanese	Greek Orthodox	Fertile	Wife is 36 and is in premature ovarian failure; currently attempting IVF with American donor eggs.	"We're trying everything possible; we'll do anything possible." He wants "just one at first, if God gives. Then maybe two or three. The gender doesn't matter."
Syrian reproductive tourist	Sunni Muslim	Fertile	Wife is 36 and is in premature ovarian failure; did "egg sharing" with a poor infertile couple who needed money; bore premature donor twins, male and female, who died in a Syrian hospital.	He would consider another cycle of egg donation "for her," but his wife is reluctant. He would like more than one child "to look like her."
Syrian reproductive tourist	Armenian Orthodox	Fertile	Wife is 45 and is pregnant with triplets from a 22-year-old "designated" unmarried, Shia Muslim donor, her friend.	"I want six! I love children! Either sex is okay, it's what God wants."

were rarely instrumental; men did not want children to work for them, to take over a family business, to care for them in their old age, or to receive their inheritance when they passed away. Although these reasons were occasionally cited, they were not common. Rather, men's major articulation

TABLE 16. Fathers and daughter preference

Nationality	Religion	Men's Comments
Lebanese, living in Panama and Brazil	Shia Muslim	"There's no difference; boys are like girls today. Girls have so much capacity, no? The President of Panama is a woman."
Lebanese	Sunni Muslim	"If I had my choice, if I could, I would have a girl as the eldest, then it doesn't matter after that. Girls are usually calmer, so then you have a calmer house. I have a friend with three boys; the house is moving around! My wife's sister has three boys; the house is moving from its place! If I had all girls, this would be no problem for me, really."
Lebanese	Maronite Catholic	"I don't care what I have, but I would like a girl, because the girl is good for the family, not the boy, and I'm not good for my family! The girl opens the door, the boy doesn't. Girls are affectionate! I love them so much. I love children so much."
Syrian	Alawi Muslim	"This mentality about carrying the [family] name is mostly among parents in Saudi Arabia. Even if I have all daughters, they are equal in importance to boys; they are given by God. Now they retrieved four eggs; imagine them being all girls! In my family, there are no girls, so when my wife goes to my parents, they cuddle her a lot because they don't have a daughter. I would like a daughter, but I'm not a fanatic about the sex of the child."
Lebanese, lived in Russia	Shia Muslim, but secular	"I want a girl now. I really want a girl. We go to all the shops for children. I pay for my [ICSI] son's clothes, but then I buy girls' clothes, too, and take them home and leave them, or give them as presents for our friends. Girls are so nice. Here, in my view, the girl helps the family more than the son. She helps her father and mother more than the son. In my mind, in my feeling, in my society, the girl loves the family more than the son. She loves her mother and father. The girl is more softhearted. Not that I don't like boys. Children are all the same; they all come from God. But the girl, if there's a choice, now I want a girl!"
Lebanese	Shia Muslim	"In my village, I'm known as one who loves children. For the children in my family, I buy clothes, and I spoil them. In truth, I'm a very nice uncle. I'd like to have a child, only one child, and I like girls more than boys. Maybe in Eastern culture, it will make a man feel like he's more of a man if he has more children. But, in my opinion, if there are too many children, it will have a bad effect on the child."
Lebanese	Maronite Catholic	"I want two children, a boy and a girl. A girl for me, and a boy for her. I like girls. If I want to have somebody open the door for me, it's the girl, not the boy."
Syrian	Roman Catholic	"I prefer girls, because they take care of their parents more than the boy."

Table 16 Fathers and daughter preference *(continued)*

Lebanese Armenian	Armenian Orthodox	"Two would be good, a boy and a girl. But if I have only one, I like the girl, I prefer a girl. The girls, it's not that they're more loving than boys. But if life was under the hands of girls, it would be better! This is why I like my wife so much! Women don't think to hurt people or life in general. They think of having a good life and family and this is something positive. If women are not good, there's a reason for it."
Lebanese	Maronite Catholic	"I want a child, and I like girls. I feel I want a girl. It's not like I'm dying for a child every time I see a girl. But, yes, I love girls; I prefer girls. If I make IVF, I want one girl and one boy. But me, I would like first to have a girl. I want her to be the oldest. In my family, I had an older sister, and our sister is like my mother. She's about 60 years old, and she's like my mother. Girls take care of their families. I see how she helps my mother even now. In general, I prefer a girl in the house, because she's more affectionate to her mother and father."
Lebanese	Sunni Muslim	"I'd take either boys or girls, but a daughter is better than a son. She's affectionate, and she's closer to her parents. I have a sister who has girls, and I love them better than my brother's sons. Every day, I'm surrounded by nieces and nephews, and I love my nieces more."
Lebanese	Maronite Catholic	"I prefer a girl. I love girls! And we've lived, me and my brothers, as all boys. There's a need for us to have girls now."
Lebanese	Maronite Catholic	"We would like to have twins—girls, not boys. She would like to dress them up. Boys just take jeans and t-shirts and go. If it will be girls, this will be better, because I see how the boys treat their parents, and I see how the girl treats them better."
Lebanese	Shia Muslim	"If God gives me a girl, I will keep her by my side and I won't let her marry!"

of child desire was entirely affective. Men told me how much they "loved," "adored," and "were crazy" about kids—the kind of responses I would never expect to hear from men in my own country.

In fact, I can only adequately express Middle Eastern men's love of children by referring to my own family's experiences. When my son, Carl, was fifteen months old, we took him to Egypt, where I conducted my first study of Middle Eastern assisted reproduction. My American, but Egyptian-looking, multiracial husband was simply amazed by Egyptian men's behavior toward our child. Almost without exception, men wanted to learn Carl's name, hold him in their arms, offer him sweets and other goodies, talk to him in Arabic, and occupy him completely during the times when

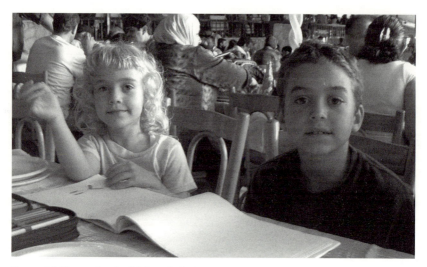

FIGURE 16. The author's children in Lebanon

we ate at family restaurants. In short, our little son Carl was a "major hit" in Egypt, and he has never been doted upon in such a way at any other time in his life.

Similarly, when our daughter Justine was four years old and was in a serious "princess phase," we took the family to Lebanon for my study of male infertility. With shining golden locks, a shy smile, and various forms of princess attire, Justine was a "magnet" for Lebanese men, who would often cross streets in the middle of deadly traffic just to elicit a smile from her, touch her pretty hair, and ask her for a "little kiss" on their cheeks (rarely reciprocated, I am afraid). Justine was our "golden girl" in Lebanon—so much so, in fact, that we worried that our son Carl, seven years old at the time, would become jealous because of all the male attention toward his sister (figure 16).

As I continue to travel back and forth between the United States and the Middle East, I am always struck by the "happy family feeling" of the airplanes, packed with men, women, and their children. Fathers carry their children up and down the aisles, change their diapers, help to feed them, kiss and caress them to sleep in the adjacent seats, and generally participate with their wives in the childcare. Each and every airplane flight only serves to reconvince me of Middle Eastern men's love for children. This is why having a child—even if by donor eggs—is such a poignant dream for most Middle Eastern men and their infertile wives.

Conclusion

This chapter on egg donation has captured many contemporary aspects of technological and masculine emergence in the Middle East. As we have seen, both Muslim and Christian men are taking pioneering moral stances regarding egg donation and adoption in order to satisfy their wives, whom they love and to whom they appear to be kind and loyal. Clearly, some Middle Eastern men today are choosing egg donation as a way to remain in long-term, loving marriages to their infertile wives, even if such dona- tion is not viewed within their religions as a morally acceptable route to parenthood. Nonetheless, in Lebanon, donor egg technologies are facili- tating conjugal commitments vis-à-vis hopes for technological and marital salvation.

As we have also seen in this chapter, some Muslim and Christian Middle Eastern men may be fairly secular, even nonreligious. Others may be religiously pious, but they, too, have made individual moral decisions about scientific technologies and practices that are not condoned by their religions. That Middle Eastern Muslim men may choose practices that, as they put it, "go against the religion" is rarely observed in Western discourse, which tends to impugn all Muslim men as religious fundamentalists and fanatics. As seen in this chapter, we need to know more—much more— about Muslim men, including their actual religious practices and think- ing, in order to interrogate the stereotypes that have served to vilify them. Similarly, the lives, experiences, and local moral worlds of Middle Eastern Christian men also need to be brought into our scholarship. The existence of minority Christian populations, who interact with fellow Muslims in Middle Eastern IVF clinics and beyond, is a reality that is equally obscure.

In Lebanon, physicians who are helping couples to conceive egg-donor babies are both Muslim and Christian. Together, these practitioners have responded to Shia *fatwas*, which have opened the door to egg donation in the country. The IVF physician community itself is invoking a variety of novel solutions to overcome egg-donor recipients' concerns about es- tablishing kinship in the absence of biological connection. As shown in Morgan Clarke's fascinating work,[28] physicians are encouraging patients to invoke traditional Islamic notions of legal guardianship and inheritance rights through gifts and bequests. Older mothers who bear egg-donor children are also encouraged to establish kinship connections through *rida'*, or "milk kinship," whereby a mother becomes "biologically" related to a child through the practice of breastfeeding.

However, not all Lebanese physicians have been as creative or sanguine about egg donation. In fact, the most politically powerful opponent of egg donation happens to be Shia Muslim IVF physician, who has repeatedly attempted to introduce legislation banning all forms of third-party reproductive assistance in the country. Despite significant support among Sunni political groups, the bill has never been passed, probably because of a combination of multisectarian resistance and postwar exhaustion and apathy.[29]

Furthermore, it is very important to reiterate that most cycles of IVF occurring in Lebanon today still do *not* involve egg donation. Sperm donation, embryo donation, and surrogacy are even rarer. Third-party reproductive assistance is widely acknowledged as an option of "last resort"—a kind of "necessary evil" or "act of desperation"—when all else fails. Today in Lebanon, the vast majority of Sunni IVF patients do not accept third-party reproductive assistance of any kind, and there are many Shia and Christian patients who do not as well. Egg donation, when undertaken, is usually hidden under conditions of doctor-patient confidentiality. In other words, men such as Eyad who accept egg donation for their wives are different from most, and can be seen as enacting a kind of religious dissent, or at least a form of resistance to the moral status quo.

Even if egg donation in the twenty-first-century Middle East remains uncommon, it is no longer unusual. It is now advertised on clinic Web sites and is known to exist by most infertile Middle Eastern couples. Egg donation is but one of many forms of technological emergence that are changing the moral and medical landscape of the Middle East. But, from a gender perspective, egg donation is a special technology, serving to save infertile marriages, conceive beloved children, and bring forth desired daughters. At the end of the day, the "emergent masculine" Middle Eastern men who take the moral plunge into egg donation are doing it "for her"—for the wives and future daughters in their lives—with love and compassion in their hearts.

Emergent Masculinities in the Middle East

Rethinking Masculinity in the Middle East

On the day I began to write this conclusion, a *Newsweek* magazine arrived on the stands. The cover attracted my attention. A little boy peers over the left shoulder of a muscular man, whose face cannot be seen, but whose back is bare. The headline shouts: "MAN UP! The Traditional Male Is an Endangered Species. It's Time to Rethink Masculinity." The second cover story advertised "The Tea Party Tempest." Flipping through the actual magazine, I found a quote on the Qur'an burning that had threatened to take place on September 11, 2010, in Florida; an essay on "Our State of Disgrace: A New Religion Book and the Mosque," which points to an American religious landscape peopled by "zealots and prophets"; the story about the American Tea Party, in which Dinesh D'Souza endorses Newt Gingrich's theory that "Obama is a Kenyan Mau Mau *mufti*"; and then the cover story on "men's lib," which tells us that it is time for a "New Macho" and suggests that "many deadline anthropologists are down on men."[1]

I am not sure what a "deadline anthropologist" is, actually. Anthropologists are generally known for taking years to conduct their painstaking research and to write their lengthy ethnographies. Furthermore, I was not aware that many colleagues in my field are "down on men." In fact, there are relatively few ethnographic accounts of men's lives, and for the most part, those that have been published are sympathetic, or at least relativistic—not critical in nature.

Nonetheless, what was striking to me about this particular issue of *Newsweek* was its concordance with many of the themes in my own research. More specifically, this issue of the magazine focused on masculinity, the Middle East, and religion. Had the three themes been brought into conversation in any meaningful way, this would have been quite remarkable, indeed. Had there been a final article on infertility and new assisted reproductive technologies in the science section, the thematic overlap would have been virtually complete.

My point is about the significance and timeliness of these topics and the need to rethink masculinity not only in America but in the Middle East as well. This rethinking is especially crucial, because so many Americans are, in fact, Islamophobic, carrying with them pernicious stereotypes about Middle Eastern men as particularly dangerous, loathsome, and fanatical. If there is one goal that I hope to have achieved in this book, it is to have provided readers with a more realistic and humanizing portrayal of Middle Eastern men's lives, through a form of person-centered, empirically based ethnography that elucidates men's reproductive life stories, as told in their own words.[2] Through such stories, we can come to appreciate Middle Eastern men not only *as men* but as *good men*, who are facing the twenty-first century in thoughtful, respectful, and locally moral ways.

Throughout this volume, I have argued for recognition of Middle Eastern men's *emergent masculinities*, a term that attempts to capture all that is new and transformative in men's embodied personhood. I began this book with the story of Hamza—my infertile driver, a returned labor migrant, a Shia Muslim, a Hizbullah sympathizer, a devoted husband, and eventually the father of a beloved ICSI daughter. Hamza is a living example of the gender transformations that I have attempted to theorize in this volume. Hamza, like so many other men in the Middle East today, is enacting masculinity in ways that defy both patriarchy and neo-Orientalist assumptions. Men such as Hamza are living moral lives with and without religious guidance. They are enacting joyful marital relations with and without children. And they are embracing new reproductive technologies with and without third-party reproductive assistance.

I would like to reiterate some basic features of Hamza's story, as well as those of other men in my study, which I believe are more generally true of Middle Eastern men in the twenty-first century. First of all, Middle Eastern men work hard, often *emigrating* for periods of their lives, in order to eventually marry and set up a *nuclear family household*. They desire *romantic love, companionship*, and *sexual passion* within a lifelong, *monogamous marriage* surrounded by a sphere of *conjugal privacy*. *Fatherhood* of two to four children—a mixture of sons and *desired daughters*—is wanted as much for joy and happiness as for patrilineal continuity, patriarchal power, or old-age security. If infertility threatens fatherhood, it is typically viewed as a *medical condition* to be overcome through invasive forms of *high-tech assisted reproduction* rather than as a sign of *diminished manhood*. Today, male infertility is being equated with other emerging diseases such as diabetes, which are deemed *hereditary*, and thus beyond men's individual control. In a region with *high rates of male infertility*, men often have friends and *male relatives* who are struggling with infertility. The modern-day treatment quest—which often includes *repeated semen analysis, clinic-based masturbation, testicular needlework, genital surgeries*, and other forms of embodied agony—is men's badge of honor, signifying the ways men suffer for reproduction and love. Their feelings of *sympathy and sacrifice*—of doing all of this "for her" are prominent motivating factors in emergent marital subjectivities in the Middle East today.

Gender scripts surrounding conjugality are also being reworked in complex ways as *ICSI and other assisted reproductive technologies* reach wider and wider audiences in the Middle Eastern region. The very growth of a *booming Middle Eastern IVF industry*—for example, with nearly 250 IVF clinics between the three Middle Eastern countries of Turkey, Iran, and Egypt—bespeaks not only regional *pronatalism* but also the physical, financial, and emotional commitments of thousands upon thousands of married couples. Increasingly, Middle Eastern couples are remaining together in *long-term childless marriages*, while trying repeated rounds of IVF and ICSI in the hopes of achieving parenthood.

When these assisted reproductive technologies fail, as they often do, some men are turning to *third-party reproductive assistance*, especially *egg donation*, to overcome their wives' infertility. Accessing donor eggs may require *reproductive tourism* (a.k.a. *cross-border reproductive care*), as well as the services of *traveling foreign egg donors* who may be American. Shia Muslim men have been permitted to employ gamete donation by *male Shia clerics*, who themselves may be *agents of moral change*. Even *sperm donation*—a globally stigmatized technology still shrouded in secrecy—has been authorized by at least one prominent Shia *fatwa*. As a result, it is now being employed by some men in two Middle Eastern countries, *Iran and Lebanon*.

Middle Eastern men who are resorting to gamete donation are not only Shia Muslims. Indeed, Sunni Muslim, Druze, and Christian men are *challenging religious orthodoxies*—sometimes "going against the religion"—to pursue assisted reproductive technologies that have been religiously forbidden to them. Resisting religious authority takes *great moral courage*, especially when certain aspects of these technologies have been deemed sinful (even sending one to hell). Whereas some Sunni Muslim men are defying the *Sunni ban on gamete donation*, Middle Eastern Catholic men are rejecting the *Vatican's ban on assisted reproduction*. This includes *male Catholic IVF physicians* in Lebanon, who are following the Shia lead in now offering both IVF/ICSI *and* gamete donation to their patients. *Middle Eastern Christian men*, whose voices are rarely heard in popular and scholarly discourses, have been among the most prominent advocates of both gamete donation and *adoption* as ways to build a family. Sunni Muslim men, too, are considering adoption and egg donation as *alternative forms of family formation*. Shia Muslim men, for their part, are major participants in the *support and fostering of orphans*.

These changes in men's attitudes, expectations, and practices of manhood and family life are indicative of what is being called "ideational change" in the Middle East.[3] To wit, total fertility rates have fallen across the region, nuclear families are becoming the socially accepted norm, levels of education for both men and women, but especially women, are rising, and assumptions about son preference and men's patriarchal rights are being questioned. This "new Arab family"—to use the term coined by anthropologist Nicholas Hopkins[4]—no longer resembles the Middle Eastern family of a generation ago. These emergent changes in family life are being followed by several Middle Eastern anthropologists, who have formed the Arab Families Working Group (AFWG) led by pioneering Lebanese American scholar Suad Joseph.[5] I look forward to seeing what AFWG researchers will discover about Arab families in the new millennium.

Just as other anthropologists are speaking of "the new Arab family," I would like to coin the term *the new Arab man*. *New Arab men* are rejecting the assumptions of their Arab forefathers, including what I call the *four notorious Ps—patriarchy, patrilineality, patrilocality, and polygyny*. According to the men in my studies, these four Ps are becoming a thing of the past. Instead, emergent masculinities in the Middle East are characterized by resistance to patriarchy, patrilineality, and patrilocality, which are being undermined. Polygyny is truly rare, just as it was in the past, according to Cambridge scholar Basim F. Musallam, the leading historian of Middle Eastern family formation.[6] Certainly, polygyny is not a common strategy today to overcome childlessness or a social norm that contemporary Middle Eastern men strive for. Although most Middle Eastern men want to father their own children, taking a second wife is not viewed as "the solution" to infertility. Instead, men seek to help their infertile wives find appropriate treatment. Middle Eastern men today also realize that they themselves may be infertile.

A GLOBAL MALE INFERTILITY CRISIS?

Why are so many Middle Eastern men infertile? Is there, in fact, a Middle Eastern "epidemic" of male infertility? And, if so, is this part of a more global "male infertility crisis"? In her book, *Exposing Men: The Science and Politics of Male Reproduction*, Cynthia R. Daniels examines claims by Danish researchers that global sperm counts are declining precipitously.[7] More specifically, in 1992 a team of Danish scientists reported that global sperm counts had dropped by rates of more than 40 percent over the previous fifty years. This "big drop theory" led to moral panic. Media and government agencies began declaring a male fertility "crisis," even announcing the potential "end of the human race."[8] As Daniels points out, proving or disproving this big drop theory was difficult, given that measurement of male reproductive health has been woefully inadequate throughout the twentieth century. Nonetheless, once this notion of declining male fertility rates leaked into the public and scholarly imagination, a range of theorized causes began to be investigated, with environmental chemicals, or so-called toxic exposures, at the top of the list.[9] Many other causes of male infertility have also been speculated. These include, *inter alia*, maternal use of drugs during pregnancy; the use of plastic diapers on male infants; the use of phytoestrogen-rich, soy-based formulas to feed male infants; increased rates of sexual activity among young men; the shift from boxer to jockey shorts (the so-called "jockey shorts hypothesis"); the rise of male obesity and dietary changes in men; increased use of drugs and alcohol, as well as male smoking in some societies; the shift from factory to sedentary work; the use of hard bicycle seats; the use of hot tubs and saunas (which overheat the testicles); and "even the advent of feminism and the decline of war!"[10]

More than two decades later, this "big drop theory" remains unproved.[11] Nonetheless, there is increasing scientific evidence that environmental pollutants—especially a class of widely used chemicals known as "endocrine disruptors"—are affecting both male and female reproductive health deleteriously, by altering the human hormones that control fertility.[12] Furthermore, reproductive epidemiological evidence strongly suggests that other environmental toxins such as lead—the heavy metal found in paint and in air-polluted cities where leaded gasoline is still used (e.g. Mexico City, Cairo, Damascus)—are, in fact, "spermatotoxic," leading to lower sperm counts in men with high levels of lead in their bodies (e.g., traffic policemen).[13]

I have always been curious about these purported causes of male infertility. With my training in both medical anthropology and reproductive epidemiology, I have been able to pursue some interesting leads, asking men a series of questions about their perceived "risk factors" for male infertility. I have published a series of ten articles on these subjects,[14] mostly with my Lebanese colleagues who have helped me with the data collection and analysis.

What have we found with respect to male infertility? First and quite fortunately, Lebanese, Syrian, and Palestinian men are *not* carrying toxic loads of heavy metals in their bodies.[15] This was determined in my colleague Jerome Nriagu's toxic metal laboratory at the University of Michigan. There, he and his assistants searched for a suite of nine toxic metals in a collection of blood samples that more than 200 men in my study willingly donated for the purposes of my research. Quite amazingly, in the post-9/11 environment in which we live, I carried these blood samples in a large, Rubbermaid cooler all the way back from Beirut to Detroit over sixteen hours and eight airport checkpoints—without ever being questioned or inspected!

Once the heavy metal analysis was completed, I and my Lebanese research assistants contacted all of the men in my study to convey their "healthy" results. Many of the men in my study were extremely curious to know what was "in" their blood, worrying, as they did, that "chemicals" in the air, food, and water were at least partly responsible for their male infertility. Thus, they were quite grateful for this health-edifying information.

Our second finding was that men in the Middle East would be much better off if they did not smoke. Like lead, smoking has been shown to be spermatotoxic, immobilizing human spermatozoa.[16] In my earliest Egyptian work, I was able to determine that men who smoked traditional water pipes were at an increased risk of being infertile.[17] Unfortunately, since the new millennium, waterpipe smoking has become increasingly fashionable across the Middle Eastern region, with entire families sharing the *nargila* (also called *argila, shisha, mu'assal* and, in English, hubble bubble or hooka) as an enjoyable family pastime. Cigarettes—and, perhaps even more so, waterpipe tobacco—contain a range of chemical toxins, such as nicotine, carbon monoxide, cadmium, and other mutagenic compounds, some of which may impair sperm motility and morphology.[18] Unfortunately, male smoking is widespread across the region, with Lebanon having among the highest rates of smoking in the Arab world. In Lebanon, by age nineteen, approximately 52.6 percent of men are already smoking.[19] In my study, 45 percent of men were current cigarette smokers (41% of the infertile men, 49% of the fertile men). However, the recent increase in *nargila* smoking by many men in my study meant that fully two-thirds (67%) were regular users of tobacco products. Among cigarette smokers, furthermore, the majority were heavy smokers, consuming one to three packs a day. This was as true among infertile men in the study as among fertile ones. In fact, few infertile men made any association between their infertility and their smoking, even though physicians had often told them to quit. Quitting attempts were relatively few and far between; only twenty men in the study (twelve infertile, eight fertile) had stopped cigarette smoking altogether. As most men told me, they had started smoking as teenagers, continued to smoke because they enjoyed it, considered smoking to be a form of sociability and a coping mechanism, and remained unconvinced that smoking had anything to do with infertility, especially since so many of their male compatriots who smoked had fathered children.

Although most men do not deem their smoking accountable for their infertility problems, this does not mean that they do not engage in self-blame. In fact, many infertile Middle Eastern men in my study felt guilt—guilt toward their wives whom they had "deprived" of children, guilt about their sexual pasts, and guilt over what they perceived to be their own infertility-inducing behaviors. These included, *inter alia*, overwork, weight gain, eating too much sugar, drinking too much coffee, drinking any kind of alcohol, sedentarism, working in conditions that were either too hot or too cold, spending too much time in cars and smelling gasoline fumes, having testicles that were too small or uneven, having been"shocked"(by a spider, gunshot, bombs, etc.), wearing tight jeans, and generally being too "stressed out"(by"work stress,""family stress,""economic stress,""infertility stress,"etc.). In general, this was a population of men who described themselves as living" in stress,"or *daght*, and they felt bad about the effects of this stress on their infertile bodies.

War Stories of Male Infertility

However, the major form of stress in my study was war-related stress. *Al harb,*"the war,"was the single-most cited reason for male infertility problems. Men attributed their infertility to *daght nafsi*, or war-related"psychological stress."Many of them told me that the war had affected their *hal nafsiya*, or"psychological condition,"in profoundly negative ways. Indeed, men's "war stories of male infertility" were rife with suffering, fear, and chronic anxiety. Just looking back at the men's stories in this volume, this is what we find: *Hamza's* father was killed, his family fled, he was beaten by soldiers, he was exiled from his country as a teenager, and after returning many years later, he was then subjected to the terror of the 2006 summer war, in which he made a daring and courageous attempt to move all of his family members to safety. *Ziad* was recruited into a Christian militia at the tender age of thirteen, never finishing his education as a consequence. *Karim's* family sent him to Dubai to escape the war, and he eventually married Mona, who had lost her fingers to an explosion. Karim and Mona never returned to live in their native country. *Abbas* was conscripted into the Lebanese marines when still a high school sophomore. Having survived the fighting, he fled to Cyprus, then the United States, returning to Lebanon once the violence had receded. *Hussain* was a Lebanese army commando, who had been on the front line throughout the fifteen-year civil war. He saw many scenes of war and carnage, claiming that he never felt fear throughout all of his years of fighting. *Waleed's* family was forced to flee from its mountain home, living mostly in Beirut bomb shelters, where Waleed developed a phobic fear of rats. Waleed's mother died within the first year, and then thirty of his family members were killed. Waleed was grazed by a bullet and developed an addiction to antianxiety medications. He married late in life because of wartime disruptions and fears that his family is now"dying out." *Shaykh Ali* and his two brothers were imprisoned in Iraq by Saddam Hussein during the First Gulf War. His brothers were killed in prison, but Shaykh Ali survived three years of torture, eventually being released and fleeing to Syria, then Lebanon. He was granted political asylum in the United States, where he leads a lonely existence as an azoospermic, divorced gas station attendant. *Ibrahim* was living in Kuwait at the time of the First Gulf War. As a Palestinian, he was kidnapped and beaten by angry Kuwaitis. So was *Eyad*, who underwent the same kidnapping and torture along with his two Palestinian brothers. Eyad fled with his family to Syria, seeking safe haven. But, without employment there, he was forced to return to Dubai alone. Eventually, he married his Palestinian childhood sweetheart, Lubna, from whom he had been separated since the beginning of the Lebanese civil war. As a Palestinian refugee, Lubna has lived her entire life in a UN-supported refugee camp in southern Lebanon and is legally prevented from joining her husband in the UAE, where he does not have citizenship rights. *Hasan* was an early member of the Shia "resistance" in southern Lebanon, which would eventually become Hizbullah. He was captured by the Israelis in 1983 and imprisoned in solitary confinement. He underwent many interrogations, including three administrations of electricity to his genitals. Upon his release in a prisoner swap, he was involved in a major car accident on war-torn roads, breaking twenty-four bones, entering a coma, and requiring brain surgery. Amazingly, he lived to tell his tale. "We lived our life in war," he said, "and we suffered a lot."

Hasan uttered a simple truth: war causes profound human suffering. Most of the Lebanese, Palestinian, and Iraqi men whom I have interviewed since the beginning of the new millennium have stories of suffering to tell. Most of these men were the victims of violence, not the perpetrators of it. When choosing which stories to include in this volume, I did not purposely select stories of men who had been affected by war. Rather, the sad reality is that most of the men in my study had been exposed directly to political violence. This included the Lebanese civil war (1975–90), the subsequent Israeli occupation of southern Lebanon (1990–2000), the First Gulf War (1990–91), the U.S.-led war in Iraq (2003–present), and the summer war between Israel and Hizbullah in Lebanon (2006).

As a result of these perpetual wars in the Middle East, men whom I met had been wounded, sometimes as fighters, but mostly as civilians. They often showed me their bullet and shrapnel wounds, pointing to where they were still carrying metal debris in their bodies. Several men had been kidnapped and threatened with death. Even more had been imprisoned and tortured. Some had lost family members, including their parents when they were still young children. In a few very poignant cases, men's entire families had been wiped out in massive bombing raids, usually by the Israelis in southern Lebanon. Most of the Lebanese men in my study had been exposed to bombing and life in bomb shelters. Some had had their homes destroyed. Families had often been forced to flee to safer havens, and in many cases, families with financial means simply left the country altogether. When entire families were unable to emigrate, they often sent their sons out of the country to prevent them from being killed.

The fact that Middle Eastern men attribute their male infertility problems to war is not so far-fetched. In two papers written with my Lebanese colleagues,[20] we have been able to show that exposure to war events significantly increases male risk of infertility, probably through stress-related testosterone suppression.[21] In my study, men who were infertile had a 57 percent increased odds of exposure to one or more war-related events, as compared to fertile men in the study. Furthermore, the men who had suffered the harshest exposures to war (through combat, kidnapping, torture, and displacement) were the most likely to be infertile. In short, my study suggests that Middle Eastern men are right about *al harb*. War diminishes their fertility, not only during the midst of the violence but also in its aftermath. That war has destroyed lives and *men's fertility* is an indigenous etiology that seems to hold up well against the epidemiological evidence.

As I have suggested in my Society for Medical Anthropology presidential address, "Medical Anthropology against War,"[22] we anthropologists need to become much more involved in antiwar activism, and in studying the embodied health effects of political violence when it happens. This is perhaps particularly true for the Middle East, where political conflicts stretch across the region from Western Sahara to Afghanistan, and many countries in between.[23] At the time of this writing, the United States is still involved in its wars in Iraq and Afghanistan, with no decisive victory or clear end in sight in either nation.

THE ICSI REVOLUTION?

War in the Middle East has probably increased male infertility on a population level. However, war is probably *not* the major reason why so many Middle Eastern men are azoospermic, or have extremely low sperm counts and poor motility. As shown in chapter 4, these severe cases tend to run in families and are probably genetically based. Men in my study were usually able to note familial patterns of male infertility, calling them *wirathi*, or "hereditary." As my Lebanese colleagues and I have argued,[24] family clustering of male infertility cases is probably genetically related to generational patterns of consanguineous marriage. Marriage to cousins likely increases the chances for genetic defects, including microdeletions of the Y chromosome linked to male infertility.[25] If most male infertility is, indeed, genetically based, then the use of ICSI as the major technological solution to overcome male infertility problems is also ethically questionable.[26] Through the use of ICSI, male offspring will also be infertile, requiring the intervention of ICSI generation after generation.[27] To prevent this from happening, some IVF practitioners are recommending the PGD-assisted "culling" of all male embryos in severe male infertility cases, before they are ever implanted. This way, only female offspring, who do not carry the Y chromosome, are born to such infertile men.[28]

Furthermore, recent research suggests that male reproductive tract abnormalities—including undescended testicles, hypospadias (a birth defect in which the opening of the urethra is on the underside, rather than at the end, of the penis), and poor semen quality—are more prevalent in male children conceived through assisted reproduction, regardless of genetic defects in their fathers' sperm.[29] This is because assisted reproduction is associated with use of artificial hormones, higher rates of prematurity, low birth weight, and multiple gestation, which are indirect risk factors for the development of male genital malformations (from the disruption of gonadal development during fetal life).[30] ICSI in particular increases the risk for hypospadias, which may require surgical repair during infancy.[31]

This then brings us to an important question: Has ICSI been a "revolutionary" technology, a "panacea" for male infertility, a form of technological "assistance," a way to give nature a "helping hand"? Or has it been something much less positive: a form of "false hope," a deleterious "eugenic" technology, or a means of "stratified reproduction"?[32]

Neither philosopher nor bioethicist, I find it difficult to pronounce an answer to these questions. Many feminist scholars before me have attempted to "theorize infertility,"[33] by condemning the assisted reproductive technologies for their negative gender effects.[34] My colleague Charis Thompson urges caution in this regard.[35] As she points out, the ethnography of infertility clearly demonstrates the power of assisted reproductive technologies such as ICSI to generate hope, fulfill desire, and "make parents" of infertile couples.[36] Sarah Franklin, one of the earliest ethnographers of assisted reproduction,[37] has recently written the history of the nearly 5 million test-tube babies born because of IVF and ICSI.[38]

In this regard, ICSI is a "hope technology,"[39] creating the "only hope" for most infertile men, especially those with serious cases. The emergence of ICSI in the Middle Eastern region in the mid-1990s led to an immediate boom in demand for this technology—a demand that has never waned. IVF clinics today are filled with ICSI-seeking couples. Baby photos prominently displayed on clinic walls, including in the OR where ICSI is performed, "keep hope alive" for these couples (figure 17). ICSI is by far the most common assisted reproductive technology now undertaken in the Middle East, because ICSI increases the chances of fertilization—the creation of "ICSI embryos." Many men in my study hoped for the chance to create these "elusive embryos."[40] As one man in my study told me, "I will try again and again and again. I will never lose hope." Or, as another man put it, "I will try until I die."

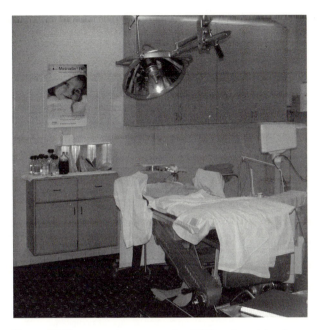

FIGURE 17. The operating room, after ICSI embryo transfer, with baby photo in background

Unfortunately, some infertile Middle Eastern men may never produce an ICSI embryo, because ICSI cannot guarantee conception. As with IVF, overall ICSI success rates are usually less than 40 percent, even in the world's best centers.[41] Depending upon other factors, such as age-related egg quality and the severity of the male infertility, ICSI success rates can be significantly less. For example, of the 220 men in my Lebanese study, 177 of them had already undertaken ICSI. Among these 177 men, there was a grand total of 434 ICSI attempts—274 among the infertile men and 160 among the fertile men with infertile wives. Yet, there were only eighteen ICSI children born to these men, including thirteen ICSI sons and five ICSI daughters (including one set of female twins). Thus, the so-called "take-home baby rate" was astonishingly low—only 4 percent. This low rate of ICSI success increased considerably if all conceptions were considered, including current pregnancies (7), ectopic pregnancies (9), miscarriages and stillbirths (29), and neonatal deaths (4). In this case, 66 conceptions took place after 434 ICSI attempts, for a pregnancy rate (as opposed to a "take-home baby rate") of 29 percent. This makes the overall success of ICSI in this Middle Eastern population seem closer to global standards. Nonetheless, most of these ICSI conceptions ended in heartbreak and suffering, including life-threatening ectopic pregnancies among men's wives, the stillbirth of seven sets of twins, and the deaths of three ICSI sons (including one with Down syndrome) and one ICSI daughter (due to a congenital heart defect). Recounting their losses, men often wiped tears from their eyes. As the mother of stillborn twin daughters, my heart ached for them.

Furthermore, some men—especially the "repeaters"—had spent small fortunes on their ICSI attempts. The average number of ICSIs was 2.5, but a few men in my study had undertaken ICSI more than ten times. When I asked men to estimate how much they had spent on their ICSI quests, those who were able to calculate averaged $17,000, with total costs ranging from $1,500 to $100,000. These costs are exceedingly high for the Middle East, if it is considered that most men in my study made well under $12,000 per year. In the United States, by comparison, the average cost of one ICSI cycle is more than $12,000, and the cost of making one "take-home baby" reaches nearly $70,000.[42]

Because of the costs of repetition, ICSI is an incredibly expensive technology, which many of the men in my study could ill afford. Some of them had used up their life savings; some had borrowed against their future retirement benefits; others had taken out bank loans; some had sold land; some of their wives had sold bridal gold; and, in many cases, men were relying on family financial aid, particularly from wealthier relatives in the diaspora. Some men had literally impoverished themselves in their ICSI quests. Others had waited years to save the requisite money for a single ICSI cycle. In a few cases, men told me matter-of-factly that they could afford only one ICSI. Thus, they were praying to God that their single attempt would succeed.

ASSISTED REPRODUCTION ACCESS AND ACTIVISM

These issues of cost and access are becoming growing global concerns.[43] The European Society of Human Reproduction and Embryology (ESHRE), which is the major assisted reproduction professional organization in Europe, convened a meeting on "Developing Countries and Infertility" in Arusha, Tanzania, in December 2007, which was followed by publication of a special issue of *Human Reproduction* in 2008.[44] It was noted that only 48 of the 191 member states of the World Health Organization have medical facilities that offer IVF and ICSI.[45] Most of the countries with the world's largest populations (i.e., China, India, Pakistan, Indonesia) offer less than 1 percent of the total projected need for assisted reproductive technologies, given their rates of infertility. Latin America—which is one of the few regions of the world to provide a collaborative registry of clinics and numbers of IVF and ICSI cycles—is characterized by limited access to these technologies and a high number of multiple births (nearly 50%)

because of the high number of embryos transferred in an attempt to im prove success rates.[46] Furthermore, the mean cost of a single IVF cycle in an international survey of twenty-five countries ranged from $1,300 in Iran to $6,400 in Hong Kong.[47] In all of these countries, the cost of a single cycle was more than half of an average individual's annual income. This concern over global inequities in cost and access to assisted reproductive technologies has been highlighted in a series of recent articles,[48] including one from the *Bulletin of the World Health Organization* entitled "Mother or Nothing: The Agony of Infertility."[49]

As I have argued in my earlier work, assisted reproductive technologies provide an example par excellence of "stratified reproduction."[50] Namely, technologically assisted reproduction is largely restricted to global elites, whereas the infertile poor, who are at highest risk of infertility, are de valued as reproducers. What I have called *arenas of constraint*—economic, cultural, and practical—serve to limit access to these technologies for most infertile couples, in the Middle East as elsewhere.[51] My colleague Rob ert Nachtigall notes that "relatively few of the world's infertile men and women can be said to have complete and equitable access to the complete range of infertility treatments at affordable levels."[52]

This is also true of Middle Eastern men and women. For those who are unable to afford or to otherwise access IVF and ICSI, they may receive either no infertility care or, more likely, substandard care that is ineffec tive and even iatrogenic (i.e., a form of physician-induced harm). In the Middle Eastern region, varicocelectomies, which are genital surgeries to remove varicose veins (i.e., varicoceles) on the testicles, are a case in point. This form of "genital cutting"—about which I have written extensively elsewhere[53]—has been deemed ineffective and obsolete by the World Health Organization and a number of prominent Western researchers who have reviewed the existing evidence.[54] Nonetheless, varicocelectomy con tinues to be widely performed as a purported "male infertility surgery" for men across the Middle Eastern region.

For example, in my earlier Egyptian IVF study, 17 percent of the men had undergone a varicocelectomy to purportedly overcome their male in fertility problems.[55] Some had undergone this surgery twice, because of the failure of a previous repair or a recurrence of the varicocele. In at least one case, the surgery itself caused the iatrogenic outcome of obstructive azoospermia, or lack of any sperm in the ejaculate due to a blockage of the epididymis caused by the surgery. As I was to discover in my more recent Lebanese study, 55 of the 120 infertile men—exactly 45 percent— had undergone varicocelectomies. Four of these men had undergone the operation twice, and one man a staggering three times![56] Twenty-two of these men (18%) had had both testicles manipulated in the surgery; sometimes, they stood to show me the incision scars in both their right and left inguinal areas. Five men suffered from serious complications, including formation of a hydrocele (i.e., "bag of water" forming around the testis) that required second surgeries. The vast majority of these infertile men who had undergone varicocelectomy noted, with defeat and anger, that the varicocelectomy was not successful, leading to no improvement in their low sperm counts. Furthermore, three of the infertile men in the study had been induced to undergo varicocelectomy surgeries to supposedly overcome azoospermia—a complete absence of sperm that is clearly *not* caused by a varicocele.

These high figures among the infertile men were less surprising than the figures from *fertile* men in my Lebanese study. Stunningly, 18 percent of these men had also undergone varicocelectomy, in six cases before marriage. Apparently, physicians had convinced them that small varicoceles detected on routine exams could lead to future male fertility impairments; thus, they became convinced of the need for surgery. Those who had undergone varicocelectomy following marriage considered it their male contribution to the infertility treatment quest. Ultimately, three of the fertile men suffered complications from varicocelectomies, including hydroceles necessitating additional surgery.

The high percentage of varicocelectomy surgeries among *both* infertile and fertile Middle Eastern men might make sense if varicocelectomies could *truly* improve low sperm counts or prevent low sperm counts from developing. However, the efficacy of varicocelectomy as a therapeutic and preventive surgery has been seriously questioned by the World Health Organization.[57] Instead, the problematics of varicocelectomies in the Middle East are suggestive of perverse economic incentives, whereby varicocelectomies are aggressively promoted by urologists through false advertisements of an infertility "cure." Unfortunately, there is no "cure" for male infertility.[58] Barring sperm donation or adoption, which are generally forbidden in the Middle East, ICSI is the only real solution to male infertility problems.

The question, therefore, is: How can access to ICSI be increased among Middle Eastern men of lesser financial means? Egypt provides a good role model in this regard. Over the past twenty-five years, Egypt has supported a thriving assisted reproduction sector, with approximately fifty IVF clinics serving an infertile population estimated at 15 percent of all married couples (or about 15.5 million persons among a total population of approximately 80 million).[59] Five of these clinics are located in government hospitals and receive some state funding to offset expenses for the infertile poor. The busiest clinic is located in Al Azhar University, Egypt's oldest and most famous institute of religious learning, under the auspices of the Al Azhar International Islamic Center for Population Studies and Research. The clinic was started by Gamal I. Serour, director of Al Azhar's Islamic Center and current president of the International Federation of Gynaecology and Obstetrics (FIGO). Designed to serve the needs of Egypt's infertile poor, the clinic provides generously subsidized IVF cycles—at $600 per cycle—to hundreds of lower-income couples each year.

The Egypt example is instructive. Egypt is a resource-poor, developing country, which has long been generally regarded as seriously overpopulated. Nonetheless, Egypt has managed to bring down its population growth rates while, at the same time, experimenting with state subsidization of infertility care, including the provision of assisted reproductive technologies. Why has Egypt moved in this direction? A combination of cultural and political factors appears to provide the answer. Culturally, Egypt is a pronatalist, Sunni Muslim country, where couples are encouraged to marry and raise families. Politically, the country hosted the famous "Cairo conference" (a.k.a. the International Conference on Population and Development [ICPD]) in 1994, where "prevention and appropriate treatment of infertility, where feasible" was mentioned as an issue for future action.[60] Furthermore, Egypt has produced a remarkable cadre of highly trained IVF physicians, as well as two FIGO presidents. One of these former presidents, Mahmoud Fathalla, has argued, through the prism of reproductive rights, that "family planning must also mean planning *for* families."[61]

Nearly twenty years post-Cairo, the meaning of reproductive rights is being examined through a prism that includes infertility and the ARTs as part of a political platform of health care equity and social justice.[62] In 2009 ESHRE convened a second meeting, this time in Genk, Belgium, to examine "Social Aspects of Accessible Infertility Care in Developing Countries."[63] Similarly, a group called "Friends of Low-Cost IVF" (LCIVF) is in the process of being formed in North America. Meeting for the first time at the 2010 annual American Society for Reproductive Medicine (ASRM) meeting in Denver, Colorado, the LCIVF board of directors is attempting to chart a future where the costs of IVF and ICSI can be brought down to more affordable levels around the world, perhaps through endowment funds to help subsidize infertile couples, efforts to lower the costs of pharmaceuticals, and other creative strategies. Together, ESHRE and LCIVF are addressing the very meaning of "reproductive rights." Does reproductive rights mean only the right to *control* fertility? Or should a more expansive notion of reproductive rights encompass the right to *facilitate* fertility when fertility is threatened? For millions of infertile couples, achieving full reproductive rights around the globe may mean achieving access to IVF, ICSI, and other assisted reproductive technologies.

ISLAMIC TECHNOSCIENCE, ADVOCACY, AND REVOLUTION

To my knowledge, I am the first social scientist to be included in the LCIVF movement as a member of the board of directors. I am honored, as I have spent my entire scholarly life attempting to pinpoint the arenas of constraint surrounding ART access among infertile couples in the Middle East.[64] In recent years, I have also been called upon in a way that I never anticipated when I began this research in the Middle East so many years ago. Namely, I am now considered something of an "expert" on the Islamic perspectives regarding assisted reproduction. I am not Muslim, and I am completely secular. However, because my research has taken me into the intricacies of Islamic thinking in both the Sunni- and Shia-dominant countries, I am occasionally called upon to provide information, counseling, and expert testimony for infertile Muslim couples.

In terms of information, I receive email inquiries from around the world, asking for clarification of *fatwa* decisions, including the differences between Sunni and Shia authorities regarding gamete donation. In a few cases, I have had quite lengthy exchanges with individuals and couples who are contemplating egg or sperm donation, especially if they are Sunni Muslim and ambivalent about taking this major step. In this regard, I am sometimes asked to send a copy of the Shia *fatwa* permitting these donor technologies. I am also asked by some couples to send my various research papers, and I make informational referrals to my Iranian colleagues, who are more aware of the contemporary intricacies of assisted reproduction practices in that country.

In the past few years, I have also been asked to meet with infertile Muslim couples in local IVF clinics, in situations where they are having difficulty deciding on their options. Although I am not a professional psychotherapist and do not offer any kind of directive counseling, I do pass along information, including some sense of the general trends I have observed over the years of my research. This would include the fact that gamete donation is taking place in the Middle East and that some Sunni Muslim couples are pursuing this option, even if it is banned in their home countries. In addition, I am currently working with my local Yale IVF physician colleague, Dr. Pasquale Patrizio, to assist an Iraqi refugee couple in accessing ICSI on a "humanitarian" basis within our own university's medical system.

Finally, in 2009, I was called to New York City to testify on behalf of an azoospermic infertile Pakistani man who was seeking political asylum and citizenship rights in the United States. An illegal immigrant, he and his wife had used donor sperm in the United States and had produced a beautiful son, now two years old. The husband feared deportation back to Sunni-dominant Pakistan, given Pakistan's strict Islamic *hudud* laws that would regard sperm donation as a major sin, carrying severe, even life-threatening penalties for him and his family. I testified on this man's behalf, arguing for the right of the family to seek asylum on these grounds. At the time of this writing, the outcome of the case is still pending.

The various forms of activism and advocacy that I have described here will only increase, in my view, with the widespread emergence of newer forms of assisted reproduction. For example, preimplantation genetic diagnosis (PGD) has entered the Middle East in the new millennium. Despite some men's professed preferences for daughters, as seen in chapter 8, the danger still exists that PGD will be used extensively for "son selection" in a region where men are patrilineally pressured to produce male offspring. According to FIGO president Gamal Serour, this trend is already beginning to emerge in the first clinics to use PGD in Jordan and Saudi Arabia.[65]

Moreover, if human reproductive cloning ever becomes a reality, it will raise other major ethical dilemmas around the world. But these dilemmas will play out in particular "local moral" ways within the Middle East. Most important in this regard, both Iran's Ayatollah Khamene'i and Lebanon's Sayyid Fadlallah (who died on July 4, 2010) have condoned reproductive cloning for their followers. Given that cloning bypasses the need for third-party reproductive assistance, the Middle East may be one of the first regions of the world to eagerly embrace human reproductive cloning, despite the current regional anti-cloning declaration made by the Islamic Organization for Medical Sciences.

Similarly, if DNA paternity testing is eventually taken up in the Middle East—as it has been in parts of Latin America[66]—it could cause a moral maelstrom within the IVF industry. As shown by Palestinian Bedouin anthropologist Aref Abu-Rabia, paternity suits without the benefit of DNA testing already occur in tribal societies in the Middle East, often being settled by traditional tribal judges on the basis of the facial features and other characteristics of the child in question.[67] According to Abu-Rabia, another common Bedouin means of establishing paternity (and other "truth claims") is "ordeal by fire," in which men are asked to lick a red-hot iron or other fiery substance.

Presumably, DNA testing will become a less physically torturous means of settling future paternity disputes, even though the emotional pain may be unbearable, as shown in the work of anthropologist Claudia Fonseca in Brazil.[68] When DNA testing eventually becomes a routine part of the Middle Eastern biotechnological environment, men who are concerned about the mixing of gametes in IVF laboratories may turn to DNA testing as a kind of follow up check. What are now still idle threats on the part of some Lebanese men may, in fact, become a reality once this technology gains a firm foothold in the region. The results could be either quite heartening—confirming the great care that is taken in Middle Eastern IVF labs to keep gametes (and *nasab*) separate—or quite shocking, revealing as-yet-unacknowledged physician and laboratory negligence. My prediction is that the emergence of a medical malpractice industry would quickly follow suit. Some physicians and embryologists would go to jail—or suffer worse penalties. The resultant loss of legitimacy for the Middle Eastern assisted reproduction industry might then become permanent.

All of these are futuristic scenarios in the world of Islamic technoscience. They are topics that need to be taken up by future medical anthropology scholars of the region. Meanwhile, my own goal has been to reveal the contemporary world of Islam and assisted reproduction at the beginning of the new millennium. In particular, my aim has been to reveal the role of men—clerics, physicians, and patients—in shaping this local moral world.

As we have seen, Middle Eastern men have their own reproductive issues and concerns, which may or may not be connected to women's reproductive health and well-being. This is an insight that is long overdue in the new millennium. Reconceiving Middle Eastern masculinities requires scholarship that brings men back into the reproductive imaginary as, on the one hand, sufferers and victims, and on the other, as progenitors, partners, fathers, decision makers, protectors, friends, companions, nurturers, lovers, and sentient human beings. My research shows that Middle Eastern men are often heavily involved and invested in many aspects of the reproductive process, from impregnation to parenting. The feminist assertion that men contribute only "patriarchy to procreation"—which I have regrettably promoted in some of my earlier work—now seems to me both patently unfair and untrue. Unseating patriarchy in the Middle East means rethinking our own scholarly polemics—mine included—as the reality of men's lives is empirically revealed.

Indeed, as I put the finishing touches on my book, Egyptians—mostly young men using social media technology—have ousted their dictatorial ruler, Hosni Mubarak, through means of peaceful protest. These Egyptian protestors'"Facebook Revolution for Democracy" was spurred by the "Jasmine Revolution" in neighboring Tunisia, where brutal dictator Zine el-Abidine Ben Ali was forced into exile in Saudi Arabia. On this day, February 11, 2011, as I write my final paragraphs, it is unclear how Egypt's democratic aspirations will be realized, or whether other Middle Eastern countries will follow in a similar path. But, in my view, the most important moral of this story is that ordinary men—and women—in the Middle East can change their social worlds. As Asef Bayat, professor of sociology and Middle Eastern studies at Leiden University writes in his prescient book, *Life as Politics: How Ordinary People Change the Middle East* (published in fall 2010 before the fall of Beni Ali and Mubarak),

> The essays compiled in this volume are about agency and change in the Muslim Middle East, the societies in which religion seems to occupy a prominent position. More specifically, they focus on the configuration of sociopolitical transformation brought about by internal social forces, by collectives and individuals. Here I focus on the

diverse ways in which the ordinary people ... strive to affect the contours of change in their societies, by refusing to exit from the social and political stage controlled by authoritarian states, moral authority, and neoliberal economies, discovering and generating new spaces within which they can voice their dissent and assert their presence in pursuit of bettering their lives.[69]

Bayat calls his theoretical framing *the art of presence*—or the "story of agency in times of constraints."[70]

If Bayat's book is about the art of presence in the Middle East, then my book is about *the art of emergence*. Just as ordinary Middle Eastern men are changing their sociopolitical worlds, these men are also changing their personal lives, interjecting new notions of manhood, gender relations, and intimate subjectivities into their ways of being. These emergent masculinities defy conventional gender stereotypes, can be found across faith traditions, challenge prevailing moral authorities, and employ emerging technoscientific innovations. Indeed, emergent masculinities in the Middle East today go hand in hand with emergent technologies—from Twitter and Facebook to testicular sperm aspiration and ICSI. Yet, while social media-driven revolutions in the Middle East have gained global media attention, reproductive technology revolutions have not. Here at the end of my book, I would like to argue that ICSI, too, is changing the Middle East in unprecedented ways, creating many new possibilities for marital, gender, and family relations. As the reproductive life histories in this book have shown, ICSI has brought with it hopes and dreams for the high numbers of infertile men in the Middle East. Indeed, ICSI has emerged as *the* major assisted reproductive technology in a region that can now boast one of the strongest and largest assisted reproduction industries in the world.

What else do these men's reproductive life histories tell us? Their stories suggest that, in the Middle East today, emergent masculinities entail love, tenderness, and affection, as well as untold sacrifice and suffering, all elements of contemporary manhood that go unnoticed and unappreciated, particularly when set against the tropes of violent hypermasculinity that characterize ongoing Western Orientalist discourse. It is my hope that *The New Arab Man* has moved us one step closer to understanding how Middle Eastern men encounter their reproductive trials and tribulations. Through these encounters, Middle Eastern men such as Hamza are living proof that manhood is being transformed in the Middle East, as men themselves reconceive their masculinity.

Acknowledgments

A s I write these words of thanks on May 25, 2010, exactly nineteen years have passed since I received my PhD in anthropology at the University of California, Berkeley, in a lovely commencement ceremony at Zellerbach Hall. I am grateful to that institution for launching my career in Middle Eastern medical anthropology, and to my wonderful mentors, Nelson Graburn and Ira Lapidus at Berkeley, and Joan Ablon and Frederick Dunn at University of California, San Francisco, who helped me to become the person I am today.

It has been a wondrous journey since then over two decades and ten Middle Eastern nations. I cannot begin to express the gratitude I feel toward my Middle Eastern interlocutors—those men and women who have shared their reproductive trials and tribulations with me. In particular, I owe a profound debt of gratitude to more than three hundred men from many Middle Eastern nations and backgrounds who took me into their reproductive lives and confidences. May they all be blessed with the ICSI children they so desire.

Over the years of my research, many Middle Eastern IVF physicians, embryologists, nurses, and staff members have helped me to recruit sometimes reluctant male patients into this study. I am grateful to all of them, including Antoine Abu Musa, Hassan Aly, Johnny Awwad, Michael Hasan Fakih, Walaa Georges, Walid Ghutmi, Najwa Hammoud, Antoine Hannoun, Jumana Husseini, Azhar Ismail, Hannah Ismail, Da'ad Lakkis, the late Mohammed Mehanna, Zaher Nassar, Khaled Sakhel, Gamal Serour, Hanady Sharara, Pankaj Shrivastav, Abdel-Hamid Wafik, Mohamed Yehia, Salah Zaki, Khaled Zeitoun, and Tony Zreik. Two American IVF physicians, Robert Nachtigall of the University of California, San Francisco, and Pasquale Patrizio of the Yale Fertility Center, have also been wonderful colleagues. I am especially grateful to Pasquale for his help with this book's detailed medical glossary.

I also want to thank my beloved Egyptian research assistant, Taysir Salem, as well as my five Lebanese research assistants, Abbass Fakih, Mary Ghanem, Najwa Hammoud, Azhar Ismail, and Hanady Sharara, for their participation in many aspects of my study, from patient recruitment to translation and cultural contextualization. I am especially grateful to Najwa for her dedicated efforts in patient recruitment and to Mary for her help in converting me from the Egyptian dialect to Lebanese Arabic. In Lebanon, the American University of Beirut provided me and my family with a fine home and institutional affiliation, particularly during the unsettling initiation of an American-led war in Iraq. I owe special thanks to Rima Afifi, Iman Nuwayhid, and Huda Zurayk, who cordially welcomed me and my whole family into the AUB Faculty of Health Sciences community.

The research upon which this book is based was generously supported by the National Science Foundation's Cultural Anthropology Program, where both Stuart Plattner and Deborah Winslow have been responsive and encouraging program officers. In addition, the U.S. Department of Education's Fulbright-Hays Faculty Research Abroad Program has provided me with monumental support, by allowing me and my family to live in three different Middle Eastern countries—Egypt, Lebanon, and the United Arab Emirates—for periods totaling nearly three years.

The research for this book was conceived and later carried out while I was a faculty member at the University of Michigan. I am particularly grateful to Noreen Clark for hiring me; Judith Irvine, Sherman James, Timothy Johnson, Michael Kennedy, Abigail Stewart, Mark Tessler, Fawwaz Ulaby, and Marc Zimmerman for being such supportive chairs and directors; Marya Ayyash, Susan Barrera, and Alissa Surges for providing superlative staff support while I directed UM's Center for Middle East and North African Studies; Beth Talbot and Pauline Kennedy for their dedicated administrative assistance, including with grant preparation and logistics; and the Institute for the Humanities, where much of this book was written while I was the Helmut F. Stern Professor in 2007–8. I am particularly grateful to my colleagues at the Institute for the Humanities, who provided valuable feedback on the prologue and introduction to this book. I also benefited from membership in the Adoption, Infertility, and Gender Study Group of the Institute for Research on Women and Gender, where we read much of the infertility literature together. At UM, I shared my research findings and ideas with a host of good colleagues and friends, including Linda Chatters, Paul Edwards and Gabrielle Hecht, Gottfried Hagen, Nancy Hunt, Yi and Richard Keep, Laura McCloskey, Mark Padilla, Holly Peters-Golden, Lauren and Geoffrey Phelps, Mary Piontek, Elizabeth Roberts, Leslie Stanton and Steven Whiting, Melissa Valerio, Caroline and Fong Wang, and Norm and Barbara Yoffee. I was also surrounded by a top-notch group of UM graduate students, several of whom have read and commented on parts of this manuscript. They include Kate Allen, Nicole Berry, Sallie Han, Lisa Harris, Laura Heinemann, Alyson Jones, Loulou Kobeissi, Jessaca Leinaweaver, Kate McClellan, Emily McKee, Molly Moran, Carla Stokes, Eric Stein, Mandy Terc, Cecilia Tomori, Emily Wentzell, and Nariman Zarzour.

I have been most fortunate to work closely on this project with five of my UM graduate students whom I hired as research assistants. Under my supervision and that of my colleague Jerome Nriagu, Luke King and Loulou Kobeissi undertook all of the epidemiological data entry and analysis. Luke King analyzed blood sample results, subsequently receiving his master's of public health degree and coauthoring an article with us on reproductive toxicology in Lebanon. Loulou Kobeissi painstakingly entered all of the reproductive history data and analyzed it from an epidemiological perspective, subsequently receiving her doctoral degree and coauthoring several articles with me and our colleagues in Lebanon. Emily Wentzell undertook a critical literature review, read several of the chapters, and generally helped me work through the masculinities literature. She also became my postdoctoral fellow at Yale and is now one of my main intellectual collaborators and coauthors. Mikaela Rogozen-Soltar has been my primary reader and bibliographer for this book, providing incredibly useful editorial feedback. Molly Moran helped me to put the final pieces in place. All of these talented students have helped me to "birth" this manuscript. I cannot thank them enough.

At Yale University, where I moved in 2008, I have been embraced enthusiastically and supportively by President Richard Levin, Vice President Linda Lorimer, Provost Peter Salovey, Associate Provosts Charles Long, Emily Bakemeier, and Frances Rosenbluth, and Ian Shapiro, the Henry R. Luce Director of the Whitney and Betty MacMillan Center for International and Area Studies, where I have chaired the Council on Middle East Studies (CMES). At Yale, I have had the opportunity to present parts of this manuscript to colleagues at CMES, the Department of Anthropology, the Global Health Working Group at the MacMillan Center, and the Medical History Program in the School of Medicine, where I received valuable feedback. At Yale, my research and writing has benefited from a supportive community of women colleagues and scholars, many of whom have become good friends as well. They include Julia Adams, Betsy Bradley, Judith Chevalier, Kamari Clarke, Jane Edwards, Inderpal Grewal, Mary Hu, Catherine Panter-Brick, Sally Promey, Nancy Ruther, Sallama Shaker, Helen Siu, and Laura Wexler. I am also surrounded by a wonderful and impressive group of junior colleagues in both Middle East Studies and Anthropology. Jafari Allen, Sean Brotherton, Narges Erami, Kaveh Khoshnood, and Mike McGovern deserve credit for crucial insights and literature suggestions that improved this manuscript immensely. I am particularly grateful to my fellow medical anthropologist, Sean Brotherton, who read most of the manuscript and made incisive comments. Thanks also go to our great faculty support team of Jennifer DeChello and Constance Buskey, who assisted me with photographs and permissions, and to Peter Kersten of Getty Images for his quick and helpful responses.

Beyond Yale, I am deeply indebted to a global community of anthropology scholars, who are also my dearest friends and who nurture my intellect and my soul. They include Aditya Bharadwaj, Daphna Birenbaum-Carmeli, Astrid Blystad, Mia Fuller, Zeynep Gurtin, Robert Hahn, Susan Martha Kahn, Karen Marie Moland, and Nefissa Naguib. I am most grateful to

Soraya Tremayne, who has literally shaped my worldview on the subject of Islam and ARTs over the past decade. She has become my primary interlocutor and coeditor, as well as a dear friend. Together, Soraya and I also traveled to Iran, where we were kindly hosted by Mohamad Mehdi Akhondi and Pegah Ebadi of the Avesina Research Center and University of Tehran. I am also eternally grateful to Mohammad Jalal Abbassi-Shavazi for the invitation to speak at the Iranian conference on "Embryo and Gamete Donation," and to Soheila Shashahani for her cordial hospitality and rug shopping expedition! I also want to thank Iran's Royan Institute, and particularly Reza O. Samani, for the great honor of receiving the 2010 Royan Epidemiology and Ethics Prize for my work. Unfortunately, due to pragmatic and political circumstances, I was unable to travel to Iran in late 2010 to receive that award.

Soraya and I are most fortunate to have had the opportunity to bring together a group of remarkable junior colleagues, all of whom work on assisted reproductive technologies in the Islamic world. They include Morgan Clarke, Thomas Eich, Shirin Garmaroudi, Zeynep Gurtin, Sandra Houot, Mansooreh Saniei, and Robert Tappan. I cannot thank Morgan Clarke enough for reading every word of this manuscript, helping to sharpen its arguments, clarify its fine points, and fine-tune its Arabic transliterations. His publications have been invaluable to my own work as well and are widely referenced in virtually every chapter of this book.

I have presented my research at a number of other universities, where I have received especially helpful feedback. These include AUB, Cambridge, Columbia, Harvard, King's College London, McGill, Oxford, Princeton, University of Bergen, University of California, Los Angeles, University of Manchester, and University of Pennsylvania. I want to thank Joao Biehl, Jude Browne, Wendy Chavkin, Jeannette Edwards, Linda Garro, Marie Griffiths, Sondra Hale, Hsain Iliahane, Firoozeh Kashani-Sabet, Arthur Kleinman, Ellen Mortensen, Iman Nuwayhid, Tobias Rees, Avi Shlaim, Susan Slyomovics, and Marilyn Strathern for their kind invitations and incredibly useful commentaries on my work. At Yale, I presented the prologue and introduction of the book to the Department of Anthropology and the Council on Middle East Studies, with incisive comments and encouragement offered by my peers.

I also want to thank those anthropologists whose theoretical and ethnographic work particularly inspires me. They include Arjun Appadurai, Joao Biehl, Suad Joseph, Arthur Kleinman, Margaret Lock, Rayna Rapp, Susan Slyomovics, and Marilyn Strathern. My entrée into the world of the "new masculinity studies" has been greatly enhanced by the work of R. W. Connell and by my colleagues Matthew Dudgeon, Matthew Gutmann, Lahoucine Ouzgane, and Richard Parker. The Middle East anthropologists Kamran Asdar Ali, Rhoda Kanaaneh, Diane King, Daniel Monterescu, and

Julie Peteet have also written path-breaking ethnographic pieces on various aspects of Middle Eastern manhood, from which I have drawn.

Over the past thirty years, I have been very fortunate to befriend a number of remarkable Middle Eastern men, who have shaped my thinking on many of the issues described in this volume. They include Abdulla and Khaled Al-Khalifa from Bahrain; Hassan Aly, Emad Esmat, Moharram Khalifa, Hatem Nabih, Mohymen Saddeek, Ali Sadek, and Khaled Zeitoun from Egypt; Mohammad Jalal Abbassi-Shavazi and Kaveh Khoshnood from Iran; Amaar Al-Hayder from Iraq; Gilbert Doumit from Lebanon; Mokhtar Ghambou from Morocco; and Iyad al-Khouri and Khaled Al-Saai from Syria. Thanks to all of them for being kind friends and defiers of the many pernicious stereotypes described in these chapters.

Several of my closest colleagues and friends, including Daphna Birenbaum-Carmeli, Sam Gedjenson, Nefissa Naguib, Sallama Shaker, and Soraya Tremayne, read parts of this manuscript, providing invaluable feedback. Many of the finishing touches were added to this book while I served as the first Diane Middlebrook and Carl Djerassi Visiting Professor in the Centre for Gender Studies at the University of Cambridge. I thank Jude Browne, Lesley Dixon, and Zeynep Gurtin for making my time at Cambridge simply amazing. I hope that the truly inspirational octogenarian, Carl Djerassi, is pleased with this book, given his own invention of the oral contraceptive and his several books and plays about intracytoplasmic sperm injection (ICSI), the assisted reproductive technology highlighted in this volume.

I want to thank Joao Biehl, Adriana Petryna, and Ian Shapiro for leading me to Princeton University Press, where I have had the great fortune to work with Fred Appel, the Anthropology and Religion senior editor, his assistant, Diana Goovaerts, and Terri O'Prey, production editor. I also want to thank Angel Foster and two anonymous readers, who provided excellent and compelling reviews.

I am sustained by a wonderful and talented community of friends in Connecticut, including John Casso and Mark Serchuk, Judy Chevalier and Steve Podos, Laura Davis and David Soper, Jo Handelsman and Casey Nagy, Betsy Henley-Cohn and Sam Gejdenson, Denise and Mark Gibson, Leslie Jacobsen and Jonathan Feinstein, Kiki and Ted Kennedy, Wendy Lewis and Tom Cleveland, Frances Rosenbluth and Ian Shapiro, and Sallama Shaker and Ghaleb Abdul-Rahman. A number of awesome women have also nurtured my spirit: Reesa Gringorten, Yun-Yang Lin, and Kathy Muench, who made beautiful music with me; Nancy Horn and Catherine Tesluk, who listened to my concerns and suggested solutions; Denise Samperi, who kept our house clean and fed my family while I was on leave at Cambridge; Amira and Kira, our affectionate cats; and the beautiful "Queen Rania," a disabled female raccoon who lives under our back porch and who visited me every day while I wrote this book, gradually mending in the process as I fed her fruits and baked goods. Rather than being a Yale "tiger mom," I am a "raccoon mom," as I tease my children.

My final thanks go to those nearest and dearest, including my oldest friend, Kristina Austin Nicholls, and my brothers, Lowell and Roger Inhorn, all of them caring, compassionate physicians who have helped me and my friends on many occasions. This book is dedicated to my parents, Shirley and Stanley Inhorn, now in their eighties, who continue to be smart as whips and excellent sounding boards. From my father, I received a keen sense of organization and scholarly discipline, as well as the love of the academic life. When I was a little girl, my father traveled as a public health doctor to Latin America with his University of Wisconsin anthropology colleagues. This was before there was a "medical anthropology," but it piqued my curiosity and, in some senses, sent me on my own future path. From my mother, I received the love of storytelling, spelling, and writing, as well as the ability to bake and to throw a fun and comfortable dinner party for people from around the world. My mother chose not to finish her own PhD in biochemistry, in a day when women in science were rare. She went on to be a devoted mom, who typed many papers in the days before computers and was the outstanding piano accompanist for me and my brothers, all string players in our father's "Inhorn Family Quartet." To both of my parents, I say "thank you," as well as "sorry" for the many worries I have put you through when I've taken myself and your grandchildren to the Middle East during unsettling times.

My *usra*—the little family that I have produced—is my pride and joy. My husband, Kirk Hooks, has done what few other American husbands would ever do, namely, encourage me in my anthropological career, including in three long periods of residence together in the Middle East, and in many weeks spent "holding down the fort" at home while I journeyed abroad. He is my human dictionary, my incisive grant reviewer, my fellow traveler, my reproductive "partner" in every sense of that term. He read every chapter of this book as I churned them out. Our children, Carl and Justine, continue to thrill us with their personalities, interests, and accomplishments. They have come to appreciate the Middle East for all of its beauties and for the kind Middle Eastern people whom they have met along the way. Indeed, Middle Eastern men have delighted over our children, showing them the kind of interest and affection that is rare for American men. Together, as a family, we dedicate this book to our driver, whom we shall call "Hamza" for the sake of anonymity, and to all of the other kind and compassionate Middle Eastern men whose stories deserve to be told and heard.

Appendix: The Assisted Reproduction *Fatwas*

Because the initial Al Azhar *fatwa* has been so profoundly important and authoritative for the majority of the world's Muslims, it is reproduced here, in a close translation (from classical Arabic into English) intended to convey the original language of its writing, as well as the style of religious-legal reasoning and analogy used to make prescriptive and proscriptive statements regarding IVF and related technologies. Furthermore, as will be clear throughout the *fatwa*, many references to Qur'anic passages and other scriptural sources are cited. It is important to note here that this *fatwa* was obtained by the author once it had already been translated from Arabic into English under the auspices of the Ford Foundation in Cairo, Egypt.[1]

1. Introduction

Lineage and relationship[s] of marriage are graces of Allah to mankind, highly appreciated, and they are [the] basis of judgment."It is He who has created man from water, then He has established relationships of lineage and marriage, for thy Lord has power over all things." (Furqan, or the Criterion 59) Therefore, origin preservation is a most essential objective of Islamic law.

In this concern, Scholar Elghazali stated:"Allah's goal is to prevent harm and cause welfare; however, human beings are to gain their benefit upon accomplishment of objectives. The benefit is to observe targets of Islamic law, which are five: to preserve beings' religion, themselves, [their] minds, descendants and money. Hence, any act implying preservation of these five fundamentals is a benefit, and, on the contrary, any act which jeopardizes them is then a harm."

Therefore, Allah permitted marriage and prohibited fornication to preserve the origins. "And among His signs is this, that He created for you mates from among yourselves, that ye may dwell in tranquility with them, and he has put love and mercy between your (hearts); verily, in that are signs for those who reflect." (Rum, or The Roman Empire 21)

"Nor come nigh to adultery: For it is a shameful (deed), and an evil, opening the road (to other evils)." (Esraa, or Children of Israel 32)

A legitimate child will grow and be raised by his parents in the best manner they can afford, while an illegitimate one is a shame for the mother and her people, neglected in the community and will then turn into a disease.

Islamic scholars discussed illegitimate children in books of Islamic law, [and] explained that they are human beings who deserve to be brought up properly and taken care of so as to stimulate what is best in them and avoid their evilness."And if any one saved a life, it would be as if he saved the life of the whole people." (Maida, or The Table 31)

As for proper origin[s], Islam is highly concerned[,] and hence it was coded in a way to call for marriage and guarantee stability of the family. Generally, Islam organized people's life in an appropriate pattern with justice and equity.

There are [a] few rules set by Islam to ensure appropriateness of origin which will be represented in the following:

Adultery is forbidden.

A compulsory period during which a divorcee should not remarry ('idda) (to ensure she is not already pregnant, which confuses father's identification).

Adoption is forbidden (by Qur'anic definition) for purposes of origin protection and family rights' preservation."Nor has He made your adopted sons your sons. Such is (only) your mouths. But God Tells (you) the truth, and He shows the (right) way. Call them by (the names of) their fathers: that is more just in the sight of God. But if ye know not their fathers' (names, call them) your brothers in faith, or your *maulas*." (Ahsab, or The Confederates 4,5)

In this, Islam is not to approve [of one] who has no origin, or force him on others.

Islam, [which] organized relations of a man and woman, emphasized that it should be in [the] form of proper marriage, so as to protect origins and respect a sperm from which a child is created."Now let man but think from what he is created! He is created from a drop emitted from between the backbone and the ribs." (Tariq, or The Night Visitant 5,6,7)"Verily, we created man from a drop of mingled sperm." (Dahr, or Time. Insan, or Man 2)

However, a sperm is not to acquire shape until it is introduced into a woman's womb ready to receive it, and that could be through a sexual body contact (intercourse). The child then will be called after his father, [if] the aspect of marriage is present. However, there are cases where a man's sperm could be introduced to a woman's womb through means other than body contact.

Islamic scholars elaborated in their books on this issue, and mentioned several examples where a woman was able to get and introduce a husband's or a master's sperm into her womb, which consequently will require a waiting period ('idda) before she remarries and creates a lineage.

In light of the above mentioned, we will discuss several issues in the following:

Marriage's noble objective is reproduction, so as to preserve mankind; moreover, body contact among husband and wife is based on natural desire.

Thus, body contact (intercourse) is the basic and only means allowing a sperm to reach the proper location as per Allah's will. If pregnancy could not occur through normal body contact (intercourse) due to some illness, it is then permissible to impregnate a woman by her husband's sperm through medical assistance (provided they are undoubtedly her husband's and not [that of] any other man or animal). A waiting period is then necessary and lineage is proved based on the previously mentioned examples.

If the husband is impotent, it is unlawful to have a stranger donate sperm. This consequently will confuse origins; furthermore, the method implies adultery which is strictly unlawful by [both the] Qur'an and Sunna (what has been taken from Prophet Muhammad, peace be upon him). If a woman's ovum to be impregnated by a man's sperm (not the husband), then the sperm donor's wife acts as surrogate, it is then considered adultery (confuses origins) as well as unlawful.

However, even though it is the husband's sperm which is not to acquire shape unless by Allah's permission upon unity with the wife's ovum, and since this aspect is not present in the case discussed, the wife then is not the husband's tilth as she should be as Allah says: "Your wives as a tilth unto you." (Baqara, or The Heifer 222) A woman shall not be pregnant unless through a normal legal intercourse with her husband or by introducing his sperm into her womb to acquire shape as Allah says: "He makes you, in the wombs of your mothers, in stages one after another, in three veils of darkness." (Zumaror, or The Crowds)

Hence, in the case discussed, the ovum is not the wife's, which implies unlawful adultery.

2. In Vitro Fertilization

[If] a wife's ovum is impregnated by her husband's sperm outside the womb in a tube, then implanted back to the womb with no doubts or confusion about sperm donor (human or animal) due to medical requirements [such] as illness of the husband or wife which might affect their relation.

However, if a trustworthy physician recommends in vitro fertilization and shall be responsible for its appropriateness, then it is permissible and obligatory as a treatment for a woman who has pregnancy impediments. Furthermore, Prophet Muhammad, peace be upon him, mentioned the necessity to seek remedy for any disease, and sterility is a disease that might be curable; therefore to seek lawful treatment is then permissible.

If the case was full surrogacy, in which an animal's womb will be used temporarily to bear and allow an impregnated ovum [to] go partially through stages of growth which are mentioned in the Qur'an: "Then we placed him as (a drop of) sperm in a place of rest, firmly fixed, then we made the sperm into a clot of congealed blood, then of that clot we made a lump [fetus], then we made out of that lump bones and clothed the bones with flesh, then we developed out of it another creature. So blessed be God, the best to create!" (Muminun, or The Believers 13,14) It will definitely acquire characteristics of the bearing animal according to genetics factors which were previously proven by the Qur'an. "Should he not know he that created?" (Mulk, or The Dominion 14) Our Prophet, peace be upon him, instructed us to choose the best woman as a wife for the sake of our children and to avoid beautiful women who grew up in a corrupted environment for genetic purposes as well as [for] ensuring a healthy atmosphere to bring up children.

The above mentioned clarifies even more how an animal's surrogacy is to affect the born creature, who will not be of a human nature. Therefore, a person who uses this method is to ruin Allah's creation. Allah says: "So fear God as much as ye can." (Tagabun, or The Mutual Loss and Gain 16)

According to Islamic law, one of the fundamentals is to prioritize harm prevention, then well being provision.

We conclude that this method of medically assisted reproduction [animal surrogacy] is an absolute cause of evil, therefore unlawful. As for the father who accepts one of the previously mentioned unlawful means of medically assisted reproduction, he is to be considered one who lost his dignity. Any child who is begotten through one of the stated cases is illegitimate, [if] it is certain that the sperm donor is not the father (adultery). Accordingly, the child is a foundling and is to be called after his mother.

Concerning the position of a physician who undertakes one of the unlawful cases, Islam allowed lawful treatment and the physician being the means to do so according to his experience. He is then responsible in case of negligence or seeking an unlawful (by Islam) method. Therefore, a physician responsible for medically assisted reproduction should study the method thoroughly [so] that it should not be unlawful, or else he will be sinning, for whatever led to an unlawful act is consequently unlawful. [Both the] Qur'an and Sunna indicated a very important principle, which is to cause harm prevention. "Revile not ye those whom they call upon besides God, lest they out of spite revile God in their ignorance." (Anam, or The Cattle 108) The principles are very clear as per the aforementioned verse; it calls not to curse polytheist Gods in order not to allow them to take it as a cause and curse Allah. Prophet Muhammad, peace be upon him, said: "May Allah damn alcohol, [a] person who drinks it, who offers it, who sells it, who buys it, who squeezes it, who carries it, and whom it is carried for." That proves one should not even assist in an unlawful act. Another example is that Islam forbids a man to study a woman's beauty or be alone with a woman, since that could be an atmosphere that causes adultery.

We herein conclude that based on the above mentioned verses of the Qur'an, definitions of the Sunna and examples, a physician who conducts a medically assisted reproduction in an unlawful form is at fault and his earning is bad.

A physician should only offer lawful treatment to a husband and wife wishing to have a legitimate child and establish a family. Furthermore, it is emphasized that medically assisted reproduction is only lawful among a husband and a wife, but to use such experiments so as to improve [the] race is absolutely unlawful. Instead of establishing a sperm bank taken from [the] best selection of men, then use it to impregnate also well-selected women, Islam instructed [us] to choose the best of either husband or wife in all aspects (health, ethics, mind, and so forth). It set lawful criteria to keep a strong and healthy human generation.

Finally, a human being is not to be taken as a means of experiment[ation], for Allah put him in a respecting position. "O ye who believe, give your response to God and his Apostle, when he calleth you to that which will give you life, and know that God cometh in between a man and his heart, and that it is he to whom ye shall (all) be gathered and fear tumult or oppression, which affecteth not in particular (only) those of you who do wrong: And know that God is strict in punishment." (Anfal, or The Spoils of War 24, 25).

The *Fatwa* of Ayatollah Ali Hussein al-Khamene'i

Ayatollah Khamene'i, who succeeded Ayatollah Khomeini after his death as the "leader of the revolution," was promoted in 1994 to the rank of *marja' al-taqlid*, or "source of emulation," defining him as a person embodying the highest principles of religious legitimacy and thus guaranteeing him a large following of Shia disciples. To that end, Ayatollah Khamene'i now regularly issues *fatwas* on a variety of subjects, often in answer to questions about new topics not mentioned in the Islamic scriptures. As shown here, his *fatwa* is presented in a question-and-answer format, quite different from the Al Azhar *fatwa* just cited. Unlike the Al Azhar *fatwa*, the author obtained this *fatwa* in an Arabic-language anthology of *fatwas* issued by Ayatollah Khamene'i. The translation of the Khamene'i *fatwa* from Arabic into English is as follows, with additional bracketed phrases by the author for the purposes of clarification in English:[2]

1. Questions

   a. Is IVF acceptable in case the sperm and egg came from the legally married couple?

   b. Suppose it is acceptable, could a foreign doctor do the operation? Would the newborn be considered the child of the married couple who collected the sperm and egg?

   c. Suppose IVF is not acceptable, could it be an exception when it comes in the form of a "marriage savior"?

2. Answer

Doing the IVF operation is acceptable under the cited circumstances. However, one should avoid getting involved in issues that are considered *haram* [forbidden] in Islamic Law—i.e., the foreign [presumably male] doctor should not perform the IVF procedure if it involves touch or gaze [of the woman's genitals].

3. Question

In some marriages where the woman does not have any eggs necessary for fertilization to occur, the couples are sometimes forced to separate or face marital and psychological disputes because their case is untreatable and they can't have any children. In this case, would it be acceptable to make use of another woman's egg and fertilize it with the husband's sperm outside of the uterus and then transfer the embryo back into the wife's uterus?

4. Answer

Although egg donation is not in and by itself legally forbidden, the newborn would be considered to be the child of the person who collected the sperm [the husband] and the egg donor, as well as the surrogate [infertile] mother. It follows that both the sperm collector [the husband] and egg donor have to apply the exceptions cited within the religious codes regarding parenting.

5. Questions

   a. If the sperm was taken from the husband and, after his death, it was fertilized by the wife's egg and implanted in her uterus, would this be considered legal?

b. Would the newborn be considered the husband's son and would he bear his name legally?

c. Does the child inherit from the owner of the sperm [the dead husband]?

6. Answer

It is okay to do the cited procedure and the newborn would be considered the child of the egg and uterus bearer and the sperm owner [dead husband], but he would not inherit anything from him.

7. Question

Is it okay to fertilize a woman's egg with a donor sperm in case her husband has some infertility problems, and then implant the fertilized embryo back into her uterus?

8. Answer

It is legally not forbidden to fertilize a woman's egg with a donor sperm in and by itself, but the opposite gender [infertile man] should avoid touching or seeing the [female] child [naked], as these are considered *haram*. In any case, a child born this way would not carry the name of his father, but rather that of the sperm owner [the donor] and the egg and uterus carrier. However, in such instances, one should abide by the exceptions that have to do with inheritance and veiling issues.

Glossary of Arabic Terms

ahlan wa-sahlan: Welcome.

al harb: The war, usually referring to the Lebanese civil war (1975–90).

alf alf mabruk: A million congratulations.

Al-Ka'ba: The stone circumambulated by pilgrims to Mecca, Saudi Arabia, the most sacred site in Islam.

Ana mish ragil: "I am not a man" (Egyptian dialect).

Ana da'if: "I am weak"; a reference to male infertility.

'aql: Intellectual reasoning.

'aqam: Infertility; sometimes used to denote erectile dysfunction as well.

'asabi: Nervous.

asmar shway: Slightly brown.

bint 'amm: Father's brother's daughter.

bint 'amma: Father's sister's daughter.

bizri: Seeds; a reference to sperm in Levantine dialect.

da'f: Weakness.

daght: Pressure, stress.

daght nafsi: Psychological stress.

da'if: Weak.

daman: Health insurance provided through the Lebanese National Social Security Fund (NSSF).

didan: Worms; a reference to sperm in Egyptian dialect.

Druze: A Shia Muslim subsect, many of whose adherents live in the mountainous regions of central Lebanon.

duktura (f.): Doctor.

fatwa: Religious proclamation outlining which attitudes and practices are *halal* (permitted) or *haram* (prohibited); a nonlegally binding but authoritative Islamic religious opinion, offered by an Islamic cleric who is considered to be an expert concerning the Islamic scriptures and jurisprudence.

fiqh: Islamic jurisprudence.

habiba (f.): Loved one.

habibi/ habibti (m./f.): "My love" or "my loved one," but also understood as "my dear," "my dear friend," or simply "my friend."

Hadith: Narrations of the words and deeds of the Prophet Muhammad.

hal nafsiya: Psychological condition.

halal: Permitted.

hamdu-lillah: Praise be to God.

haraka: Movement, motility; used in reference to sperm.

haram: Prohibited.

harami: Thief.

hasad: Envy; evil eye.

hasanat: Good deeds.

hayawanat al-minawi: Spermatic animals; a reference to sperm in some dialects of Arabic.

hijab: Islamic headscarf.

hubb: Love.

hudud: Islamic law stating the limits ordained by God.

ibn haram: Son of the forbidden; bastard.

'idda: Waiting period required to establish pregnancy.

Ijtihad: Religious reasoning.

ikhtilat al-ansab: Mixture of (genealogical) relations.

insha'Allah: God willing.

insha'Allah khayr: Formulaic expression of divine intervention said as an expression of good luck within Lebanese clinics.

jallabiya: Traditional male robe.

jihad: Mandate to defend the religion when it is threatened by outside forces.

kafalat al-yatim: Guardianship of orphans.

kafil: Guardian.

katb al-kitab: Marriage contract.

khalas: Over; finished.

kufr: Apostasy.

laqit: An abandoned orphan or foundling; these orphans are considered to be the illegitimate offspring of unmarried persons.

madrasa: School.

ma fi shi abadan: There is nothing wrong at all.

mahram: Someone forbidden to you in marriage (e.g., a woman's brother), affecting gender comportment in family life (e.g., no requirement to veil before him).

majlis: Council; the term used for the Iranian parliament.

makruh: A practice that is reprehensible and should be avoided but is not absolutely prohibited (*haram*).

marad: Disease; sickness.

marja' al-taqlid: Source of emulation, usually contracted to *marja'*; Shia religious authority of the highest rank; source of guidance for lay Shia Muslims.

mash Allah: What God wills.

miskin: Poor one.

mufti: A jurist who interprets Islamic law.

mut'a: Also called *sigheh* in Iran; a fixed-term contract of temporary marriage in Shia Islam.

nafsiya: Mental life; psychology.

nargila: Traditional water pipe; also called hookah or hubble bubble (in English) or *argila, shisha, mu'assal* (in Arabic).

nasab: Filiation; lineage; relations by blood; genealogy.

nasib: Destiny; fate.

qaraba: Relation; closeness; kinship.

Qur'an: The sacred writings of Islam revealed by God to the Prophet Muhammad.

Rajul: Man.

rida': Milk kinship.

rizq: God's bounty or sustenance, believed to be inherent in the birth of every child.

rujula: Manhood or masculinity (*rujuli* in Lebanese dialect).

Sayyid: Descendant of the Prophet Muhammad.

Shafi'i: One of the four schools of Islamic jurisprudence within the Sunni branch of Islam.

Shaykh: Honorific term for an elder, an Islamic scholar, or a person of royal lineage.

Shari'a: Body of religious law.

Shia: The minority branch of Islam, constituting slightly more than 10 percent of the world's Muslim population.

sifah al-maharim: Incest; having sex with those prohibited to you.

Sunna: The way of the Prophet Muhammad.

Sunni: The majority branch of Islam, constituting 80 to 90 percent of the world's Muslim population.

Tabanni: Adoption.

tifl unbub: Baby of a tube; test-tube baby (in Levantine dialect).

tahlil bizri: Sperm analysis.

takafful: Guardianship or sponsorship, whereby an adult supports the living expenses of a child, often in an orphanage; the care of orphans.

umma: Community of the faithful.

'umra: A pilgrimage by Muslims to Mecca, Saudi Arabia, which can be undertaken at any time of the year.

usra: Nuclear family.

walad al-zina: Son of illicit sex; out-of-wedlock bastard.

walla marra: Not once.

wiratha: Heredity.

wirathi: Hereditary.

zakat: Charity to the less fortunate, a religious duty.

zina: Illicit sexuality in Islam, including adultery.

Glossary of Medical Terms

assisted reproduction (a.k.a. assisted conception): A number of advanced medical techniques to aid fertilization, thereby achieving pregnancy in couples with infertility; in vitro fertilization (IVF) is the best known of the assisted reproduction techniques.

assisted reproductive technology (ART): All fertility treatments in which both eggs and sperm are handled; in general, ART procedures involve surgically removing eggs from a woman's ovaries, combining them with sperm in the laboratory, and returning them to the woman's body or donating them to another woman; IVF is the best-known ART.

asthenozoospermia: The condition in which a male has poor sperm motility (i.e., movement); normally, at least 50 percent of sperm should be motile.

azoospermia: The condition in which a male has complete absence of sperm in the ejaculate.

congenital bilateral absence of the vas deferens: An inherited condition in males where the tubes that carry sperm out of the testes (the vas deferens; see below) fail to develop properly; although the testes usually develop and function normally, sperm cannot become part of the semen because the vas deferens is missing; as a result, men with this condition are unable to father children unless they use assisted reproductive technologies; this condition is one of the signs of cystic fibrosis, an inherited disease of the mucus glands (see below); when absence of the vas deferens occurs alone, it is considered a mild, genital form of cystic fibrosis.

cross-border reproductive care (a.k.a. reproductive tourism; see below): Movements of individuals and couples who are seeking assisted reproductive technologies (ARTs) from a country or jurisdiction where ARTs are unavailable to another country or jurisdiction where they can obtain the treatment they need.

cyropreservation: Freezing of tissue or cells in order to preserve these for future use; sperm samples and excess embryos are routinely frozen for future ART cycles; more recently, eggs and ovarian tissue have also been cryopreserved.

cystic fibrosis: An inherited disease that causes thick, sticky mucus to build up in the lungs and digestive tract; it is one of the most common chronic lung diseases in children and young adults, and may result in early death; males with cystic fibrosis are infertile because of congenital absence of the vas deferens (see above).

diagnostic laparoscopy: A surgical procedure that allows a health care provider to view a woman's reproductive organs; several gynecological problems can be diagnosed (and treated) this way.

donor insemination (DI): The process by which sperm from a male donor is placed into the reproductive tract of a female for the purpose of impregnation without sexual intercourse; DI is used in cases where the male partner produces no sperm or the woman has no male partner (i.e., single women, lesbians); in the Middle East, donor insemination is practiced only in cases of male infertility and only in two countries, Iran and Lebanon.

donor technologies: All forms of third-party reproductive assistance, including sperm donation, oocyte (egg) donation, embryo donation, and gestational surrogacy; in the Middle East, donor technologies are used in only two countries, Iran and Lebanon.

ectopic pregnancy: A complication of pregnancy in which the embryo implants outside the uterine cavity; most ectopic pregnancies occur in the fallopian tube (so-called tubal pregnancies), but implantation can also occur in the cervix, ovaries, and abdomen; with rare exceptions (abdominal pregnancies), ectopic pregnancies are not viable; an ectopic pregnancy is a potential medical emergency, and, if not recognized and treated properly, can lead to death.

egg donation (aka oocyte donation): The process by which a woman provides one or several (usually ten to fifteen) eggs (ova, oocytes) for purposes of assisted reproduction or biomedical research.

embryo: A fertilized egg that has begun cell division, first called a pre-embryo (or pre-implantation embryo), and then an embryo at the completion of the pre-embryonic stage, which is considered to end at about day fourteen; in general, the term embryo is used to describe the early stages of fetal growth, from conception to the eighth week of pregnancy.

embryo disposition: Decisions about the future use of excess embryos produced through ART cycles; choices include cryopreservation (freezing), disposal, donation to other couples, or donation to medical research.

embryo donation: Excess embryos produced in one couple's ART cycle are donated to other couples for their use; in the Middle East, embryo donation is currently practiced in only one country, Iran.

endometriosis: A female gynecological condition in which the tissue that behaves like the cells lining the uterus (endometrium) grows in other areas of the body, causing pain, irregular bleeding, and possible infertility.

epididymis: A narrow, tightly coiled tube connecting the efferent ducts from the rear of each testicle to the vas deferens (see below); spermatozoa formed in the testis undergo maturation in the epididymis before exiting the body through ejaculation.

erectile dysfunction (a.k.a. impotence): The inability of a man to attain or sustain a penile erection.

European Society for Human Reproduction and Embryology (ESHRE): Formed in 1985, the main European professional organization to promote interest in, and understanding of, reproductive biology and medicine; ESHRE does this through facilitating research and subsequent dissemination of research findings in human reproduction and embryology to the general public, scientists, clinicians, and patient associations; it also works to inform politicians and policy makers throughout Europe.

fine-needle aspiration (FNA): A technique involving the insertion of a thin needle into the testes of an azoospermic man in an attempt to collect testicular tissue and possibly detect mature sperm.

follicle stimulating hormone (FSH): A hormone synthesized and secreted by gonadotrophs of the anterior pituitary gland in the brain; FSH regulates the development, growth, pubertal maturation, and reproductive processes of the body.

gamete: A mature sexual reproductive cell, either a sperm or egg, which unites with another cell to form a new organism.

gamete donation: Donation of sperm or eggs from one human or couple to another.

high-order multiple pregnancy (HOMP): Triplets, quadruplets, and beyond, often the result of an ART cycle or treatment with fertility drugs.

human cloning: Autonomous, asexual reproduction, involving the creation of a genetically identical copy of a human; human cloning is ethically controversial and widely banned; it has yet to be successfully achieved in humans, despite its success in other mammals.

human embryonic stem cell (hESC): Pluripotent stem cells derived from the inner cell mass (ICM) of the blastocyst, an early-stage embryo; isolating the inner cell mass results in destruction of the human embryo, which raises ethical issues; nonetheless, under defined conditions, embryonic stem cells are capable of propagating themselves indefinitely, thereby producing limitless numbers of themselves for continued research, regenerative medicine, and tissue replacement after injury or disease.

hydrocele: The presence of fluid within the scrotum (the sac that contains the testicles), sometimes occurring as a complication of varicocelectomy (see below); the main symptom is a painless, but swollen scrotum.

hypospadias: A birth defect in males in which the opening of the urethra is on the underside, rather than at the end, of the penis; in moderate to severe cases, it requires surgical correction during infancy.

hysteroscopy: The inspection of the uterine cavity by a lighted scope with access through the cervix; hysteroscopy allows for the diagnosis of intrauterine pathology and serves as a method for surgical intervention inside the uterus.

iatrogenesis: Inadvertent adverse effects or complications caused by or resulting from medical treatment or advice; physician-induced harm.

idiopathic: Any disease that is of uncertain or unknown origin.

impotence: See erectile dysfunction.

infertility: The failure of a couple to conceive a pregnancy after trying to do so for at least one full year; in *primary infertility*, pregnancy has never occurred; in *secondary infertility*, one or both members of the couple have previously conceived, but are unable to conceive again after a full year of trying; the World Health Organization considers the diagnosis of infertility to occur after two years of trying to conceive.

International Conference on Population and Development (ICPD) (a.k.a. the "Cairo Conference"): A conference coordinated by the United Nations in Cairo, Egypt, September 5–13, 1994; its resulting Programme of Action is the steering document for the United Nations Population Fund (UNFPA); infertility was included in the ICPD program, along with a variety of population issues, including infant mortality, birth control, family planning, the education of women, and protection for women from unsafe abortion services.

intracytoplasmic sperm injection (ICSI): A variant of in vitro fertilization (IVF), developed in Belgium in 1991, in which a single sperm is injected directly into an egg to "aid" fertilization; the procedure was designed to overcome male infertility problems, although it is now beginning to supplant IVF because of improved fertilization rates; the procedure is carried out in IVF laboratories under a high-powered microscope using multiple micromanipulation devices; although ICSI is considered safe and effective for overcoming male infertility, it may carry an increased risk for the transmission of selected genetic abnormalities to offspring, either through the procedure itself or through the increased inherent risk of such abnormalities in parents requiring the procedure.

intrauterine insemination (IUI): The process by which sperm is placed into the reproductive tract of a female for the purpose of impregnation by means other than sexual intercourse; in humans, it is an assisted reproductive technology, using either sperm from the woman's male partner or sperm from a sperm donor in cases where the male partner produces no sperm or the woman has no male partner (i.e., single women, lesbians); generally in IUI, "washed sperm" that have been removed from most other components of the seminal fluids are injected directly into a woman's uterus.

in vitro fertilization (IVF): A process by which egg cells are fertilized by sperm outside the body, or in vitro; the process involves hormonally controlling the ovulatory process, removing oocytes (eggs) from the woman's ovaries and letting sperm fertilize them in a fluid medium in a laboratory, the resulting embryo is then transferred to the patient's uterus with the intent to establish a successful pregnancy; IVF is the most well-known ART, invented in 1978 with the first successful birth of a "test tube baby," Louise Brown; Robert G. Edwards, the doctor who developed the treatment, was awarded the Nobel Prize in Physiology or Medicine in 2010.

motility: Movement of the sperm, required for successful fertilization.

multifetal pregnancy: A pregnancy with twins, triplets, or beyond; the incidence has increased dramatically over the past two decades, mainly because of the widespread use of ovulation induction agents and assisted reproductive technologies (ARTs); twin and higher order pregnancies have long been associated with an increased risk of maternal complications as well as a high prevalence of prenatal and neonatal morbidity and mortality.

multifetal pregnancy reduction (MPR) (a.k.a. selective reduction): A procedure of selective therapeutic abortion, which, in recent years, has become both clinically and ethically accepted as a therapeutic option in pregnancies with three, four, or more fetuses and in multifetal pregnancies in which one or more of the fetuses have congenital abnormalities; in cases of twin and triplet gestations, however, this option remains controversial; although several techniques of MPR have been reported, the most popular is the injection of potassium chloride into the fetal heart through the mother's abdomen at ten to twelve weeks' gestation.

mumps orchitis: An inflammation of one or both testicles, most commonly associated with the virus that causes mumps; at least one-third of males who contract mumps after puberty develop orchitis, and most will go on to experience male infertility.

non-obstructive azoospermia: The condition in which a male has complete absence of sperm in the ejaculate because sperm production is severely disturbed or absent; the testes are abnormal, atrophic, or poorly developed, and FSH levels (see above) tend to be elevated; causes include congenital and genetic issues, undescended testicles, mumps orchitis, surgery, cancer radiation, and other causes; men with unexplained non-obstructive azoospermia need to undergo a chromosomal and genetic evaluation and ultimately may need a testicular biopsy to clarify the diagnosis.

obstructive azoospermia: A form of male infertility in which the passage of sperm out of the testes, where they are produced, is somehow blocked, leading to azoospermia (see above); obstructive azoospermia can be caused by congenital absence of the vas deferens (see above), or a vasectomy; furthermore, sexually transmitted infections such as chlamydia and gonorrhea may cause inflammation of the epididymis, thereby obstructing the tubules conducting mature sperm out of the testes into the vas deferens (see below).

oligoasthenozoospermia: The condition in which a male with a low sperm count will also have poor sperm motility.

oligozoospermia: The condition in which a male has semen with a low concentration of sperm (low sperm count); for many decades, sperm concentrations of less than 20 million sperm per milliliter were considered low or oligozoospermic; recently, however, the World Health Organization (WHO) reassessed sperm criteria and established a lower reference point, less than 15 million, consistent with the fifth percentile for fertile men.

oocyte (a.k.a. ovum, egg): The female gamete in many sexually reproducing organisms, including humans.

oocyte donation: See egg donation (above).

ooplasm transfer (OT): An experimental fertility technique that involves injecting a small amount of ooplasm from eggs of fertile women into eggs of usually older women whose fertility is compromised; the modified egg is then fertilized with sperm and implanted in the uterus of the woman attempting to achieve pregnancy; children born from this procedure have been reported to possess cytoplasmic organelles called mitochondria from both their biological mother and the ooplasmic donor, a condition referred to as mitochondrial heteroplasmy.

percutaneous epididymal sperm aspiration (PESA): One of the surgical sperm harvesting techniques used for retrieving sperm in patients with obstructive azoospermia (see above), especially following vasectomy; a small needle is inserted through the skin of the scrotum to collect sperm from the epididymis, where sperm are usually stored after production in the testes; PESA is now also widely used to extract sperm for intracytoplasmic sperm injection (ICSI) (see above).

preimplantation genetic diagnosis (PGD): A technique used to identify genetic defects in embryos created through in vitro fertilization (IVF) before their transfer into the uterus; when one or both genetic parents has a known genetic abnormality, the testing is performed on one of the cells of the embryo to determine if it also carries a genetic abnormality; controversial uses of PGD include sex selection and the creation of "savior siblings" for children with life-threatening illnesses.

premature ovarian failure (POF) (a.k.a. premature menopause): The loss of function of the ovaries before age forty.

reproductive tourism (a.k.a. fertility tourism, reproductive tourism): See cross-border reproductive care (above).

sexually transmitted infection (STI): An illness that has a significant probability of transmission between humans by means of human sexual behavior, including vaginal intercourse, oral sex, and anal sex; a person may be infected and may potentially infect others, without showing signs of disease.

spermatogenesis: The process by which spermatozoa (see below) are produced; in mammals, it occurs in the male testes in a stepwise fashion, and for humans takes approximately sixty-four days; spermatogenesis is highly dependent upon optimal conditions for the process to occur correctly and is essential for sexual reproduction.

spermatozoa: The mature male gametes in many sexually reproducing organisms, including humans.

sperm donation: The provision (or donation) by a man, known as a sperm donor, of his sperm, known as donor sperm, with the intention that it be used to impregnate a woman who is not usually the man's sexual partner in order to produce a child.

surrogacy: An arrangement in which a woman carries and delivers a child for another couple or person; she may be the child's genetic mother by contributing her own egg (traditional surrogacy), or she may carry the pregnancy to delivery after another couple's embryo is transferred to her uterus (gestational surrogacy).

teratozoospermia: The condition in which a male has abnormally shaped sperm, which can negatively affect fertility by preventing sperm from adhering to the ovum; these abnormalities may include heads that are large, small, tapered, or misshapen, or tails that are abnormally shaped.

testicular sperm aspiration (TESA): One of the surgical sperm harvesting techniques used for retrieving sperm in patients with azoospermia (see above); using a local anesthetic, a small needle and a special syringe are used to extract sperm directly from the testicles to be used for diagnosis and/or sperm freezing.

testicular sperm extraction (TESE): One of the surgical sperm harvesting techniques used for retrieving sperm in patients with azoospermia (see above); sperm are extracted from testicular tissue obtained through a small incision in the scrotum and in the testicles (see testicular biopsy).

testicular biopsy: One of the surgical sperm harvesting techniques used for retrieving sperm in patients with azoospermia (see above); using local or general anesthesia, a testicular biopsy removes a small sample of tissue from one or both testicles and examines it under a microscope to evaluate the presence of sperm and a man's ability to father a child.

third-party reproductive assistance (a.k.a. donation): See donor technologies (above).

undescended testicle (a.k.a. cryptorchidism): One or both testicles fail to move into the scrotum before birth; common in premature infants and in about 3–4 percent of full-term infants; testicles that do not descend by the time the child is one year old should be surgically descended into the scrotum to reduce the chances of permanent damage to the testicles, including both male infertility and testicular cancer.

varicocele: An abnormal enlargement of the vein that is in the scrotum draining the testicles; a varicocele occurs when the valves within the veins along the spermatic cord do not work properly; this is essentially the same process as varicose veins, which are common in the legs; the backflow of blood and increased pressure may lead to damage to the testicular tissue, causing male infertility.

varicocelectomy: The surgical correction of a varicocele, which is present in approximately 40 percent of men with infertility; although varicocelectomy is the most common male infertility surgery, including in the Middle East, the effectiveness of varicocelectomy has been intensely debated and is no longer recommended by many infertility specialists or the World Health Organization.

vas deferens: Part of the male anatomy involved in transport of sperm from the epididymis (see above) in anticipation of ejaculation.

Notes

PROLOGUE: HAMZA, MY INFERTILE DRIVER

1. All names in this volume are pseudonyms.

INTRODUCTION: RECONCEIVING MIDDLE EASTERN MANHOOD

1. Ouzgane 2006.
2. Inhorn et al. 2010.
3. Inhorn and Patrizio 2009.
4. Inhorn 2008.
5. Shaheen 2008.
6. Abu-Lughod 1986.
7. Abu-Lughod 1991.
8. Abu-Lughod 1989.
9. As a board member of the Middle East Studies Association (MESA), editor of the *Journal of Middle East Women's Studies* (*JMEWS*), and chair of the Yale Council on Middle East Studies (CMES), I organized this conference theme with MESA president Suad Joseph, who is also an anthropologist. We are very grateful to Bonnie Rose Schulman, who is JMEWS managing editor and CMES program coordinator, for assisting us with the conference planning.
10. Mahdavi 2008.
11. Inhorn 1994, 1996, and 2003.
12. Ali 1996; Boddy 1989, 2007; Clarke 2009; Delaney 1991; Fadlalla 2007; Good 1994; Ivry 2009; Kahn 2000; Kanaaneh 2002; Loeffler 2007; Morsy 1993; Onder 2007; Pliskin 1987; Raz 2005; Sanai 2011; Teman 2010.
13. The Diana Forsythe Prize, given by the Council on the Anthropology of Science, Technology, and Computing (CASTAC) of the American Anthropological Association, celebrated ten years of award-winning science and technology ethnographies at the 2009 AAA Annual Meeting in Philadelphia.
14. Gutmann 1997.
15. Ben-Ari 1998; Cornwall and Lindisfarne 1994; Jones 2006; Kanaaneh 2005, 2008; Lupton and Barclay 1997; Monterescu 2006, 2007; Nashif 2008; Ouzgane and Morrell 2005; Pringle 2005; Townsend 2002.
16. Brandes 1981, 2003; Carillo 2002; Gonzalez-Lopez 2005; Gutmann 1996, 2003, 2007; Hirsch 2003; Lancaster 1992; McKee Irwin 2003; Padilla 2007; Parker 1991, 1998.
17. Gutmann 1997, p. 386, emphasis added.
18. Gutmann 2007.
19. De Beauvoir 1975.
20. Inhorn et al. 2009.
21. Inhorn 2006a.

22. Reed 2005; Townsend 2002.

23. Kilshaw 2009.

24. Gutmann 2007.

25. Gay Becker's *The Elusive Embryo* (2000) was one of the few ethnographies to include men, as both infertile users of ARTs and donor insemination, and as partners to infertile women.

26. A new ethnography by my former student and colleague, Emily Wentzell, based on her PhD thesis (Wentzell 2009), is forthcoming.

27. Eager 2007; Haberland and Measham 2002; Sen et al. 2002.

28. Hartmann 2002; Roberts 1998.

29. Inhorn and Birenbaum-Carmeli 2010.

30. Petchesky et al. 2001.

31. Spar 2006.

32. Inhorn and van Balen 2002.

33. Inhorn 2009a.

34. My mother was deeply offended and reported the incident to me. However, her answer to my relative about the social suffering of infertility and my quest for understanding this in the Middle East failed to resonate with my relatives.

35. Dudgeon and Inhorn 2003, 2004.

36. Greene 2000.

37. Schneider and Schneider 1995.

38. Basu 1996.

39. Greene and Biddlecom 2000.

40. Inhorn 2006a.

41. Greene and Biddlecom 2000.

42. Ibid.

43. Examples include Ahmed 1992; Charrad 2001; Hatem 1986; Kandiyoti 1991, 1994; Mernissi 1987, 1991; Mir-Hosseini 2002; Moors 1996; Sabbah 1984.

44. Suad Joseph 1993, 1994, 1999, 2000, 2004, 2009.

45. Examples include Boddy 1994; El Guindi 1999; Gole 1997; Gruenbaum 2000; MacLeod 1993; Mernissi 1987, 1991; Saadawi 1980; Sedghi 2007; Wikan 2008; Zuhur 1992a.

46. Examples include Abu-Lughod 1986, 1993; Al-Ali 2007; Al-Ali and Pratt 2009; cooke 1996; Grima 2005; Kapchan 1996; Makdisi 1990.

47. Examples include Al-Ali 2000; Brodsky 2003; Esfandiari 1997; Hale 1996, 1997; Moghadam 2003; Peteet 2005; Shahidian 2002; White 2003.

48. A 2009 American Anthropological Association panel "Having Relations: Gender Enactment in Female/Male Interactions," organized by Emily A. Wentzell in Philadelphia, explored this lacuna within anthropology.

49. Lagrange 2000.

50. Kanaaneh 2008; Kaplan 2000, 2005; Peteet 2005; Sinclair-Webb 2000.

51. Massad 2008.

52. Aghacy 2009.

53. Shaheen 2008.

54. Ghoussoub and Sinclair-Webb 2000.

55. Sinclair-Webb 2000, p. 8.

56. Ibid.

57. Ghoussoub 2000, p. 230.

58. Sinclair Webb 2000, p. 9.

59. Storrow 2005. The three books are: *Quest for Conception: Gender, Infertility, and Egyptian Medical Traditions* (1994); *Infertility and Patriarchy: The Cultural Politics of Gender and Family Life in Egypt* (1996); and *Local Babies, Global Science: Gender, Religion, and In Vitro Fertilization in Egypt* (2003).

60. Inhorn 1996, pp. 3–4.

61. Ouzgane 2006.

62. Ouzgane and Morrell 2005.

63. Inhorn 2006b.

64. Inhorn 2005.

65. Inhorn 1996, p. 46.

66. Inhorn 2003.

67. My PhD is from the Joint Program in Medical Anthropology at the University of California, Berkeley/University of California, San Francisco. My Master's of Public Health (MPH) degree in Epidemiology is from the UC-Berkeley School of Public Health.

68. Langness and Frank 1981; Singer 2005.

69. The best recent example is Biehl 2005; see also Frank 2000.

70. Hollan 2001, p. 48.

71. Biehl et al. 2007, p. 1.

72. Abraham and Shryock 2000.

73. World Health Organization 2010.

74. In a few cases, other family members, such as a mother, a mother-in-law, a father-in-law, a brother, or a child, were present.

75. From 2001–8, I was a professor at the University of Michigan. While in Lebanon from January–August 2003, I was a visiting research professor at the American University of Beirut, Faculty of Health Sciences. My project was reviewed and approved by institutional review boards (IRBs) at both universities.

76. The issue of tape-recording will be taken up in chapter 2. Suffice it to say here that most men were not comfortable speaking to a tape recorder, even if they agreed to speak to the anthropologist. This was also true in my earlier studies of infertility and IVF in Egypt; IVF was considered "top secret" at the time (see Inhorn 2003 and 2004a).

77. Blood can be used as a biomarker of heavy metal toxicity. Some heavy metals, such as lead, are spermatotoxic, leading to male infertility (see Inhorn et al. 2008a).

78. Inhorn 2004a.

79. Lloyd 1996.

80. Inhorn 2003, 2004a.

81. Inhorn and Fakih 2006.

82. Inhorn and Shrivastav 2010.

83. Inhorn 2006c.

84. Franklin 2007.

85. Riska 2003; Rosenfeld and Faircloth 2006.

86. Inhorn 1994, 2005, 2006b.

87. World Health Organization 2010.

88. Becker 2002.

89. Tournaye 2002.

90. Professor Mohamed Yehia introduced ICSI to Egypt in 1994, a story that is told in my book, *Local Babies, Global Science: Gender, Religion, and in Vitro Fertilization in Egypt*.

91. Becker 2000.

92. Ola et al. 2001.

93. Moore 2008.

94. Bentley and Mascie-Taylor 2000; Bittles and Matson 2000.

95. Friese et al. 2006, 2007.

96. Becker 1994, 1997; Friese et al. 2006, 2007; Kirkman 2003.

97. Wentzell and Salmerón 2009; Inhorn and Wentzell 2011.

98. Two of the senior physicians with whom I worked in Lebanon had trained at Yale and one at Harvard. Another was trained in Japan. Several of the physicians and embryologists had also received training in Michigan.

99. Hoodfar 1995; Garmaroudi, in press; Saniei, in press; Najmabadi 2005; Tober 2004, 2008; Tremayne, in press.

100. Inhorn 1994.

101. Williams 1978, p. 123.

102. Connell 1995.

103. Inhorn 2005, 2006b.

104. Myntti et al. 2000, pp. 169–170.

105. Kleinman 2006; 1997, p. 45.

106. Kleinman and Kleinman 1992.

107. Asad 1986, p. 14.

108. Brockopp 2003; Brockopp and Eich 2008; Sachedina 2009; Serour 1991, 1994.

109. Lotfalian 2004.

110. Lotfalian 2004, p. 6; see Huntington 1996.

111. Blyth and Landau 2004.

112. Hess 1994, p. 16.

113. Inhorn and Tremayne, in press.

114. Gelvin 2005, p. 292.

115. Ouzgane 2006, p. 1.

116. Ouzgane 2006, p. 2.

117. Ouzgane 2006, p. 6.

118. Ibid.

CHAPTER 1: HEGEMONIC MASCULINITY

1. Inhorn and Wentzell, 2011.

2. Carrigan et al. 1985; Connell 1990, 1993, 1995, 2001; Connell and Messerschmidt 2005. See Gramsci 1971.

3. Williams 1978.

4. Inhorn 2005, 2006b.

5. Carrigan et al. 1985.

6. Connell 1995.

7. Carrigan et al. 1985.

8. Connell 1995.

9. Ibid.

10. Connell 1993.

11. Connell 1995, p. 37.

12. Connell 1993.

13. Connell and Messerschmidt 2005, p. 848.

14. Connell 1993, p. 602.

15. Demetriou 2001, p. 355.

16. Demetriou 2001.

17. Donaldson 1993, pp. 645–46.

18. Connell and Messerschmidt 2005.

19. Connell 1993, p. 601.

20. Inhorn and Wentzell 2011.

21. Connell 1995.

22. Inhorn and Wentzell 2011.

23. Connell and Messerschmidt 2005, p. 830.

24. Connell and Messerschmidt 2005, p. 854.

25. Connell and Messerschmidt 2005, p. 848.

26. Ibid.

27. Connell and Messerschmidt 2005, p. 849.

28. Connell and Messerschmidt 2005, p. 851.

29. Connell and Messerschmidt 2005, p. 846.

30. Connell and Messerschmidt 2005, p. 854.

31. Connell et al. 1982.

32. I am grateful to Mikaela Rogozen-Soltar (2010) for introducing me to the concept of "self-stereotypy," or how cultural groups produce and disseminate indigenous stereotypes. I would like to call this form of self-stereotyping *indigenous Orientalism.*

33. Said 1978; Said and Hitchens 2001.

34. Inhorn and Fakih 2006.

35. Massad 2008.

36. Sobo 1995.

37. Wajahat 2010.

38. Wajahat 2010, p. 2.

39. Connell and Messerschmidt 2005.

40. Inhorn 1996.

41. Williams 1978. I thank my colleague, Mike McGovern, for leading me to this reference.

42. Williams 1978, p. 125, emphasis in original.

43. Williams 1978, p. 123.

44. Padilla 2007.

45. Gutmann 1996, 2003, 2007; Gonzalez-Lopez 2005; Hirsch 2003; Wentzell 2009.

46. McLelland and Dasgupta 2005; Taga 2004.

47. Baird 2010, p. 24.
48. Ibid.
49. Inhorn 2003, chap. 7; Lock 1993; Van Wolputte 2004.

CHAPTER 2: INFERTILE SUBJECTIVITIES

1. Greil and McQuillan 2010.
2. Vayena et al. 2002.
3. Irvine 1998.
4. Boerma and Zaida 2000; van Balen and Inhorn 2002.
5. Devroey et al. 1998.
6. Inhorn and Birenbaum-Carmeli 2010.
7. Inhorn 2004b.
8. Maduro and Lamb 2002.
9. Mundigo 1998, 2000.
10. Becker 2000, 2002; Greil 1991.
11. Upton 2002.
12. Van Balen and Inhorn 2002.
13. Lloyd 1996.
14. Brown 1993, p. 1675.
15. Webb and Daniluk 1999.
16. Webb and Daniluk 1999, p. 15, emphasis in original.
17. Moynihan 1998.
18. Abbey et al. 1991; Daniluk 1988; Greil 1991, 1997; Greil et al. 1990a, 1990b; Nachtigall et al. 1992.
19. Throsby and Gill 2004.
20. Greil and McQuillan 2010.
21. Birenbaum-Carmeli et al. 2000; Carmeli and Birenbaum-Carmeli 1994; Goldberg 2009.
22. Carmeli and Birenbaum-Carmeli 1994.
23. Carmeli and Birenbaum-Carmeli 1994, p. 674.
24. Goldberg 2009, pp. 215–16.
25. Greil et al. 2009.
26. Greil et al. 2009, p. 148.
27. Ibid.
28. Greil et al. 2009, p. 146.
29. Ibid.
30. Greil et al. 2009, p. 154.
31. Inhorn 2005, 2006b.
32. Inhorn 2003.
33. Population Reference Bureau 2010.
34. Kandiyoti 1991, 1994, 1998; King and Stone 2010; Obermeyer 1999; Ouzgane 1997.
35. Joseph 1993, 1994, 1999.
36. Lindisfarne 1994; Sinclair-Webb 2000.
37. Inhorn 2006b.
38. Ali 2000; Lindisfarne 1994; Ouzgane 1997.

39. Ouzgane 1997, p. 3.
40. Ghoussoub and Sinclair-Webb 2000.
41. Ouzgane 1997, p. 4.
42. Ghoussoub and Sinclair-Webb 2000.
43. Lloyd 1996.
44. Lloyd 1996, p. 435.
45. Ibid.
46. Lloyd 1996, p. 434.
47. Lloyd 1996, p. 452.
48. Inhorn 1994, 1996, 2003.
49. Inhorn 2004a.
50. Clarke and Inhorn 2011.
51. This has also been noted by Helene Goldberg for Israel (2009).
52. Abu-Musa et al. 2008; Inhorn 2004b; Kobeissi et al. 2008.
53. Inhorn 2004a, 2004b, 2005.
54. World Health Organization 2010; Patrizio and Inhorn, forthcoming.
55. Inhorn 1996, 2006b.
56. Delaney 1991.
57. Kanaaneh 2002.
58. Inhorn and Birenbaum-Carmeli 2008.
59. Inhorn 1996, 2006b.
60. Goffman 1963.
61. Inhorn 2005, 2006b.
62. Inhorn 1994, 2003.
63. Van Balen and Inhorn 2002.
64. Greil et al. 2009.
65. Inhorn 1996.

Chapter 3: Love Stories

1. Hatem's story, as well as parts of this chapter, are also found in my chapter in *Love and Globalization: Transformations of Intimacy in the Contemporary World*, ed. Padilla et al. (2007).

2. See *Infertility and Patriarchy* (1996) for my examination of "conjugal connectivity" among the Egyptian poor. See *Local Babies, Global Science* (2003) for similar sentiments among the Egyptian urban elite.

3. Ahearn 2001; Cole and Thomas 2009; de Munck 1998; Hirsch and Wardlow 2006; Jankowiak 2008; Padilla et al. 2007; Povinelli 2006.

4. Jankowiak and Fischer 1992, p. 149.

5. Jankowiak and Fischer 1992, p. 150.

6. Ibid.

7. De Munck 1996.

8. De Munck 1996, p. 698.

9. Smith 2001.

10. Larkin 1997.

11. Povinelli 2006.

12. Trawick 1990.

13. Trawick 1990, p. 91.

14. Soueif 2000, pp. 386–87.

15. Knysh 2000.

16. Knysh 2000, p. 9.

17. Musallam 1983.

18. Charrad 2001.

19. Ibid.

20. Charrad 2001, p. 35.

21. Charrad 2001, p. 38.

22. Charrad (2001) reports rates of 2 percent, whereas Omran and Roudi (1993) report regional rates of 3–4 percent.

23. Serour 1996.

24. Omran and Roudi 1993.

25. Fluehr-Lobban 2004.

26. Parker-Pope 2010.

27. Bennett and Ellison 2010.

28. Singerman and Ibrahim 2004.

29. Inhorn 1996.

30. Inhorn 2003.

31. Baron 1991; Musallam 2009.

32. Abu-Lughod 2002.

33. Inhorn 1996, 2003.

34. Joseph 1993, 1994, 1999.

35. Charrad 2001.

36. Moghadam 2004.

37. Parker-Pope 2010.

38. Becker 1997; Greil 1991; Greil et al. 1990a 1990b; Peterson et al. 2011.

39. Inhorn 1996.

40. Inhorn 2003.

41. Parker-Pope 2010.

42. Ibid.

43. Some Christian men explained that marital annulments or divorces in civil court could be obtained but with "great difficulty" and "high cost." As a result, marital dissolutions among Christians are rare in the Middle East.

44. Sometimes men were embarrassed to have forgotten their actual wedding dates, although they always knew the length of marriage. To retrieve the information, some men checked their medical records or engravings on their wedding rings. Some men were funny, quipping, "Don't tell my wife. She'll kill me!"

45. Parker-Pope 2010.

46. Baron 1991.

47. Musallam 2009.

48. Musallam 2009, p. 197.

CHAPTER 4: CONSANGUINEOUS CONNECTIVITY

1. Bittles and Matson 2000; Chan 2007; Kurinczuk 2003; Ola et al. 2001.

2. Consanguineous marriage, known as "cousin marriage" in popular parlance, is usually defined as the intermarriage of two individuals who have at least one ancestor in common, the ancestor being no more distant than a great-great grand-parent. The progeny of such consanguineous marriages are usually referred to as inbred (Gunaid et al. 2004). Abbas's story, as well as parts of this chapter, can be found in my coauthored chapter (Inhorn et al. 2008b) in *Anthropology and Public Health: Bridging Differences in Culture and Society*, ed. Hahn and Inhorn (2008). Tables 9–11 can be found in my coauthored article, "Consanguinity and Family Clustering of Male Infertility in Lebanon," *Fertility and Sterility* 91 (2009):1104–9.

3. Joseph 1993, 1994, 1999.
4. Joseph 1993, 1994.
5. Joseph 1999, pp. 121–22.
6. Ibid.
7. Johnson and Joseph 2009.
8. Yount and Rashad 2008.
9. United National Development Programme 2002.
10. United National Development Programme 2002, pp. 15–16.
11. Kassak et al., n.d.
12. Joseph 2009.
13. United National Development Programme 2002.
14. United National Development Programme 2002, p. 2.
15. Ibid.
16. Ibid.
17. Inhorn 2003, 2009a.
18. Inhorn 2003.
19. Inhorn 1994, 1996, 2003.
20. Al-Gazali et al. 1997; Gunaid et al. 2004; Hamamy et al. 2005; Jurdi and Saxena 2003; Saadat et al. 2004; Shavazi et al. 2006; Sueyoshi and Ohtsuka 2003.
21. Inhorn et al. 2008b, 2009.
22. Baccetti et al. 2001; Latini et al. 2004.
23. Maduro and Lamb 2002, p. 2197.
24. Maduro et al. 2003; Maduro and Lamb 2002.
25. Chan 2007; Krausz et al. 2003.
26. Baccetti et al. 2001.
27. Birenbaum-Carmeli 2004.
28. Teebi 2010.
29. Rajab and Patton 2000; Zlotogora 1997.
30. Mumtaz et al. 2007; Tamim et al. 2003.
31. Alkhalaf et al. 2002; Kumtepe et al. 2009; Mohammed et al. 2007.
32. Bittles et al. 1991, 2002.
33. Bittles et al. 1991, 2002.
34. Bittles et al. 1991.
35. Ottenheimer 1996.
36. Bittles et al. 1991; Eickelman 1989.
37. Hussain and Bittles 2004; Shavazi et al. 2006.

38. Bittles et al. 1991; El-Hazmi et al. 1995; Gunaid et al. 2004; Jurdi and Saxena 2003; Rajab and Patton 2000; Shah 2004; Tremayne 2006.

39. Gunaid et al. 2004.

40. Inhorn 1996.

41. Bittles et al. 2002; Hussain and Bittles 2004.

42. Gunaid et al. 2004; Jurdi and Saxena 2003.

43. Al Abdulkareem and Ballal 1998; Shah 2004.

44. Gunaid et al. 2004.

45. Saxena et al. 2004; Jabbra 2004.

46. Some pious Muslim men will not shake the hand, or otherwise touch, a woman who is not a relative, on the assumption that illicit sexual feelings might emerge through such touch. See also Deeb 2006.

47. This clinic was still performing zygote intrafallopian transfer (ZIFT), in which fertilized zygotes are surgically placed in a woman's fallopian tubes, thereby increasing the risk of an ectopic, or tubal pregnancy. ZIFT is no longer practiced in most Western countries.

48. I could not help but think that Waleed's younger brother is gay, although I did not pose this question to Waleed, especially in his highly emotional state.

49. Inhorn 2003.

50. Hussain 1999, 2002.

51. Al-Gazali 2005; Panter-Brick 1991; Raz et al. 2003.

52. Kumtepe et al. 2009, p. 465.

53. Franklin and Roberts 2006.

54. Serour 2008.

55. Endometriosis is a painful disease in which tissue behaving like the cellular lining of the uterus (the endometrium) grows outside the uterine cavity, mostly on the ovaries. The condition is painful, and may cause irregular bleeding and infertility in women.

56. Clarke 2007b.

57. Ibid.

CHAPTER 5: MASTURBATION AND SEMEN COLLECTION

1. Testicular transplants are being done only as autografts on men who have been medically castrated for testicular cancer treatment. They are not being done in male infertility cases, or from one human to another.

2. Parts of this chapter are based on my article, "Masturbation, Semen Collection, and Men's IVF Experiences: Anxieties in the Muslim World," *Body and Society* 13 (2007):37–53, in a special issue on "Islam, Body, and Health."

3. Bourdieu 1977.

4. Giami 2010.

5. Kahn 2000; Birenbaum-Carmeli et al. 1995; Carmeli and Birenbaum-Carmeli 1994.

6. In Israel, orthodox Jewish men who are prohibited from masturbating are given special condoms with perforations. Following intercourse, the condoms are removed, and the semen is squeezed through the perforation into a collection cup

(Kahn 2000, 2002). I have never heard of such a practice in the Muslim Middle East, including for religiously pious Muslim men.

7. Traina et al. 2008.

8. Boivin et al. 1999; Daniluk 1988; Greil et al. 1990a; Hurwitz 1989; Inhorn 2005; Rantala and Koskimies 1988; Takefman et al. 1990; Van Zyl 1987a, 1987b.

9. Rantala and Koskimies 1988.

10. Khuri 2001; Musallam 1983.

11. Musallam 1983, p. 33.

12. Ibid.

13. Khuri 2001.

14. Khuri 2001, p. 22.

15. Musallam 1983, p. 33, emphasis in original.

16. Ibid.

17. Ibid.

18. Khuri 2001, p. 83.

19. Ibid.

20. Many Islamic jurists have ruled that it is legally permissible for men to be masturbated by their wives, because a man has "a right to enjoyment of her hand as he has to the rest of her body" (Musallam 1983, p. 34). However, these same jurists mentioned nothing about the masturbation of women by their husbands (Khuri 2001).

21. Khuri 2001.

22. Khuri 2001, pp. 84–85. Al-Ka'ba is the stone circumambulated by pilgrims to Mecca.

23. Khuri 2001, p. 85.

24. Ibid.

25. Khuri 2001, p. 84.

26. Khuri 2001, p. 86.

27. Inhorn 1994, 2003.

28. Crapanzano 1973; Delaney 1991; Good 1980; Greenwood 1981.

29. Inhorn 1994.

30. This transliteration reflects the colloquial Arabic pronunciation in Lebanon.

31. Dialmy 2010; Siraj 2006.

32. Inhorn 2005.

33. Anonymous, n.d.

34. Inhorn 2005.

35. Ibid.

36. Ibid.

37. Inhorn 2004a.

38. Kanaaneh (2002) reports that satellite television has now brought Turkish "soft porn" shows into Palestinian homes in the Galilee region of Israel.

39. Inhorn 2003.

CHAPTER 6: ISLAM AND ASSISTED REPRODUCTION

1. Serour 2008.

2. Qur'an 42:49–50.

3. Inhorn 1994, 2003; Lotfalian 2004.

4. Gurtin, in press.

5. Moghimehfar and Nasr-Esfahani, n.d.

6. Inhorn 2003; Serour 1996, 2008; Serour and Dickens 2001.

7. Brockopp 2003; Brockopp and Eich 2008; Inhorn 1994; Musallam 1983.

8. Parts of this chapter are based on my article, "Making Muslim Babies: IVF and Gamete Donation in Sunni Versus Shi'a Islam," *Culture, Medicine, & Psychiatry* 30 (2006):427–50.

9. As noted by Iqbal and Noble (2009:108), "A *fatwa* is a legal pronouncement made by a *mufti*, a scholar capable of issuing judgements on Islamic law (*sharia*). These are neither binding nor legally enforceable, but provide invaluable insight when gauging Islamic opinions on a given topic. Fatwas can be published in daily newspapers and periodicals or broadcast on radio or television."

10. Lane and Rubinstein 1991; Zuhur 1992b.

11. Inhorn et al. 2010.

12. Inhorn 1994, 1996, 2003 2006d; Inhorn and Tremayne, in press.; Serour 1996, 2008; Serour et al. 1990, 1995.

13. Gamal I. Serour, personal communication, July 30, 2007.

14. Serour 1996, 2008; Serour and Dickens 2001.

15. Serour 1994, 1996, 2008; Serour and Dickens 2001; Serour et al. 1990, 1991, 1995; Serour and Omran 1992.

16. To date, no cases of imprisonment or capital punishment of Middle Eastern IVF physicians, for witting or unwitting negligence, have occurred, except for one case in Turkey, where the IVF physician was imprisoned. According to Gamal Serour, capital punishment is theoretically possible.

17. Moosa 2003, p. 23.

18. Meirow and Schenker 1997.

19. Meirow and Schenker 1997, p. 134.

20. The notable exceptions are Iran, Sudan, and Somalia, where Islamic law has been imposed on all citizens (including non-Muslims) in matters other than family law. Sudan, however, has recently divided into two countries.

21. Inhorn 2009a.

22. Inhorn 2010, pp. 130–31.

23. Ibid.

24. Eich 2006, p. 1.

25. Clarke 2006a, 2009.

26. Cole 2002; Hoodfar 1995; Najmabadi 2008; Tober 2004; Tremayne 2005, 2006, 2008.

27. Zuhur 1992a.

28. Haeri 1989.

29. Ibid.

30. Clarke 2009.

31. Tremayne 2009.

32. Clarke 2006a, 2009.

33. Houjaij et al. 2000.

34. Houjaij et al. 2000, pp. 8–9.

35. Clarke 2006a; Clarke and Inhorn 2011.

36. Eich 2002; Moosa 2003; Mohamed Yehia, personal communication, 2010.

37. Franklin 2007.

38. Tremayne 2009.

39. Garmaroudi, in press.

40. Tremayne 2005, 2006, 2008, in press.

41. Tremayne, in press.

42. Garmaroudi, in press.

43. Soraya Tremayne, personal communication, July 23, 2004.

44. Inhorn 2006e.

45. Clarke 2006a, 2009.

46. Clarke 2006a.

47. Ibid.

48. Abbasi-Shavazi et al. 2008; Inhorn and Tremayne, in press.

49. Demographics of Lebanon, http://en.wikipedia.org/wiki/Demographics_of_Lebanon.

50. Ouzgane 2006.

51. Asad 2003.

52. Clarke 2009; Clarke and Inhorn 2011.

53. "Ayatollah" is the term used for clerics in Iran, a Farsi-speaking country. Ayatollah is not a common clerical term of reference in the Arabic-speaking world. Rather, "Sayyid" is the term used for clerics who are descendants of the Prophet Muhammad, and the term "Shaykh" is often used for those who are not prophetic descendants.

54. This was directed at the anthropologist, who, at that time, was a professor at the University of Michigan.

55. He did not return to the clinic. However, the anthropologist was able to interview three other Shia clerics in Lebanon on their opinions about ARTs.

56. She is Lebanon's most famous diva and national icon.

57. The anthropologist soon learned to accommodate the uncertainties of hand shaking by never offering her hand first, and only shaking hands with those who offered theirs. Otherwise, she covered her heart with her outstretched right hand, as a sign of greeting and respect. She also hired a male research assistant in the clinic to sit through interviews in such cases. See also Deeb 2006.

58. Abbasi-Shavazi et al. 2008; Inhorn and Tremayne, in press.

59. Tremayne 2008.

60. Inhorn et al. 2010.

61. Clarke 2006a, p. 26.

62. Clarke 2009; Eich 2005, 2006; Mahmoud, in press.

63. Hoodfar 1995.

64. Lane and Rubinstein 1991.

65. Hoodfar 1995; Tober 2004.

66. Nasr 2006.

Chapter 7: Sperm Donation and Adoption

1. Many men in the study had poor dentition, with darkened and missing teeth. Their lips were often darkened or bluish as a result of heavy smoking.

2. See note 57, chapter 6. See also Deeb 2006.

3. Tremayne 2009; Reza O. Samani, personal communication, August 2010.

4. Clarke 2009.

5. Strathern 1992a.

6. Carsten 2000, 2004, 2007; Edwards et al. 1999; Franklin and McKinnon 2001; Strathern 1992b.

7. Bonaccorso 2008; Clarke 2009; Edwards 2000; Franklin 1997; Konrad 2005; Thompson 2005.

8. Strathern 1992a, pp. 27–28.

9. Bonaccorso 2008; Edwards 2000; Edwards et al. 1999; Franklin 1997; Franklin and Ragone 1998; Harrington et al. 2008; Konrad 2005; Melhuus 2007; Ragone 1994; Thompson 2005.

10. Schneider 1980.

11. Ragone 1996.

12. Becker 2000; Franklin 1997; Inhorn 2003; Ragone 1994.

13. Bharadwaj 2003; Birenbaum-Carmeli and Carmeli 2010; Storrow 2006.

14. Becker 2000; Carsten 2000.

15. Carsten 2004, 2007; Strathern 2005.

16. Collard and de Parseval 2007.

17. Becker 2000; Thompson 2005.

18. Agigian 2004; Ragone 1994; Sullivan 2004.

19. Franklin and Ragone 1998; Thompson 2001, 2005.

20. Clarke 2009.

21. Serour 1996.

22. Clarke 2006a, 2006b, 2007a, 2007b, 2008; Inhorn 2006e; Tremayne 2008.

23. Parts of this chapter are based on my article, "<~?~thinspace>'He Won't Be My Son': Middle Eastern Muslim Men's Discourses of Adoption and Gamete Donation," *Medical Anthropology Quarterly* 20 (2006):94–120.

24. Serour 1996; Sonbol 1995.

25. Sonbol 1995.

26. Ibid.

27. Ibid.

28. Clarke 2009; Inhorn 1996; King and Stone 2010.

29. King and Stone 2010.

30. Sonbol 1995, p. 60.

31. See the appendix for the full passage.

32. Inhorn 1996; Sonbol 1995; Zuhur 1992b.

33. Sonbol 1995.

34. Abbasi-Shavazi et al. 2008.

35. Ibid.

36. Janet Heindl, personal communication, July 8, 2004; Tober 2004.

37. Sonbol 1995; Inhorn 1996, 2003.

38. Sonbol 1995; Inhorn 1996, 2003.

39. Bargach 2002.

40. In the Muslim world, breastfeeding confers kinship on a child. Thus, two children who are breastfed by the same woman become "milk siblings" and are pre-

vented from ever marrying. Theoretically, an adopted or donor child could become a "member of the family" through breastfeeding, as noted in this man's comment.

41. See Inhorn 2003. These fears of "mixing" were rampant in the mid-1990s, when ICSI was first introduced in Egypt.

42. This is to avoid having an unrelated male physician gaze at a woman's genitals. Religious Shia and Sunni Muslims increasingly prefer to use female gynecologists and obstetricians.

43. Inhorn 2004a.

44. King and Stone 2010.

45. King and Stone 2010, p. 323.

46. King and Stone 2010, p. 327.

47. King and Stone 2010, p. 332.

48. Croll 2000; Obermeyer 1999.

49. Clarke 2007b, p. 382.

50. Ibid.

51. Tremayne, in press.

52. Reza O. Samani, Royan Institute, Tehran, Iran; personal communication, July 2010.

53. Becker 2002; Inhorn and Birenbaum-Carmeli 2008.

54. Becker 2002; Becker et al. 2005; Nachtigall et al. 1997, 1998. See also Birenbaum-Carmeli et al. 2000; Carmeli and Birenbaum-Carmeli 2000.

55. Becker 2002.

56. Patrizio and Inhorn, forthcoming.

Chapter 8: Egg Donation and Emergence

1. Reproductive "tourism" (a.k.a. fertility tourism, procreative tourism) has been challenged as the best term for such reproductive travel, because it ignores the difficulties and suffering of infertile couples who feel forced to leave their home countries to seek assisted reproduction. My colleagues and I have forwarded the notion of reproductive "exile" as the term that best describes the subjective experiences of reproductive travelers (see Inhorn and Patrizio 2009; Matorras 2005). In the medical literature, the term "cross-border reproductive care" (CBRC) is now being forwarded (Pennings 2002; Shenfield et al. 2010).

2. Demographics of Lebanon, http://en.wikipedia.org/wiki/Demographics_of_Lebanon.

3. Birenbaum-Carmeli and Inhorn 2009; Inhorn and Birenbaum-Carmeli 2010.

4. Inhorn 2003.

5. Traina et al. 2008.

6. Clarke 2009.

7. Heng 2007.

8. Spar 2006.

9. Surrogacy is still very uncommon in Lebanon, but surrogates are being recruited from Palestinian refugee camps and from foreign maid services. According to anthropologist Jared McCormick, a Sri Lankan "madame" has set up a service in Beirut with Sri Lankan maids serving as gestational surrogates for childless Leba-

nese couples. The Sri Lankan gestational surrogate-maids live in a home under the madame's care during the course of their pregnancies. Jared McCormick, personal communication, October 29, 2010.

10. Hourvitz 2009.
11. Inhorn 2003.
12. Rapp 1988, 1998.
13. This would occur through the practice of "milk kinship."
14. Kobeissi et al. 2008.
15. Inhorn 2003.
16. Inhorn et al. 2010; Nicholson and Nicholson 1994; Bonaccorso 2008.
17. Traina et al. 2008.
18. Catechism 2002, p. 509, as cited in Richards 2009.
19. Traina et al. 2008, p. 38.
20. Richards 2009.
21. Nachtigall et al. 2005.
22. Serour 2008.
23. Ibid.
24. Ibid.
25. Gray 2010.
26. Inhorn 1996.
27. Obermeyer 1999; van Balen and Inhorn 2002.
28. Clarke 2009.
29. Inhorn et al. 2010.

CONCLUSION: EMERGENT MASCULINITIES IN THE MIDDLE EAST

1. *Newsweek*, September 27, 2010.
2. Hollan 2001.
3. Yount and Rashad 2008.
4. Hopkins 2004.
5. Arab Families Working Group, http://www.afwg.info.
6. Musallam 2009.
7. Daniels 2006.
8. Daniels 2006, p. 32.
9. Ibid.; Schettler et al. 1999.
10. Daniels 2006, p. 48.
11. Auger 2010.
12. Bentley 2000.
13. Inhorn et al. 2008a.
14. Abu Musa et al. 2008; Bazzi et al. 2005; Inhorn et al. 2008a, 2008b, 2009; Inhorn and Buss 1993, 1994; Inhorn and Kobeissi 2006; Kobeissi et al. 2008; Kobeissi and Inhorn 2007.
15. Inhorn 2008a.
16. Calogero et al. 2009.
17. Inhorn and Buss 1994.
18. Curtis et al. 1997.
19. Nakkash et al. 2010.

20. Abu Musa et al. 2008; Kobeissi et al. 2008.

21. I thank my colleague Richard Bribiescas, a specialist in male reproductive endocrinology, for this insight. See Bribiescas 2001, 2006.

22. Inhorn 2008.

23. These would include Algeria, Iraq, Israel/Palestine, Libya, Sudan, Syria, and Yemen.

24. Inhorn et al. 2008b, 2009.

25. Baccetti et al. 2001; Latini et al. 2004.

26. Bittles and Matson 2000; Spar 2006.

27. Spar 2006.

28. I thank my colleague Pankaj Shrivistav for explaining this to me. See also Spar 2006.

29. Funke et al. 2010.

30. Ibid.

31. Ibid.

32. Ginsburg and Rapp 1995.

33. Thompson 2002.

34. Lorber 1989; Van der Ploeg 1995.

35. Thompson 2002.

36. Thompson 2005.

37. Franklin 1996.

38. Franklin, in press.

39. Franklin 1997.

40. Becker 2000.

41. Osmanagaoglu et al. 1999.

42. Chambers et al. 2009; Collins 2002; Spar 2006.

43. Ombelet 2009; Sharma et al. 2009; Vayena et al. 2009.

44. European Society for Human Reproduction and Embryology 2008, 2009a, 2009b.

45. Nachtigall 2006.

46. Zegers-Hoschild et al. 2008.

47. Collins 2002.

48. Ata and Seli 2010; Chambers et al. 2009; Ombelet 2009; Sharma et al. 2009; Vayena et al. 2009.

49. Cui 2010.

50. Inhorn 2003.

51. Ibid.

52. Nachtigall 2006, p. 874.

53. Inhorn 2007b, 2009b. Interestingly, my father, who underwent a varicocelectomy early in marriage, attributes my birth and those of my two brothers to the success of this surgery.

54. Kamischke and Nieschlag 1988; Tournaye 2002; World Health Organization 1992.

55. Inhorn 2003.

56. Inhorn 2007b, 2009b.

57. Vayena et al. 2002.

58. Maduro et al. 2003; Maduro and Lamb 2002.
59. Inhorn 2003, 2009a.
60. Van Balen and Gerrits 2001.
61. Fathalla 2002, p. 30, emphasis added.
62. European Society of Human Reproduction and Embryology 2009b; Ombelet 2009; Vayena et al. 2009.
63. European Society for Human Reproduction and Embryology 2009b.
64. Inhorn 2003, 2009a.
65. Inhorn 2010.
66. Fonseca 2009.
67. Abu-Rabia 2010.
68. Fonseca 2009.
69. Bayat 2010, p. ix.
70. Ibid.

APPENDIX: THE ASSISTED REPRODUCTION *FATWAS*

1. This *fatwa* is also found in Inhorn 2003, 2006c.
2. This *fatwa* is also found in Inhorn 2006c.

References Cited

Abbasi-Shavazi, Mohammad Jalal, Marcia C. Inhorn, Hajiieh Bibi Razeghi-Nasrabad, and Ghasem Toloo. "The 'Iranian ART Revolution': Infertility, Assisted Reproductive Technology, and Third-Party Donation in the Islamic Republic of Iran." *Journal of Middle East Women's Studies* 4 (2008):1–28.

Abbey, Antonia, Frank M. Andrews, and L. Jill Halman. "Gender's Role in Responses to Infertility." *Psychology of Women Quarterly* 15 (1991):295–316.

Abraham, Nabeel, and Andrew Shryock, eds. *Arab Detroit: From Margin to Mainstream.* Detroit: Wayne State University Press, 2000.

Abu-Lughod, Lila. *Veiled Sentiments: Honor and Poetry in a Bedouin Society.* Berkeley: University of California Press, 1986.

———."Zones of Theory in the Anthropology of the Arab World." *Annual Review of Anthropology* 18 (1989):267–306.

———. "Writing Against Culture." In *Recapturing Anthropology: Working in the Present*, edited by Richard G. Fox, 137–62. Santa Fe, NM: SAR Press, 1991.

———. *Writing Women's Worlds: Bedouin Stories.* Berkeley: University of California Press, 1993.

———."The Marriage of Feminism and Islamism in Egypt: Selective Repudiation as a Dynamic of Postcolonial Cultural Politics." In *The Anthropology of Globalization: A Reader*, edited by Jonathan Xavier Inda and Renato Rosaldo, 428–51. Malden, MA: Blackwell, 2002.

Abu-Musa, Antoine A., Loulou Kobeissi, Antoine B. Hannoun, and Marcia C. Inhorn."Effect of War on Fertility: A Review of the Literature." *Reproductive BioMedicine Online* 17 (Suppl. 1) (2008):43–53.

Abu-Rabia, Aref."Paternity Suits in Tribal Society in the Middle East." Paper presented at the World Association for Medicine and Law, Zaghreb, Croatia, August 2010.

Aghacy, Samira. *Masculine Identity in the Fiction of the Arab East since 1967.* Syracuse, NY: Syracuse University Press, 2009.

Agigian, Amy. *Baby Steps: How Lesbian Alternative Insemination Is Changing the World.* Middletown, CT: Wesleyan University Press, 2004.

Ahearn, Laura. *Invitations to Love: Literacy, Love Letters, and Social Change in Nepal.* Ann Arbor: University of Michigan Press, 2001.

Ahmed, Leila. *Women and Gender in Islam.* New Haven, CT: Yale University Press, 1992.

Al Abdulkareem A., and S. G. Ballal."Consanguineous Marriage in an Urban Area of Saudi Arabia: Rates and Adverse Health Effects on the Offspring."*Journal of Community Health* 23 (1998):75–83.

Al-Ali, Nadje S. *Secularism, Gender and the State in the Middle East: The Egyptian Women's Movement.* Cambridge, UK: Cambridge University Press, 2000.

———. *Iraqi Women: Untold Stories from 1948 to the Present.* New York: Zed Books, 2007.

Al-Ali, Nadje S., and Nicola Pratt. *Women and War in the Middle East: Transnational Perspectives.* New York: Zed Books, 2009.

Al-Gazali, L. I . "Attitudes toward Genetic Counseling in the United Arab Emirates." *Community Genetics* 8 (2005):48–51.

Al-Gazali, L. I., A. Bener, Y. M. Abdulrazzaq, R. Micallef, A. I. Al-Khayat, and T. Gaber. "Consanguineous Marriages in the United Arab Emirates." *Journal of Biosocial Sciences* 29 (1997):491–97.

Ali, Kamran Asdar. "Notes on Rethinking Masculinities: An Egyptian Case." In *Learning about Sexuality: A Practical Beginning,* edited by S. Zeidenstein and Kirsten Moore, 98–109. New York: Population Council, 1996.

———. "Making 'Responsible' Men: Planning the Family in Egypt." In *Fertility and the Male Life-Cycle in the Era of Fertility Decline,* edited by Susana Lerner, Caroline Bledsoe, and Jane I. Guyer, 119–43. Oxford, UK: Oxford University Press, 2000.

Alkhalaf, M., L. Verghese, and N. Mhuarib. "A Cytogenetic Study of Kuwaiti Couples with Infertility and Reproductive Disorders: Short Arm Deletion of Chromosome 21 is Associated with Male Infertility." *Annales de Genetique* 45 (2002):147–49.

Anonymous. "Consanguineous Marriage Affects the Sexual Function of Infertile Male." Unpublished manuscript, n.d.

Asad, Talal. "The Idea of an Anthropology of Islam." Center for Contemporary Arab Studies, Occasional Papers Series. Washington, DC: Georgetown University Center for Contemporary Arab Studies, 1986.

———. *Formations of the Secular: Christianity, Islam, Modernity.* Stanford, CA: Stanford University Press, 2003.

Ata, Baris, and Emre Seli. "Economics of Assisted Reproductive Technologies." *Current Opinions in Obstetrics and Gynecology* 22 (2010):183–88.

Auger, Jacques. "Declining Human Semen Quality and Male Fertility: Where Do We Stand Now?" *International Federation of Fertility Societies Newsletter,* Spring 2010, 3.

Baccetti, B., S. Capitani, G. Collodel, G. Cairano, L. Gambera, and E. Moretti. "Genetic Sperm Defects and Consanguinity." *Human Reproduction* 16 (2001):1365–71.

Baird, Julia. "Beyond the Bad Boys: A Quiet Revolution in Male Behavior," *Newsweek,* April 19, 2010.

Bargach, Jamila. *Orphans of Islam: Family, Abandonment and Secret Adoption in Morocco.* Lanham, MD: Rowman and Littlefield, 2002.

Baron, Beth. "The Making and Breaking of Marital Bonds in Modern Egypt." In *Women in Middle Eastern History: Shifting Boundaries in Sex and Gender,* edited by Nikki Keddie and Beth Baron, 275–91. New Haven, CT: Yale University Press, 1991.

Basu, A. M. "The International Conference on Population and Development, Cairo 1994. Is Its Plan of Action Important, Desirable and Feasible? ICPD: What about Men's Rights and Women's Responsibilities?" *Health Transition Review* 6 (1996):225–27.

Bayat, Asef. *Life as Politics: How Ordinary People Change the Middle East.* Stanford, CA: Stanford University Press, 2010.

Bazzi, Ali, Jerome O. Nriagu, Marcia C. Inhorn, and Aaron Lindner. "Determination of Antimony in Human Blood with Inductively Coupled Plasma-Mass Spectrometry." *Journal of Environmental Monitoring* 7 (2005):1251–54.

Becker, Gay. "Metaphors in Disrupted Lives: Infertility and Cultural Constructions of Continuity." *Medical Anthropology Quarterly* 8 (1994):383–410.

———. *Healing the Infertile Family: Strengthening Your Relationship in the Search for Parenthood.* Berkeley: University of California Press, 1997.

———. *The Elusive Embryo: How Women and Men Approach New Reproductive Technologies.* Berkeley: University of California Press, 2000.

———. "Deciding Whether to Tell Children about Donor Insemination: An Unresolved Question in the United States." In *Infertility around the Globe: New Thinking on Childlessness, Gender, and Reproductive Technologies,* edited by Marcia C. Inhorn and Frank van Balen, 119–33. Berkeley: University of California Press, 2002.

Becker, Gay, A. Butler, and R. D. Nachtigall. "Resemblance Talk: A Challenge for Parents Whose Children Were Conceived with Donor Gametes in the U.S." *Social Science and Medicine* 61 (2005):1300–1309.

Ben-Ari, Eyal. *Mastering Soldiers: Conflict, Emotions and the Enemy in an Israeli Military Unit.* New York: Berghahn Books, 1998.

Bennett, Jessica, and Jesse Ellison. "I Don't: The Case against Marriage." *Newsweek,* June 21, 2010, 42–45.

Bentley, Gillian R. "Environmental Influences on Infertility." In *Infertility in the Modern World: Present and Future Prospects,* edited by Gillian R. Bentley and C. G. Nicholas Mascie-Taylor, 83–152. Cambridge, UK: Cambridge University Press, 2000.

Bentley, Gillian R., and C. G. Nicholas Mascie-Taylor, eds. *Infertility in the Modern World: Present and Future Prospects.* Cambridge, UK: Cambridge University Press, 2000.

Bharadwaj, Aditya. "Why Adoption Is Not an Option in India: The Visibility of Infertility, the Secrecy of Donor Insemination, and Other Cultural Complexities." *Social Science and Medicine* 56 (2003):1867–80.

Biehl, Joao. *Vita: Life in a Zone of Social Abandonment.* Berkeley: University of California Press, 2005.

Biehl, Joao, Byron Good, and Arthur Kleinman, eds. *Subjectivity: Ethnographic Investigations.* Berkeley: University of California Press, 2007.

Birenbaum-Carmeli, Daphna. "Increased Prevalence of Mediterranean and Muslim Populations in Mutation-Related Research Literature." *Community Genetics* 279 (2004):1–5.

Birenbaum-Carmeli, Daphna, and Yoram S. Carmeli. "Introduction: Reproduction, Medicine and the State—The Israeli Case." In *Kin, Gene, Community: Reproductive Technology among Jewish Israelis,* edited by Daphna Birenbaum-Carmeli and Yoram S. Carmeli, 1–48. New York: Berghahn, 2010.

Birenbaum-Carmeli, Daphna, Yoram S. Carmeli, and R. Casper. "Discrimination against Men in Fertility Treatments: The Underprivileged Male." *Journal of Reproductive Medicine* 40 (1995):590–93.

Birenbaum-Carmeli, Daphna, Yoram S. Carmeli, and H. Yavetz. "Secrecy among Israeli Recipients of Donor Insemination." *Politics and the Life Sciences* 19 (2000):69–76.

Birenbaum-Carmeli, Daphna, and Marcia C. Inhorn. "Masculinity and Marginality: Palestinian Men's Struggles with Infertility in Israel and Lebanon." *Journal of Middle East Women's Studies* 5 (2009):23–51.

Bittles, A. H., J. C. Grant, S. G. Sullivan, and R. Hussain. "Does Inbreeding Lead to Decreased Human Fertility?" *Annals of Human Biology* 29 (2002):111–30.

Bittles, A. H., W. Manson, J. Greene, and N. A. Rao. "Reproductive Behavior and Health in Consanguineous Marriages." *Science* 252 (1991):789–94.

Bittles, A. H., and P. L. Matson. "Genetic Influences on Human Infertility." In *Infertility in the Modern World: Present and Future Prospects,* edited by Gillian R. Bentley and C. G. Nicholas Mascie-Taylor, 46–81. Cambridge, UK: Cambridge University Press, 2000.

Blyth, Eric, and Ruth Landau, eds. *Third Party Assisted Conception across Cultures: Social, Legal, and Ethical Perspectives.* London: Routledge, 2004.

Boddy, Janice. *Wombs and Alien Spirits: Women, Men, and the Zar Cult in Northern Sudan.* Madison: University of Wisconsin Press, 1989.

———. *Civilizing Women: British Crusades in Colonial Sudan.* Princeton, NJ: Princeton University Press, 2007.

Boerma, J. T., and Zaida Mgalla, eds. *Women and Infertility in Sub-Saharan Africa: A Multi-Disciplinary Perspective.* Amsterdam: Royal Tropical Institute, 2000.

Boivin, J., L. C. Scanlan, and S. M. Walker. "Why Are Infertile Patients Not Using Psychosocial Counselling?" *Human Reproduction* 14 (1999):1384–91.

Bonaccorso, Monica. *Conceiving Kinship: Assisted Conception, Procreation and Family in Southern Europe.* New York: Berghahn, 2008.

Bourdieu, Pierre. *Outline of a Theory of Practice.* Translated by Richard Nice. New York: Cambridge University Press, 1977.

Brandes, Stanley. *Metaphors of Masculinity: Sex and Status in Andalusian Folklore.* Philadelphia: University of Pennsylvania Press, 1981.

———. "Drink, Abstinence, and Male Identity in Mexico City." In *Changing Men and Masculinities in Latin America,* edited by Matthew C. Gutmann, 153–78. Durham, NC: Duke University Press, 2003.

Bribiescas, Richard. "Reproductive Ecology and Life History of the Human Male." *Yearbook of Physical Anthropology* 44 (2001):148–76.

———. "On the Evolution, Life History, and Proximate Mechanisms of Human Male Reproductive Senescence." *Evolutionary Anthropology* 15 (2006):132–41.

Brockopp, Jonathan E., ed. *Islamic Ethics of Life: Abortion, War, and Euthanasia.* Columbia: University of South Carolina Press, 2003.

Brockopp, Jonathan E., and Thomas Eich, eds. *Muslim Medical Ethics: From Theory to Practice.* Columbia: University of South Carolina Press, 2008.

Brodsky, Anne. *With All Our Strength: The Revolutionary Association of the Women of Afghanistan.* London: Routledge, 2003.

Brown, Lesley, ed. *The New Shorter Oxford English Dictionary.* Vol. 1. Oxford: Clarendon Press, 1993.

Calogero, Aldo, R. Polosa, A. Perdichizzi, F. Guarino, S. La Vignera, A. Scarfia, E. Fratantonio, R. Condorelli, O. Bonanno, N. Barone, N. Burrello, R. D'Agata, and E. Vicari. "Cigarette Smoke Extract Immobilizes Human Spermatozoa and Induces Sperm Apoptosis." *Reproductive BioMedicine Online* 19 (2009):564–71.

Carillo, Héctor. *The Night Is Young: Sexuality in Mexico in the Time of AIDS.* Chicago, IL: University of Chicago Press, 2002.

Carmeli, Yoram S., and Daphna Birenbaum-Carmeli. "The Predicament of Masculinity: Towards Understanding the Male's Experience of Infertility Treatments." *Sex Roles* 30 (1994):663–77.

———. "Ritualizing the 'Natural Family': Secrecy in Israeli Donor Insemination." *Science as Culture* 9 (2000):301–24.

Carrigan, Tim, Bob Connell, and John Lee. "Toward a New Sociology of Masculinity." *Theory and Society* 14 (1985):551–604.

Carsten, Janet. "Knowing Where You've Come From: Ruptures and Continuities of Time and Kinship in Narratives of Adoption Reunions." *Journal of the Royal Anthropological Institute* 6 (2000):637–53.

———. *After Kinship.* Cambridge, UK: Cambridge University Press, 2004.

———, ed. *Ghosts of Memory: Essays on Remembrance and Relatedness.* Malden, MA: Blackwell, 2007.

Chambers, Georgina M., Elizabeth A. Sullivan, Osaum Ishihara, Michael G. Chapman, and G. David Adamson. "The Economic Impact of Assisted Reproductive Technology: A Review of Selected Developed Countries." *Fertility and Sterility* 91 (2009):2281–94.

Chan, Peter. "Practical Genetic Issues in Male Infertility Management." Paper presented at American Society for Reproductive Medicine, October 13, 2007.

Charrad, Mounira. *States and Women's Rights: The Making of Postcolonial Tunisia, Algeria, and Morocco.* Berkeley: University of California Press, 2001.

Clarke, Morgan. "Shi'ite Perspectives on Kinship and New Reproductive Technologies." *ISIM Newsletter* 17 (2006a):26–27.

———. "Islam, Kinship, and New Reproductive Technology." *Anthropology Today* 22 (2006b):17–20.

———. "The Modernity of Milk Kinship." *Social Anthropology* 15 (2007a):297–304.

———. "Closeness in the Age of Mechanical Reproduction: Debating Kinship and Biomedicine in Lebanon and the Middle East." *Anthropological Quarterly* 80 (2007b):379–402.

———. "New Kinship, Islam and the Liberal Tradition: Sexual Morality and New Reproductive Technology in Lebanon." *Journal of the Royal Anthropological Institute* 14 (2008):153–69.

———. *Islam and New Kinship: Reproductive Technology and the Shariah in Lebanon.* New York: Berghahn, 2009.

Clarke, Morgan, and Marcia C. Inhorn."Mutuality and Immediacy between *Marja'* and *Muqallid*: Evidence from Male In Vitro Fertilization Patients in Shi'i Lebanon."*International Journal of Middle East Studies 43* (2011):409–427.

Cole, Jennifer, and Lynn Thomas, eds. *Love in Africa*. Chicago, IL: University of Chicago Press, 2009.

Cole, Juan. *Sacred Space and Holy War: The Politics, Culture and History of Shi'ite Islam*. London: I. B. Tauris, 2002.

Collard, C., and G. D. de Parseval."La gestation pour autrui: un bricolage des representations de la paternité de la maternité euro-américaines."*L'Homme* 183 (2007):1–26.

Collins, J. A."An International Survey of the Health Economics of IVF and ICSI." *Human Reproduction Update* 8 (2002):265–77.

Connell, R. W."The State, Gender and Sexual Politics: Theory and Appraisal."*Theory and Society* 19 (1990):507–44.

———."The Big Picture: Masculinities in Recent World History."*Theory and Society* 22 (1993):597–623.

———. *Masculinities*. Berkeley: University of California Press, 1995.

———. *The Men and the Boys*. Boston: Allen and Unwin, 2001.

Connell, R. W., D. J. Ashenden, S. Kessler, and G. W. Dowsett. *Making the Difference: Schools, Families and Social Division*. Sydney: George Allen & Unwin, 1982.

Connell, R. W., and James W. Messerschmidt."Hegemonic Masculinity: Rethinking the Concept."*Gender & Society* 19 (2005):829–59.

cooke, miriam. *Women and the War Story*. Berkeley: University of California Press, 1996.

Cornwall, Andrea, and Nancy Lindisfarne, eds. *Dislocating Masculinity: Comparative Ethnographies*. London: Routledge, 1994.

Crapanzano, Vincent. *The Hamadsha: A Study in Moroccan Ethnopsychiatry*. Berkeley: University of California Press, 1973.

Croll, Elisabeth. *Endangered Daughters: Discrimination and Development in Asia*. London: Routledge, 2000.

Cui, Weiyuan."Mother or Nothing: The Agony of Infertility." *Bulletin of the World Health Organization* 88 (2010):881–82.

Curtis, K. M., D. A. Savitz, and T. E. Arbuckle."Effects of Cigarette Smoking, Caffeine Consumption, and Alcohol Intake on Fecundability."*American Journal of Epidemiology* 146 (1997):1025–63.

Daniels, Cynthia R. *Exposing Men: The Science and Politics of Male Reproduction*. Oxford, UK: Oxford University Press, 2006.

Daniluk, Judith C."Infertility: Intrapersonal and Interpersonal Impact."*Fertility and Sterility* 49 (1988):982–90.

de Beauvoir, Simone. *The Second Sex*. Translated by H. M. Pasheley. New York: Knopf, 1975.

Deeb, Laura. *An Enchanted Modern: Gender and Public Piety in Shi'i Lebanon*. Princeton, NJ: Princeton University Press, 2006.

Delaney, Carol. *The Seed and the Soil: Gender and Cosmology in Turkish Village Society*. Berkeley: University of California Press, 1991.

Demetriou, Demetrakis Z. "Connell's Concept of Hegemonic Masculinity: A Critique." *Theory and Society* 30 (2001):337–61.

de Munck, Victor C. "Love and Marriage in a Sri Lankan Muslim Community: Toward a Reevaluation of Dravidian Marriage Practices." *American Ethnologist* 23 (1996):698–716.

Devroey, P., M. Vandervorst, P. Nagy, and A. Van Steirteghem. "Do We Treat the Male or His Gamete?" *Human Reproduction* 13 (1998):178–85.

Dialmy, Abdessamad. "Sexuality and Islam." *European Journal of Contraception and Reproductive Health* 15 (2010):160–68.

Donaldson, Mike. "What Is Hegemonic Masculinity?" *Theory and Society* 22 (1993):643–57.

Dudgeon, Matthew R., and Marcia C. Inhorn. "Gender, Masculinity, and Reproduction: Anthropological Perspectives." *International Journal of Men's Health* 2 (2003):31–56.

———. "Men's Influences on Women's Reproductive Health: Medical Anthropological Perspectives." *Social Science and Medicine* 59 (2004):1379–95.

Eager, Paige Whaley. *Global Population Policy: From Population Control to Reproductive Rights.* Aldershot, UK: Ashgate, 2007.

Edwards, Jeanette. *Born and Bred: Idioms of Kinship and New Reproductive Technologies in England.* Oxford, UK: Oxford University Press, 2000.

Edwards, Jeanette, Sarah Franklin, Eric Hirsch, Frances Price, and Marilyn Strathern. *Technologies of Procreation: Kinship in the Age of Assisted Conception.* London: Routledge, 1999.

Eich, Thomas. "Muslim Voices on Cloning." *ISIM Newsletter* 12 (2002):38–39.

———. *Islam und Bioethik: Eine Kritische Analyse der Modernen Diskussion im Islamischen Recht.* Heidelberg: Reichert, 2005.

———. "Changing Concepts of Kinship in the Islamic World." Paper presented at the Society for Applied Anthropology/Society for Medical Anthropology meeting, Vancouver, British Columbia, 2006.

Eickelman, Dale F. *The Middle East: An Anthropological Approach.* 2nd ed. Englewood Cliffs, NJ: Prentice-Hall, 1989.

El Guindi, Fadwa. *Veil: Modesty, Privacy, and Resistance.* Oxford, UK: Berg, 1999.

El-Hazmi, M. A., A. R. Al-Swailem, A. S. Warsy, A. M. Al-Swailem, R. Sulaimani, and A. Al-Meshari. "Consanguinity among the Saudi Arabian Population." *Journal of Medical Genetics* 32 (1995):623–26.

Esfandiari, Haleh. *Reconstructed Lives: Women and Iran's Islamic Revolution.* Baltimore, MD: Johns Hopkins University Press, 1997.

European Society of Human Reproduction and Embryology. "Developing Countries and Infertility." *Human Reproduction Special Issue* (2008) (doi:10.1093).

———. "Social Aspects of Accessible Infertility Care in Developing Countries." *Facts, Views & Vision: Issues in Obstetrics, Gynaecology and Reproductive Health in ObGyn.* Belgium: Universa Press, 2009a.

———. ESHRE Task Force on Ethics and Law. "Providing Infertility Treatment in Resource-Poor Countries." *Human Reproduction* 24 (2009b):1008–11.

Fadlalla, Amal Hassan. *Embodying Honor: Fertility, Foreignness, and Regeneration in Eastern Sudan.* Madison: University of Wisconsin Press, 2007.

Fathalla, Mahmoud. "Current Challenges in Assisted Reproduction." In *Current Practices and Controversies in Assisted Reproduction*, edited by Effy Vayena, Patrick J. Rowe, and P. David Griffin, 3–12. Geneva: World Health Organization, 2002.

Fluehr-Lobban, Carolyn. *Islamic Society in Practice*. 2nd ed. Gainesville: University Press of Florida, 2004.

Fonseca, Claudia. "Doubt Is the Mother of All Inventions: DNA and Paternity in a Brazilian Setting." In *Assisting Reproduction, Testing Genes: Global Encounters with New Biotechnologies*, edited by Daphna Birenbaum-Carmeli and Marcia C. Inhorn, 258–84. New York: Berghahn, 2009.

Frank, Gelya. *Venus on Wheels: Two Decades of Dialogue on Disability, Biography, and Being Female in America*. Berkeley: University of California Press, 2000.

Franklin, Sarah. *Embodied Progress: A Cultural Account of Assisted Conception*. London: Routledge, 1997.

———. *Dolly Mixtures: The Remaking of Genealogy*. Durham, NC: Duke University Press, 2007.

———. "Five Million Test-Tube Babies." In *Reproductive Technologies as Global Form: Ethnographies of Knowledge, Practices, and the Transnational Encounters*, edited by Michi Knecht, Maren Klotz, and Stefan Beck. Chicago, IL: University of Chicago Press, in press.

Franklin, Sarah, and Susan McKinnon, eds. *Relative Values: Reconfiguring Kinship Studies*. Durham, NC: Duke University Press, 2001.

Franklin, Sarah, and Helene Ragone, eds. *Reproducing Reproduction: Kinship, Power, and Technological Innovation*. Philadelphia: University of Pennsylvania Press, 1998.

Franklin, Sarah, and Celia Roberts. *Born and Made: An Ethnography of Preimplantation Genetic Diagnosis*. Princeton, NJ: Princeton University Press, 2006.

Friese, C., G. Becker, and R. D. Nachtigall. "Rethinking the Biological Clock: Eleventh Hour Moms, Miracle Moms and Meanings of Age-Related Infertility." *Social Science and Medicine* 63 (2006):1550–60.

———. "Older Motherhood and the Changing Life Course in the Era of Assisted Reproductive Technologies." *Journal of Aging Studies* 22 (2007):65–73.

Funke, Simone, Edina Flach, Istvan Kiss, Janos Sandor, Gabriella Vida, Jozsef Bodis, and Tibor Erti. "Male Reproductive Tract Abnormalities: More Common after Assisted Reproduction?" *Early Human Development* 86 (2010):547–50.

Garmaroudi, Shirin. "Gestational Surrogacy in Iran: Uterine Kinship in Shia Thought and Practice." In *Islam and Assisted Reproductive Technologies: Sunni and Shia Perspectives*, edited by Marcia C. Inhorn and Soraya Tremayne. New York: Berghahn, in press.

Gelvin, James L. *The Modern Middle East: A History*. New York: Oxford University Press, 2005.

Ghoussoub, Mai. "Chewing Gum, Insatiable Women and Foreign Enemies: Male Fears and the Arab Media." In *Imagined Masculinities: Male Identity and*

Culture in the Modern Middle East, edited by Mai Ghoussoub and Emma Sinclair-Webb, 227–35. London: Saqi, 2000.

Ghoussoub, Mai, and Emma Sinclair-Webb, eds. *Imagined Masculinities: Male Identity and Culture in the Modern Middle East.* London: Saqi, 2000.

Giami, Alain."'Glauque': Le recueil de sperme dans les procédures de Procréation Médicalement Assistée" [The "murky" and the production of sperm in infertility treatment]. *Ethnologie Française 41* (2011):41–48.

Ginsburg, Faye, and Rayna Rapp, eds. *Conceiving the New World Order: The Global Politics of Reproduction.* Berkeley: University of California Press, 1995.

Goffman, Erving. *Stigma: Notes on the Management of Spoiled Identity.* Englewood Cliffs, NJ: Prentice-Hall, 1963.

Goldberg, Helene. "The Sex in the Sperm: Male Infertility and Its Challenges to Masculinity in an Israeli-Jewish Context." In *Reconceiving the Second Sex: Men, Masculinity, and Reproduction,* edited by Marcia C. Inhorn, Tine Tjørnhøg-Thomsen, Helene Goldberg and Maruska La Cour Mosegaard, 203–26. New York: Berghahn, 2009.

Gole, Nilufer. *The Forbidden Modern: Civilization and Veiling.* Ann Arbor: University of Michigan Press, 1997.

Gonzalez-Lopez, Gloria. *Erotic Journeys: Mexican Immigrants and Their Sex Lives.* Berkeley: University of California Press, 2005.

Good, Byron. *Medicine, Rationality, and Experience: An Anthropological Perspective.* Cambridge, UK: Cambridge University Press, 1994.

Good, Mary-Jo DelVecchio. "Of Blood and Babies: The Relationship of Popular Islamic Physiology to Fertility." *Social Science and Medicine* 14B (1980):147–56.

Gramsci, Antonio. *Selections from the Prison Notebooks of Antonio Gramsci.* Translated by Quintin Hoare and Geoffrey Nowell Smith. New York: International Publishers, 1971.

Gray, Melissa. "Vatican Official Criticizes Award of Nobel Prize to Robert Edwards." www.cnn.com, October 5, 2010.

Greene, Margaret E. "Changing Women and Avoiding Men: Gender Stereotypes and Reproductive Health Programmes." *IDS Bulletin-Institute of Development Studies* 31 (2000):49–59.

Greene, Margaret, and Ann Biddlecom. "Absent and Problematic Men: Demographic Accounts of Male Reproductive Roles." *Population and Development Review* 26 (2000):81–115.

Greenwood, Bernard. "Perceiving Systems: Cold or Spirits? Choice and Ambiguity in Morocco's Pluralistic Medical System." *Social Science and Medicine* 15B (1981):219–35.

Greil, Arthur L. *Not Yet Pregnant: Infertile Couples in Contemporary America.* New Brunswick, NJ: Rutgers University Press, 1991.

———. "Infertility and Psychological Distress: A Critical Review of the Literature." *Social Science and Medicine* 45 (1997):1679–1704.

Greil, Arthur L., Thomas A. Leitko, and Karen L. Porter. "Infertility: His and Hers." *Gender and Society* 2 (1990b):172–99.

Greil, Arthur L., and Julia McQuillan. "'Trying Times': Medicalization, Intent, and Ambiguity in the Definition of Infertility." *Medical Anthropology Quarterly* 24 (2010):137–56.

Greil, Arthur L., Karen L. Porter, and Thomas A. Leitko. "Sex and Intimacy among Infertile Couples." *Journal of Psychology & Human Sexuality* 2 (1990a):117–38.

Greil, Arthur L., Kathleen Slauson-Blevins, and Julia McQuillan. "The Experience of Infertility: A Review of Recent Literature." *Sociology of Health and Illness* 32 (2009):140–62.

Grima, Benedicte. *The Performance of Emotion among Paxtun Women: "The Misfortunes Which Have Befallen Me."* Oxford, UK: Oxford University Press, 2005.

Gruenbaum, Ellen. *The Female Circumcision Controversy: An Anthropological Perspective.* Philadelphia: University of Pennsylvania Press, 2000.

Gunaid, A., N. Hummad, and K. Tamim. "Consanguinity Marriage in the Capital City Sana'a, Yemen." *Journal of Biosocial Sciences* 36 (2004):111–21.

Gurtin, Zeynep. "Assisted Reproduction in Secular Turkey: Regulation, Rhetoric, and the Role of Religion." In *Islam and Assisted Reproductive Technologies: Sunni and Shia Perspectives*, edited by Marcia C. Inhorn and Soraya Tremayne. New York: Berghahn, in press.

Gutmann, Matthew. *The Meanings of Macho: Being a Man in Mexico City.* Berkeley: University of California Press, 1996.

———. "Trafficking in Men: The Anthropology of Masculinity." *Annual Review of Anthropology* 26 (1997):385–409.

———, ed. *Changing Men and Masculinities in Latin America.* Durham, NC: Duke University Press, 2003.

———. *Fixing Men: Sex, Birth Control, and AIDS in Mexico.* Berkeley: University of California Press, 2007.

Haberland, Nicole, and Diana Measham, eds. *Responding to Cairo: Case Studies of Changing Practice in Reproductive Health and Family Planning.* New York: Population Council, 2002.

Haeri, Shahla. *Law of Desire: Temporary Marriage in Shi'i Iran.* Syracuse, NY: Syracuse University Press, 1989.

Hahn, Robert A., and Marcia C. Inhorn, eds. *Anthropology and Public Health: Bridging Differences in Culture and Society.* New York: Oxford University Press, 2008.

Hale, Sondra. "The New Muslim Woman: Sudan's National Islamic Front and the Invention of Identity." *Muslim World* 86 (1996):176–99.

———. *Gender and Politics in Sudan: Islamism, Socialism, and the State.* Boulder, CO: Westview Press, 1997.

Hamamy, H., L. Jamhawi, J. Al-Darawsheh, and K. Ajlouni. "Consanguineous Marriages in Jordan: Why Is the Rate Changing with Time?" *Clinical Genetics* 67 (2005):511–16.

Harrington, Jennifer, Gay Becker, and Robert Nachtigall. "Non-reproductive Technologies: Remediating Kin Structure with Donor Gametes." *Science Technology and Human Values* 33 (2008):393–418.

Hartmann, Betsy. "Charting a Path Ahead: Who Defines Women's Health and How?" Paper presented at "Defining Women's Health: An Interdisciplinary Dialogue," Harvard University, Cambridge, MA, 2002.

Hatem, Mervat. "The Enduring Alliance of Nationalism and Patriarchy in Muslim Personal Status Laws: The Case of Modern Egypt." *Gender Issues* 6 (1986):19–43.

Heng, Boon Chin. "Regulatory Safeguards Needed for the Foreign Travelling Egg Donor." *Human Reproduction* 22 (2007):2350–52.

Hess, David. "Parallel Universes: Anthropology in the World of Technoscience." *Anthropology Today* 10 (1994):16–18.

Hirsch, Jennifer. *A Courtship after Marriage: Sexuality and Love in Mexican Transnational Families.* Berkeley: University of California Press, 2003.

Hirsch, Jennifer, and Holly Wardlow, eds. *Modern Love: The Anthropology of Romantic Courtship and Companionate Marriage.* Ann Arbor: University of Michigan Press, 2006.

Hollan, Douglas. "Developments in Person-Centered Ethnography." In *The Psychology of Cultural Experience,* edited by Carmella C. Moore and Holly F. Mathews, 48–67. Cambridge, UK: Cambridge University Press, 2001.

Hoodfar, Homa. "Population Policy and Gender Equity in Post-revolutionary Iran." In *Family, Gender and Population in the Middle East: Policies in Context,* edited by Carla Makhlouf Obermeyer, 105–35. Cairo: American University Press, 1995.

Hopkins, Nicholas S., ed. *The New Arab Family.* Cairo: American University Press, 2004.

Houjaij, Ali, Barbara Labban, Mohamad Kashmar, Mazen Khalil, Mouen Khashab, Rabih Loutfi, and Walid Osta. *IVF in Lebanon: Assessment of Its Current Status.* Beirut: American University of Beirut, 2000.

Hourvitz, Ariel. "Assisted Reproduction in Women over 40 Years of Age: How Old Is Too Old?" *Reproductive BioMedicine Online* 19 (2009):599–603.

Huntington, Samuel P. *The Clash of Civilizations: Remaking of World Order.* New York: Touchstone Press, 1996.

Hurwitz, M. B. "Sexual Dysfunction Associated with Infertility: A Comparison of Sexual Function during the Fertile and Non-fertile Phase of the Menstrual Cycle." *South African Medical Journal* 76 (1989):58–61.

Hussain, R. "Community Perceptions of Reasons for Preference for Consanguineous Marriages in Pakistan." *Journal of Biosocial Sciences* 31 (1999):449–61.

———. "Lay Perceptions of Genetic Risks Attributable to Inbreeding in Pakistan." *American Journal of Human Biology* 14 (2002):264–74.

Hussain, R., and A. H. Bittles. "Assessment of Association between Consanguinity and Fertility in Asian Populations." *Journal of Health, Population and Nutrition* 22 (2004):1–12.

Inhorn, Marcia C. *Quest for Conception: Gender, Infertility, and Egyptian Medical Traditions.* Philadelphia: University of Pennsylvania Press, 1994.

———. *Infertility and Patriarchy: The Cultural Politics of Gender and Family Life in Egypt.* Philadelphia: University of Pennsylvania Press, 1996.

Inhorn, Marcia C. *Local Babies, Global Science: Gender, Religion, and in Vitro Fertilization in Egypt.* New York: Routledge, 2003.

———. "Privacy, Privatization, and the Politics of Patronage: Ethnographic Challenges to Penetrating the Secret World of Middle Eastern, Hospital-Based in Vitro Fertilization." *Social Science and Medicine* 10 (2004a):2095–3108.

———. "Middle Eastern Masculinities in the Age of New Reproductive Technologies: Male Infertility and Stigma in Egypt and Lebanon." *Medical Anthropology Quarterly* 18 (2004b):162–82.

———. "Sexuality, Masculinity, and Infertility in Egypt: Potent Troubles in Marital and Medical Encounters." In *African Masculinities: Men in Africa from the Late Nineteenth Century to the Present,* edited by Lahoucine Ouzgane and Robert Morrell, 289–303. New York: Palgrave, 2005.

———. "Defining Women's Health: A Dozen Messages from More than 150 Ethnographies." *Medical Anthropology Quarterly* 20 (2006a):345–78.

———. "'The Worms Are Weak': Male Infertility and Patriarchal Paradoxes in Egypt." In *Islamic Masculinities,* edited by Lahoucine Ouzgane, 217–37. London: Zed, 2006b.

———. "Fatwas and ARTs: IVF and Gamete Donation in Sunni V. Shi'a Islam." *Journal of Gender, Race & Justice* 9 (2006c):291–317.

———. "'He Won't Be My Son': Middle Eastern Muslim Men's Discourses of Adoption and Gamete Donation." *Medical Anthropology Quarterly* 20 (2006d):94–120.

———. "A More Open Mind toward Iran." *Chronicle of Higher Education,* June 23, 2006e.

———. "Making Muslim Babies: IVF and Gamete Donation in Sunni versus Shi'a Islam." *Culture, Medicine, and Psychiatry* 30 (2006f):427–50.

———. "Masturbation, Semen Collection, and Men's IVF Experiences: Anxieties in the Muslim World." *Body & Society* 13 (2007a):37–53.

———. "Masculinity, Reproduction, and Male Infertility Surgeries in Egypt and Lebanon." *Journal of Middle East Women's Studies* 3 (2007b):1–20.

———, ed. *Reproductive Disruptions: Gender, Technology, and Biopolitics in the New Millennium.* New York: Berghahn, 2008a.

———. "Medical Anthropology against War." *Medical Anthropology Quarterly* 22 (2008b):416–24.

———. "Right to Assisted Reproductive Technology: Overcoming Infertility in Low-Resource Countries." *International Journal of Gynecology and Obstetrics* 106 (2009a):172–74.

———. "Male Genital Cutting: Masculinity, Reproduction, and Male Infertility Surgeries in Egypt and Lebanon." In *Reconceiving the Second Sex: Men, Masculinity, and Reproduction,* edited by Marcia C. Inhorn, Tine Tjørnhøg-Thomsen, Helene Goldberg and Maruska La Cour Mosegaard, 253–78. New York: Berghahn, 2009b.

———. "Globalization and Gametes: Islam, Assisted Reproductive Technologies, and the Middle Eastern State." In *Reproduction, Globalization, and the State,* edited by C. H. Browner and C. F. Sargent, 126–37. Durham, NC: Duke University Press, 2010.

Inhorn, Marcia C., and Daphna Birenbaum-Carmeli. "Assisted Reproductive Technologies and Culture Change." *Annual Review of Anthropology* 37 (2008):177–96.

———."Male Infertility, Chronicity, and the Plight of Palestinian Men in Israel and Lebanon." In *Chronic Conditions, Fluid States: Chronicity and the Anthropology of Illness*, edited by Lenore Manderson and Carolyn Smith-Morris, 77–95. New Brunswick, NJ: Rutgers University Press, 2010.

Inhorn, Marcia C., and Kimberly A. Buss."Ethnography, Epidemiology, and Infertility in Egypt." *Social Science and Medicine* 39 (1994):671–86.

———."Infertility, Infection, and Iatrogenesis in Egypt: The Anthropological Epidemiology of Blocked Tubes." *Medical Anthropology* 15 (1993):217–44.

Inhorn, Marcia C., and Michael H. Fakih."Arab Americans, African Americans, and Infertility: Barriers to Reproduction and Medical Care." *Fertility and Sterility* 85 (2006):844–52.

Inhorn, Marcia C., Luke King, Jerome O. Nriagu, Loulou Kobeissi, Najwa Hammoud, Johnny Awwad, Antoine A. Abu-Musa, and Antoine B. Hannoun. "Occupational and Environmental Exposures to Heavy Metals: Risk Factors for Male Infertility in Lebanon?" *Reproductive Toxicology* 25 (2008a):203–12.

Inhorn, Marcia C., and Loulou Kobeissi."The Public Health Costs of War in Iraq: Lessons from Post-War Lebanon." *Journal of Social Affairs* 23 (2006):13–47.

Inhorn, Marcia C., Loulou Kobeissi, Antoine A. Abu-Musa, Johnny Awwad, Michael H. Fakih, Najwa Hammoud, Antoine B. Hannoun, Da'ad Lakkis, and Zaher Nassar."Male Infertility and Consanguinity in Lebanon: The Power of Ethnographic Epidemiology." In *Anthropology and Public Health: Bridging Differences in Culture and Society*, edited by Robert A. Hahn and Marcia C. Inhorn, 165–95. Oxford,UK: Oxford University Press, 2008b.

Inhorn, Marcia C., Loulou Kobeissi, Zaher Nassar, Da'ad Lakkis, and Michael Hassan Fakih. "Consanguinity and Family Clustering of Male Infertility in Lebanon." *Fertility and Sterility* 91 (2009):1104–9.

Inhorn, Marcia C., and Pasquale Patrizio."Rethinking Reproductive'Tourism' as Reproductive'Exile.'" *Fertility and Sterility* 92 (2009):904–6.

Inhorn, Marcia C., Pasquale Patrizio, and Gamal I. Serour. "Third-Party Reproductive Assistance around the Mediterranean: Comparing Sunni Egypt, Catholic Italy, and Multisectarian Lebanon." *Reproductive BioMedicine Online* 21 (2010):848–53.

Inhorn, Marcia C., and Pankaj Shrivistav. "Globalization and Reproductive Tourism in the United Arab Emirates." *Asia-Pacific Journal of Public Health* 22 (Suppl.) (2010):68–74.

Inhorn, Marcia C., Tine Tjørnhøj-Thomsen, Helene Goldberg, and Maruska la Cour Mosegaard, eds., *Reconceiving the Second Sex: Men, Masculinity, and Reproduction.* New York: Berghahn, 2009c.

Inhorn, Marcia C., and Soraya Tremayne, eds. *Islam and Assisted Reproductive Technologies: Sunni and Shia Perspectives.* New York: Berghahn, in press.

Inhorn, Marcia C., and Frank van Balen, eds. *Infertility around the Globe: New Thinking on Childlessness, Gender, and Reproductive Technologies.* Berkeley: University of California Press, 2002.

Inhorn, Marcia C., and Emily A. Wentzell. "Embodying Emergent Masculinities: Reproductive and Sexual Health Technologies in the Middle East and Mexico." *American Ethnologist* 38 (2011), in press.

Iqbal, Mohammad, and Ray Noble. "Islamic Identity and the Ethics of Assisted Reproduction." In *Faith and Fertility: Attitudes towards Reproductive Practices in Different Religions from Ancient to Modern Times,* edited by Eric Blyth and Ruth Landau, 86–110. London: Jessica Kingsley, 2009.

Irvine, D. S. "Epidemiology and Aetiology of Male Infertility." *Human Reproduction* 13 (Suppl.) (1998):33–44.

Ivry, Tsipy. *Embodying Culture: Pregnancy in Japan and Israel.* Brunswick, NJ: Rutgers University Press, 2009.

Jabbra, Nancy W. "Family Change in Lebanon's Biqa Valley: What Are the Results of the Civil War?" *Journal of Comparative Family Studies* 35 (2004):259–70.

Jankowiak, William R., ed. *Intimacies: Love and Sex across Cultures.* New York: Columbia University Press, 2008.

Jankowiak, William R., and Edward F. Fischer. "A Cross-Cultural Perspective on Romantic Love." *Ethnology* 31 (1992):149–55.

Johnson, Penny, and Suad Joseph. "Introduction: War and Transnational Arab Families." *Journal of Middle East Women's Studies* 5 (2009):1–10.

Jones, Adam, ed. *Men of the Global South: A Reader.* New York: Zed Books, 2006.

Joseph, Suad. "Connectivity and Patriarchy among Urban Working-Class Arab Families in Lebanon." *Ethos* 21 (1993):452–84.

———. "Brother/Sister Relationships: Connectivity, Love, and Power in the Reproduction of Patriarchy in Lebanon." *American Ethnologist* 21 (1994):50–73.

———, ed. *Intimate Selving in Arab Families: Gender, Self, and Identity.* Syracuse, NY: Syracuse University Press, 1999.

———, ed. *Gender and Citizenship in the Middle East.* Syracuse, NY: Syracuse University Press, 2000.

———. "Conceiving Family Relationships in Post-War Lebanon." *Journal of Comparative Family Studies* 35 (2004):271–93.

———, ed. "War and Transnational Arab Families." *Journal of Middle East Women's Studies* 5 (3) (2009):1–202.

Jurdi, R., and C. Saxena. "The Prevalence and Correlates of Consanguineous Marriages in Yemen: Similarities and Contrasts with Other Arab Countries." *Journal of Biosocial Sciences* 35 (2003):1–13.

Kahn, Susan Martha. *Reproducing Jews: A Cultural Account of Assisted Conception in Israel.* Durham, NC: Duke University Press, 2000.

——— . "Rabbis and Reproduction: The Social Uses of New Reproductive Technologies among Ultra-Orthodox Jews in Israel." In *Infertility around the Globe: New Thinking on Childlessness, Gender, and Reproductive Technologies,* edited by Marcia C. Inhorn and Frank van Balen, 298–314. Berkeley: University of California Press, 2002.

Kamischke, A., and F. Nieschlag. "Conventional Treatments of Male Infertility in the Age of Evidence-Based Andrology." *Human Reproduction* 13 (Suppl. 1) (1988):62–75.

Kanaaneh, Rhoda Ann. *Birthing the Nation: Strategies of Palestinian Women in Israel.* Berkeley: University of California Press, 2002.

———. "Boys or Men? Duped or Made? Palestinian Soldiers in the Israeli Military." *American Ethnologist* 32 (2005):260–75.

———. *Surrounded: Palestinian Soldiers in the Israeli Military.* Stanford, CA: Stanford University Press, 2008.

Kandiyoti, Deniz. *Women, Islam, and the State.* Philadelphia: Temple University Press, 1991.

———. "Bargaining with Patriarchy." *Gender and Society* 2 (1994):274–90.

———. "Gender, Power, and Contestations: 'Rethinking Bargaining with Patriarchy'." In *Feminist Visions of Development: Gender Analysis and Policy,* edited by Cecile Jackson and Ruth Pearson, 138–54. London: Routledge, 1998.

Kapchan, Deborah. *Gender on the Market: Moroccan Women and the Revoicing of Tradition.* Philadelphia: University of Pennsylvania Press, 1996.

Kaplan, Danny. "The Military as a Second Bar-Mitzvah: Combat Service as Initiation to Zionist Masculinity." In *Imagined Masculinities: Male Identity and Culture in the Modern Middle East,* edited by Mai Ghoussoub and Emma Sinclair-Webb, 127–46. London: Saqi, 2000.

Kassak, K. M., H. Ghomrawi, A.M.A. Osseiran, and H. Kobeissi. "The Providers of Health Services in Lebanon: I. A Survey of Physicians." Unpublished manuscript, American University of Beirut, Faculty of Health Sciences, n.d.

Khuri, Fuad I. *The Body in Islamic Culture.* London: Saqi Books, 2001.

Kilshaw, Susie. *Impotent Warriors: Perspectives on Gulf War Syndrome, Vulnerability and Masculinity.* New York: Berghahn, 2009.

King, Diane, and Linda Stone. "Lineal Masculinity: Gendered Memory within Patriliny." *American Ethnologist* 37 (2010):323–36.

Kirkman, Maggie. "Egg and Embryo Donation and the Meaning of Motherhood." *Women's Health* 38 (2003):1–18.

Kleinman, Arthur. *Writing at the Margins: Discourse between Anthropology and Medicine.* Berkeley: University of California Press, 1997.

———. *What Really Matters: Living a Moral Life amidst Uncertainty and Danger.* New York: Oxford University Press, 2006.

Kleinman, Arthur, and Joan Kleinman. "Local Worlds of Suffering: An Interpersonal Focus for Ethnographies of Illness Experience." *Qualitative Health Research* 2 (1992):127–34.

Knysh, Alexander. *Islamic Mysticism: A Short History.* Leiden: Brill, 2000.

Kobeissi, Loulou, and Marcia C. Inhorn. "Male Infertility in Lebanon: A Case-Controlled Study." *Ethnicity and Disease* 17 (Suppl. 3) (2007):33–38.

Kobeissi, Loulou, Marcia C. Inhorn, Antoine B. Hannoun, Najwa Hammoud, Johnny Awwad, Antoine A. Abu-Musa. "Civil War and Male Infertility in Lebanon." *Fertility and Sterility* 90 (2008):340–45.

Konrad, Monica. *Nameless Relations: Anonymity, Melanesia and Reproductive Gift Exchange between British Ova Donors and Recipients*. New York: Berghahn, 2005.

Krausz, C., G. Forti, and K. McElreavey. "The Y Chromosome and Male Fertility and Infertility." *International Journal of Andrology* 26 (2003):570–75.

Kumtepe, Yakup, Cagri Beyazyurek, Cigdem Cinar, Isa Ozbey, Semih Ozkan, Kadir Cetinkaya, Güvenc Karlikaya, Hale Karagozoglu, and Semra Kahraman. "A Genetic Survey of 1935 Turkish Men with Severe Male Factor Infertility." *Reproductive BioMedicine Online* 18 (2009):465–574.

Kurinczuk, J. J. "Safety Issues in Assisted Reproduction Technology: From Theory to Reality—Just What Are the Data Telling Us about ICSI Offspring Health and Future Fertility and Should We Be Concerned?" *Human Reproduction* 18 (2003):925–31.

Lagrange, Frederic. "Male Homosexuality in Modern Arabic Literature." In *Imagined Masculinities: Male Identity and Culture in the Modern Middle East*, edited by Mai Ghoussoub and Emma Sinclair-Webb, 169–98. London: Saqi, 2000.

Lancaster, Roger. *Life Is Hard: Machismo, Danger, and the Intimacy of Power in Nicaragua*. Berkeley: University of California Press, 1992.

Lane, Sandra D., and Robert A. Rubinstein. "The Use of Fatwas in the Production of Reproductive Health Policy in Egypt." Paper presented at the 90th annual meeting of the American Anthropological Association, Chicago, 1991.

Langness, L. L., and Gelya Frank. *Lives: An Anthropological Approach to Biography*. New York: Chandler and Sharp, 1981.

Larkin, Brian. "Indian Films and Nigerian Lovers: Media and the Creation of Parallel Modernities." *Africa* 67 (1997):406–40.

Latini, M., L. Gandini, A. Lenzi, and F. Romanelli. "Sperm Tail Agenesis in a Case of Consanguinity." *Fertility and Sterility* 81 (2004):1688–91.

Lindisfarne, Nancy. "Variant Masculinities, Variant Virginities: Rethinking Honour and Shame." In *Dislocating Masculinity: Comparative Ethnographies*, edited by Cornwall Andrea and Lindisfarne Nancy, 82–96. London: Routledge, 1994.

Lloyd, Mike. "Condemned to Be Meaningful: Non-response in Studies of Men and Infertility." *Sociology of Health and Illness* 18 (1996):433–54.

Lock, Margaret. "Cultivating the Body: Anthropology and Epistemologies of Bodily Practice and Knowledge." *Annual Review of Anthropology* 22 (1993):133–55.

Loeffler, Agnes. *Allopathy Goes Native: Traditional versus Modern Medicine in Iran*. London: I. B. Tauris, 2007.

Lorber, Judith. "Choice, Gift, or Patriarchal Bargain? Women's Consent to In Vitro Fertilization in Male Infertility." *Hypatia* 4 (1989):23–36.

Lotfalian, Mazyar. *Islam, Technoscientific Identities, and the Culture of Curiosity*. Washington, DC: University Press of America, 2004.

Lupton, Deborah, and Lesley Barclay. *Constructing Fatherhood: Discourses and Experiences*. London: Sage, 1997.

MacLeod, Arlene Elowe. *Accommodating Protest. Working Women, the New Veiling, and Change in Cairo*. New York: Columbia University Press, 1993.

Maduro, M. R., and D. J. Lamb. "Understanding the New Genetics of Male Infertility." *Journal of Urology* 168 (2002):2197–2205.

Maduro, M. R., K. C. Lo, W. W. Chuang, and D. J. Lamb. "Genes and Male Infertility: What Can Go Wrong?" *Journal of Andrology* 24 (2003):485–93.

Mahdavi, Pardis. *Passionate Uprisings: Iran's Sexual Revolution*. Stanford, CA: Stanford University Press, 2008.

Mahmoud, Farouk. "Controversies in Islamic Evaluation of Assisted Reproductive Technologies." In *Islam and Assisted Reproductive Technologies: Sunni and Shia Perspectives*, edited by Marcia C. Inhorn and Soraya Tremayne. New York: Berghahn, in press.

Makdisi, Jean. *Beirut Fragments: A War Memoir*. New York: Persea Books, 1990.

Massad, Joseph A. *Desiring Arabs*. Chicago, IL: University of Chicago Press, 2008.

Matorras, Roberto. "Reproductive Exile versus Reproductive Tourism." *Human Reproduction* 20 (2005):3571.

McKee Irwin, Robert. *Mexican Masculinities*. Minneapolis: University of Minnesota Press, 2003.

McLelland, Mark, and Romit Dasgupta, eds. *Genders, Transgenders, and Sexualities in Japan*. New York: Routledge, 2005.

Meirow, D., and J. G. Schenker. "The Current Status of Sperm Donation in Assisted Reproduction Technology: Ethical and Legal Considerations." *Journal of Assisted Reproduction and Genetics* 14 (1997):133–38.

Melhuus, Marit. "Procreative Imaginations: When Experts Disagree on the Meaning of Kinship." In *Holding Worlds Together: Ethnographies of Knowing and Belonging*, edited by Marianne Elisabeth Lien and Marit Melhuus, 37–56. New York: Berghahn, 2007.

Mernissi, Fatima. *Beyond the Veil: Male-Female Dynamics in Modern Muslim Society*. London: Saqi, 1987.

———. *The Veil and the Male Elite: A Feminist Interpretation of Women's Rights in Islam*. New York: Basic Books, 1991.

Mir-Hosseini, Ziba. "The Conservative–Reformist Conflict over Women's Rights in Iran." *International Journal of Politics, Culture, and Society* 16 (2002):37–53.

Moghadam, Valentine. *Modernizing Women: Gender and Social Change in the Middle East*. Boulder: Lynne Rienner, 2003.

———. "Patriarchy in Transition: Women and the Changing Family in the Middle East." *Journal of Comparative Family Studies* 35 (2004):137–62.

Moghimehfar, Farhad, and Mohamad H. Nasr-Esfahani. "Decisive Factors in Reproductive Tourism Destination Choice: Case Study of Isfahan, Iran." Unpublished manuscript, Department of Tourism Management, Allameh Tabataba'a University, Tehran, Iran, and Department of Reproduction and Development, Royan Institute Animal Biotechnology, Isfahan, Iran, n.d.

Mohammed, F., F. Al-Yatama, M. Al-Bader, S. M. Tayel, S. Gouda, and K. K. Naguib. "Primary Male Infertility in Kuwait: A Cytogenetic and Molecular Study of 289 Infertile Kuwaiti Patients." *Andrologia* 39 (2007):87–92.

Monterescu, Daniel. "Stranger Masculinities: Gender and Politics in a Palestinian-Israeli Third Space." In *Islamic Masculinities*, edited by Lahoucine Ouzgane, 123–42. London: Zed Press, 2006.

———. "Masculinity as a Relational Mode: Palestinian Gender Ideologies and Working-Class Categorical Boundaries in an Ethnically Mixed Town." In *Reapproaching Borders: New Perspectives on the Study of Israel/Palestine*, edited by Sandy Sufian and Mark LeVine, 177–98. New York: Rowman and Littlefield, 2007.

Moore, Lisa Jean. *Sperm Counts: Overcome by Man's Most Precious Fluid*. New York: New York University Press, 2008.

Moors, Annelies. *Women, Property and Islam: Palestinian Experiences, 1920–1990*. Cambridge, UK: Cambridge University Press, 1996.

Moosa, Ebrahim. "Human Cloning in Muslim Ethics." *Voices Across Boundaries*, Fall 2003, 23–26.

Morsy, Soheir A. *Gender, Sickness, and Healing in Rural Egypt: Ethnography in Historical Context*. Boulder, CO: Westview Press, 1993.

Moynihan, Clare. "Theories of Masculinity." *British Medical Journal* 317 (1998):1072–75.

Mumtaz, G., H. Tamim, M. Kanaan, M. Khawaja, M. Khogali, G. Wakim, and K. H. Yunis. "Effect of Consanguinity on Birth Weight for Gestational Age in a Developing Country." *American Journal of Epidemiology* 165 (2007):742–52.

Mundigo, A. I. "The Role of Men in Improving Reproductive Health: The Direction Research Should Take." In *Reproductive Health Research: The New Directions, Biennial Report, 1996–1997*, edited by J. van Look and P.F.A. Khanna, 124–31. Geneva: World Health Organization, 1998.

———. "Re-conceptualizing the Role of Men in the Post-Cairo Era." *Culture, Health and Sexuality* 2 (2000):323–37.

Musallam, Basim F. *Sex and Society in Islam: Birth Control before the Nineteenth Century*. Cambridge, UK: Cambridge University Press, 1983.

———. "The Ordering of Muslim Societies." In *Cambridge Illustrated History: Islamic World*, edited by Francis Robinson, 164–207. Cambridge, UK: Cambridge University Press, 2009.

Myntti, Cynthia, Abir Ballan, Omar Dewachi, Faysal El-Kak, and Mary E. Deeb. "Challenging the Stereotypes: Men, Withdrawal, and Reproductive Health in Lebanon." *Contraception* 65 (2000):165–70.

Nachtigall, Robert D. "International Disparities in Access to Infertility Services." *Fertility and Sterility* 85 (2006):871–75.

Nachtigall, R. D., G. Becker, C. Friese, and A. Butler. "Parents' Conceptualization of Their Frozen Embryos Complicates the Disposition Decision." *Fertility and Sterility* 84 (2005):431–3 4.

Nachtigall, Robert D., Gay Becker, Seline S. Szkupinski-Quiroga, and Jeanne M. Tschann. "The Disclosure Decision: Concerns and Issues of Parents of Children Conceived through Donor Insemination." *American Journal of Obstetrics and Gynecology* 178 (1998):1165–70.

Nachtigall, Robert D., Gay Becker, and Mark Wonny. "Effects of Gender-Specific Diagnosis on Men's and Women's Response to Infertility." *Fertility and Sterility* 54 (1992):113–21.

Nachtigall, Robert D., Jeanne M. Tschann, Linda Pitcher, Seline S. Szkupinski-Quiroga, and Gay Becker. "Stigma, Disclosure, and Family Functioning among Parents of Children Conceived through Donor Insemination."*Fertility and Sterility* 68 (1997):83–89.

Najmabadi, Afsaneh. "Transing and Transpassing across Sex-Gender Walls in Iran." *Women's Studies Quarterly* 36 (2008):234–43.

Nakkash, R., J. Khalil, M. Chaaya, and Rema A. Afifi. "Building Research Evidence for Policy Advocacy: A Qualitative Evaluation of Existing Smoke-Free Policies in Lebanon." *Asia-Pacific Journal of Public Health* 22 (Suppl.) (2010):168–74.

Nashif, Esmail. *Palestinian Political Prisoners: Identity and Community.* London: Routledge, 2008.

Nasr, Vali. *The Shia Revival: How Conflicts within Islam Will Shape the Future.* New York: W. W. Norton, 2006.

Nicholson, Roberto F., and Roberto E. Nicholson. "Assisted Reproduction in Latin America." *Journal of Assisted Reproduction and Genetics* 11 (1994):438–44.

Obermeyer, Carla Makhlouf. "Fairness and Fertility: The Meaning of Son Preference in Morocco." In *Dynamics of Values in Fertility Change*, edited by Leete Richard, 275–92. Oxford, UK: Oxford University Press, 1999.

Ola, B., M. Afnan, K. Sharif, S. Papaioannou, N. Hammadieh, and C.L.R. Barratt. "Should ICSI Be the Treatment of Choice for All Cases of In-vitro Conception? Considerations of Fertilization and Embryo Development, Cost Effectiveness and Safety."*Human Reproduction* 16 (2001):2485–90.

Ombelet, Willem. "Reproductive Healthcare Systems Should Include Accessible Infertility Diagnosis and Treatment: An Important Challenge for Resource-Poor Countries." *International Journal of Gynecology and Obstetrics* 106 (2009):168–71.

Omran, Abdel Rahim, and Farzaneh Roudi. "The Middle East Population Puzzle." *Population Bulletin* 48 (1993):1–40.

Onder, Sylvia Wing. *We Have No Microbes Here: Healing Practices in a Turkish Black Sea Village.* Durham, NC: Carolina Academic Press, 2007.

Osmanagaoglu, Kaan, Herman Tournaye, Michel Camus, Mark Vandervorst, Andre Van Steirteghem, and Paul Devroey. "Cumulative Delivery Rates after ICSI: A Five-Years Follow-up of 498 Patients." *Human Reproduction* 14 (1999):2651–55.

Ottenheimer, Martin. *Forbidden Relatives: The American Myth of Cousin Marriage.* Champaign, IL: University of Illinois Press, 1996.

Ouzgane, Lahoucine. "Masculinity as Virility in Tahar Ben Jelloun's Fiction."*Contagion: Journal of Violence, Mimesis, and Culture* 4 (1997):1–13.

———, ed. *Islamic Masculinities.* London: Zed, 2006.

Ouzgane, Lahoucine, and Robert Morrell, eds. *African Masculinities: Men in Africa from the Late Nineteenth Century to the Present.* New York: Palgrave, 2005.

Padilla, Mark. *Caribbean Pleasure Industry: Tourism, Sexuality, and AIDS in the Dominican Republic*. Chicago, IL: University of Chicago Press, 2007.

Padilla, Mark, Jennifer Hirsch, Miguel Munoz-Laboy, Robert Sember, and Richard G. Parker, eds. *Love and Globalization: Transformations of Intimacy in the Contemporary World*. Nashville, TN: Vanderbilt University Press, 2007.

Panter-Brick, Catherine. "Parental Responses to Consanguinity and Genetic Disease in Saudi Arabia." *Social Science and Medicine* 33 (1991):1295–1302.

Parker, Richard G. *Bodies, Pleasure, and Passions: Sexual Culture in Contemporary Brazil*. Boston: Beacon Press, 1991.

———. *Beneath the Equator: Cultures of Desire, Male Homosexuality, and Emerging Gay Communities in Brazil*. New York: Routledge, 1998.

Parker-Pope, Tara. *For Better: The Science of a Good Marriage*. New York: Dutton, 2010.

Patrizio, Pasquale, and Marcia C. Inhorn. "Ethical and Religious Challenges in Male Infertility Treatment." In *Male Infertility Practice*, edited by Nabil F. Aziz, n.d.

Pennings, Guido. "Reproductive Tourism as Moral Pluralism in Motion." *Journal of Medical Ethics* 228 (2002):337–41.

Petchesky, Rosalind, Karen Judd, and IRRAG. *Negotiating Reproductive Rights*. New York: Palgrave, 2001.

Peteet, Julie Marie. *Landscape of Hope and Despair: Palestinian Refugee Camps*. Philadelphia: University of Pennsylvania Press, 2005.

Peterson, Brennan D., Matthew Pirritano, Jessica M. Block, and Lone Schmidt. "Marital Benefit and Coping Strategies in Men and Women Undergoing Unsuccessful Fertility Treatments over a Five Year Period." *Fertility and Sterility* 95 (2011):1759–63.

Pliskin, Karen. *Silent Boundaries: Cultural Constraints on Sickness and Diagnosis of Iranians in Israel*. New Haven, CT: Yale University Press, 1987.

Population Reference Bureau. *World Population Data Sheet*. Washington: Population Reference Bureau, 2010.

Povinelli, Elizabeth A. *The Empire of Love: Toward a Theory of Intimacy, Genealogy, and Carnality*. Durham, NC: Duke University Press, 2006.

Pringle, Richard. "Masculinities, Sport, and Power: A Critical Comparison of Gramscian and Foucauldian Inspired Theoretical Tools." *Journal of Sport and Social Issues* 29 (2005):256–78.

Ragone, Helena. *Surrogate Motherhood: Conception in the Heart*. Boulder, CO: Westview Press, 1994.

———. "Chasing the Blood Tie: Surrogate Mothers, Adoptive Mothers and Fathers." *American Ethnologist* 23 (1996):352–65.

Rajab, A., and M. A. Patton. "A Study of Consanguinity in the Sultanate of Oman." *Annals of Human Biology* 27 (2000):321–26.

Rantala, M. L., and A. I. Koskimies. "Sexual Behavior of Infertile Couples." *International Journal of Fertility* 33 (1988):26–30.

Rapp, Rayna. "Moral Pioneers: Women, Men and Fetuses on a Frontier of Reproductive Technology." In *Embryos, Ethics, and Women's Rights: Exploring the New Reproductive Technologies*, edited by Amadeo F. D'Adamo, Elaine

Hoffman Baruch Jr., and Joni Seager, 101–16. New York: Haworth Press, 1988.

———. *Testing Women, Testing the Fetus: The Social Impact of Amniocentesis in America*. New York: Routledge, 1998.

Raz, A. E. *The Gene and the Genie: Tradition, Medicalization, and Genetic Counseling in a Bedouin Community in Israel*. Durham, NC: Carolina Academic Press, 2005.

Raz, A. E., M. Atar, M. Rodnay, I. Shohan-Vardi, and R. Carmi. "Between Acculturation and Ambivalence: Knowledge of Genetics and Attitudes towards Genetic Testing in a Consanguineous Bedouin Community." *Community Genetics* 6 (2003):88–95.

Reed, Richard K. *Birthing Fathers: The Transformation of Men in American Rites of Birth*. New Brunswick, NJ: Rutgers University Press, 2005.

Richards, Jim. "A Roman Catholic Perspective on Fertility Issues: Objective Truths, Moral Absolutes and the Natural Law." In *Faith and Fertility: Attitudes towards Reproductive Practices in Different Religions from Ancient to Modern Times*, edited by Eric Blyth and Ruth Landau, 35–56. London: Jessica Kingsley, 2009.

Riska, Elianne. "Gendering the Medicalization Thesis." In *Gender Perspectives on Health and Healing: Key Themes, Advances in Gender Research*, edited by M. S. Segal and V. Demos, 59–87. Oxford, UK: Elsevier, 2003.

Roberts, Dorothy. *Killing the Black Body: Race, Reproduction, and the Meaning of Liberty*. New York: Vintage, 1998.

Rogozen-Soltar, Mikaela. "Andalusian Encounters: Immigration, Islam, and Regional Identity in Southern Spain." PhD dissertation, University of Michigan, 2010.

Rosenfeld, Dana, and Christopher A. Faircloth. "Medicalized Masculinities: The Missing Link?" In *Medicalized Masculinities*, edited by Dana Rosenfeld and Christopher A. Faircloth, 1–20. Philadelphia, PA: Temple University Press, 2006.

Saadat, M., M. Ansari-Lari, and D. D. Farhud. "Consanguineous Marriage in Iran." *Annals of Human Biology* 2 (2004):263–69.

Saadawi, Nawal. *The Hidden Face of Eve: Women in the Arab World*. London: Zed, 1980.

Sabbah, Fatna. *Women in the Muslim Unconscious*. New York: Pergamon, 1984.

Sachedina, Abdulaziz Abdulhussein. *Islamic Biomedical Ethics: Principles and Application*. Oxford, UK: Oxford University Press, 2009.

Said, Edward W. *Orientalism*. New York: Vintage Books, 1978.

Said, Edward W., and Christopher Hitchens, eds. *Blaming the Victims: Spurious Scholarship and the Palestinian Question*. London: Verso, 2001.

Sanai, Aslihan. *New Organs within Us: Transplants and the Moral Economy*. Durham, NC: Duke University Press, 2011.

Saniei, Mansooreh. "Human Embryonic Stem Cell Research in Iran: The Significance of the Islamic Context." In *Islam and Assisted Reproductive Technologies: Sunni and Shia Perspectives*, edited by Marcia C. Inhorn and Soraya Tremayne. New York: Berghahn, in press.

Saxena, C., A. Kulczyck, and R. Jurdi. "Nuptiality Transition and Marriage Squeeze in Lebanon: Consequences of Sixteen Years of Civil War." *Journal of Comparative Family Studies* 35 (2004):241–58.

Schettler, Ted, Gina Soloma, Maria Valenti, and Annette Huddle, eds. *Generations at Risk: Reproductive Health and the Environment.* Cambridge, MA: MIT Press, 1999.

Schneider, David M. *American Kinship: A Cultural Account.* Chicago, IL: University of Chicago Press, 1980.

Schneider, Peter, and Jane Schneider. "Coitus Interruptus and Family Responsibility in Catholic Europe: A Sicilian Case Study." In *Conceiving the New World Order: The Global Politics of Reproduction*, edited by Faye Ginsberg and Rayna Rapp, 177–94. Berkeley: University of California Press, 1995.

Sedghi, Hamideh. *Women and Politics in Iran: Veiling, Unveiling, and Reveiling.* Cambridge, UK: Cambridge University Press, 2007.

Sen, Gita, Asha George, and Piroska Ostlin, eds. *Engendering International Health: The Challenge of Equity.* Cambridge, MA: MIT Press, 2002.

Serour, Gamal I. "Bioethics in Medically Assisted Conception Research: Dilemma of Practice and Research—Islamic Views." Proceedings of the First International Conference on Bioethics in Human Reproduction Research in the Muslim World, December 10–13, 1991, Al Azhar University, Cairo, 234–42.

——— . "Islam and the Four Principles." In *Principles of Health Care Ethics*, edited by R. Gillon, 75–91. London: John Wiley, 1994.

——— . "Bioethics in Reproductive Health: A Muslim's Perspective." *Middle East Fertility Society Journal* 1 (1996):30–35.

——— . "Islamic Perspectives in Human Reproduction." *Reproductive BioMedicine Online* 17 (Suppl. 3) (2008):34–38.

Serour, G. I., M. A. Aboulghar, and R. T. Mansour. "Bioethics in Medically Assisted Conception in the Muslim World." *Journal of Assisted Reproduction and Genetics* 12 (1995):559–65.

Serour, G. I., and B. M. Dickens. "Assisted Reproduction Developments in the Islamic World." *International Journal of Gynecology and Obstetrics* 74 (2001):2.

Serour, G. I., M. El Ghar, and R. T. Mansour. "In Vitro Fertilization and Embryo Transfer: Ethical Aspects in Techniques in the Muslim World." *Population Sciences* 9 (1990):45–54.

——— . "Infertility: A Health Problem in the Muslim World." *Population Sciences* 10 (1991):41–58.

Serour, G. I., and A. R. Omran, eds. *Ethical Guidelines for Human Reproduction Research in the Muslim World.* Cairo: International Islamic Center for Population Studies and Research, 1992.

Shah, Nasra M. "Women's Socio-economic Characteristics and Marital Patterns in Rapidly Developing Muslim Society, Kuwait." *Journal of Comparative Family Studies* 35 (2004):163–83.

Shaheen, Jack. *Guilty: Hollywood's Verdict on Arabs after 9/11.* New York: Olive Branch Press, 2008.

Shahidian, Hammed. *Women in Iran: Emerging Voices in the Women's Movement.* Westport, CT: Greenwood, 2002.

Sharma, S., S. Mittal, and P. Aggarwal. "Management of Infertility in Low Resource Countries." *British Journal of Obstetrics and Gynecology* 116 (Suppl. 1) (2009):77–83.

Shavazi, M.J.A., P. McDonald, and M. Hosseini-Chavoshi. "Modernization and the Cultural Practice of Consanguineous Marriage: A Study of Four Provinces of Iran." Paper presented at the European Population Conference, Liverpool, England, June 21–24, 2006.

Shenfield, F., J. de Mouzon, G. Pennings, A. P. Ferraretti, A. N. Andersen, G. de Wert, V. Goossens, and ESHRE Taskforce on Cross Border Reproductive Care. "Cross Border Reproductive Care in Six European Countries." *Human Reproduction* 25 (2010):1361–68.

Sinclair-Webb, Emma. "Our Bulent Is Now a Commando: Military Service and Manhood in Turkey." In *Imagined Masculinities: Male Identity and Culture in the Modern Middle East,* edited by Mai Ghoussoub and Emma Sinclair-Webb, 65–91. London: Saqi, 2000.

Singer, Merrill. *The Face of Social Suffering: Life History of a Street Drug Addict.* Long Grove, IL: Waveland Press, 2005.

Singerman, Diane, and Barbara Ibrahim. "The Cost of Marriage in Egypt: A Hidden Variable in the New Arab Demography." In *The New Arab Family,* edited by Nicholas S. Hopkins, 80–116. Cairo: American University of Cairo Press, 2004.

Siraj, Asifa. "On Being Homosexual and Muslim: Conflicts and Challenges." In *Islamic Masculinities,* edited by Lahoucine Ouzgane, 202–16. London: Zed, 2006.

Smith, Daniel Jordan. "Romance, Parenthood, and Gender in a Modern African Society." *Ethnology* 40 (2001):129–51.

Sobo, Elisa J. *Choosing Unsafe Sex: AIDS-Risk Denial among Disadvantaged Women.* Philadelphia: University of Pennsylvania Press, 1995.

Sonbol, Amira el Azhary. "Adoption in Islamic Society: A Historical Survey." In *Children in the Muslim Middle East,* edited by Fernea Elizabeth Warnock, 45–67. Austin: University of Texas Press, 1995.

Soueif, Ahdaf. *The Map of Love: A Novel.* New York: Random House, 2000.

Spar, Deborah L. *The Baby Business: How Money, Science, and Politics Drive the Commerce of Conception.* Boston: Harvard Business School Press, 2006.

Storrow, Richard F. "The Handmaid's Tale of Fertility Tourism: Passports and Third Parties in the Religious Regulation of Assisted Conception." *Texas Wesleyan Law Review* 12 (2005):189–211.

———. "Marginalizing Adoption through the Regulation of Assisted Reproduction." *Capital University Law Review* 35 (2006):479–516.

Strathern, Marilyn. *Reproducing the Future: Anthropology, Kinship and the New Reproductive Technologies.* Manchester, UK: Manchester University Press, 1992a.

———. *After Nature: English Kinship in the Late Twentieth Century.* Cambridge, UK: Cambridge University Press, 1992b.

Strathern, Marilyn. *Kinship, Law and the Unexpected: Relatives Are Always a Surprise*. Cambridge, UK: Cambridge University Press, 2005.

Sueyoshi, S., and R. Ohtsuka. "Effects of Polygyny and Consanguinity on High Fertility in the Rural Arab Population in South Jordan." *Journal of Biosocial Sciences* 35 (2003):513–26.

Sullivan, Maureen. *Family of Women: Lesbian Mothers, Their Children, and the Undoing of Gender*. Berkeley: University of California Press, 2004.

Taga, Futoshi. "East Asian Masculinities." In *Handbook of Studies on Men and Masculinities*, edited by Michael S. Kimmel, Jeff R. Hearn, and R. W. Connell, 129–40. New York: Sage, 2004.

Takefman, J. E., W. Brender, J. Boivin, and T. Tulandi. "Sexual and Emotional Adjustment of Couples Undergoing Infertility Investigation and the Effectiveness of Preparatory Information." *Journal of Psychosomatic Obstetrics and Gynecology* 11 (1990):275–90.

Tamim, H., M. Khogali, H. Beydoun, I. Melki, and K. Yunis. "Consanguinity and Apnea of Prematurity." *American Journal of Epidemiology* 158 (2003):942–46.

Teebi, Ahmed S., ed. *Genetic Disorders among Arab Populations*. 2nd ed. Heidelberg: Springer-Verlag, 2010.

Teman, Elly. *Birthing a Mother: The Surrogate Body and the Pregnant Self*. Berkeley: University of California Press, 2010.

Thompson, Charis M. "Strategic Naturalizing: Kinship in an Infertility Clinic." In *Relative Values: Reconfiguring Kinship Studies*, edited by Sarah Franklin and Susan McKinnon, 175–202. Durham, NC: Duke University Press, 2001.

———. "Fertile Ground: Feminists Theorize Infertility." In *Infertility around the Globe: New Thinking on Childlessness, Gender, and Reproductive Technologies*, edited by Marcia C. and Frank van Balen, 52–78. Berkeley: University of California Press, 2002.

———. *Making Parents: The Ontological Choreography of Reproductive Technologies*. Cambridge, MA: MIT Press, 2005.

Throsby, Karen, and Rosalind Gill. "It's Different for Men." *Men and Masculinities* 6 (2004):330–48.

Tober, Diane M. "Shi'ism, Pragmatism, and Modernity: Islamic Bioethics and Health Policy in the Islamic Republic of Iran." Paper presented at the University of Michigan, Ann Arbor, 2004.

———. "Fewer Children, Better Life or as Many as God Wants." *Medical Anthropology Quarterly* 20 (2008):50–71.

Tournaye, Herman. "Gamete Source and Manipulation." In *Current Practices and Controversies in Assisted Reproduction*, edited by Effy Vayena, Patrick J. Rowe, and P. David Griffin, 83–101. Geneva: World Health Organization, 2002.

Townsend, Nicholas. *The Package Deal: Marriage, Work and Fatherhood in Men's Lives*. Philadelphia, PA: Temple University Press, 2002.

Traina, Cristina, Eugenia Georges, Marcia C. Inhorn, Susan Kahn, and Maura A. Ryan. "Compatible Contradictions: Religion and the Naturalization of Assisted Reproduction." In *Altering Nature*, vol. II: *Religion, Biotechnol-*

ogy, and Public Policy, edited by B. Andrew Lustig, Baruch A. Brody, and Gerald P. McKenny, 15–85. New York: Springer, 2008.

Trawick, Margaret. *Notes on Love in a Tamil Family*. Berkeley: University of California Press, 1990.

Tremayne, Soraya. "The Moral, Ethical and Legal Implications of Egg, Sperm and Embryo Donation in Iran." Paper presented at "Reproductive Disruptions: Childlessness, Adoption, and Other Reproductive Complexities," University of Michigan, Ann Arbor, 2005.

———. "Whither Kinship? New Assisted Reproduction Technology Practices, Authoritative Knowledge and Relatedness—Case Studies from Iran." Paper presented at "Gamete and Embryo Donation," University of Tehran, Iran, 2006.

———. "Law, Ethics, and Donor Technologies in Shia Iran." In *Assisting Reproduction, Testing Genes: Global Encounters with New Biotechnologies*, edited by Daphna Birenbaum-Carmeli and Marcia C. Inhorn, 144–63. New York: Berghahn, 2009.

———. "The 'Down Side' of Gamete Donation: Challenging 'Happy Family' Rhetoric in Iran." In *Islam and Assisted Reproductive Technologies: Sunni and Shia Perspectives*, edited by Marcia C. Inhorn and Soraya Tremayne. New York: Berghahn, in press.

United Nations Development Programme. "National Human Development Report: Lebanon, 2001–2002; Globalization—Towards a Lebanese Agenda." Beirut, 2002.

Upton, Rebecca L. "Perceptions of and Attitudes toward Male Infertility in Northern Botswana: Some Implications for Family Planning and AIDS Prevention Policies." *African Journal of Reproductive Health* 6 (2002):103–11.

van Balen, Frank, and Trudie Gerrits. "Quality of Infertility Care in Poor-Resource Areas and the Introduction of New Reproductive Technologies." *Human Reproduction* 16 (2001):215–19.

van Balen, Frank, and Marcia C. Inhorn. "Introduction: Interpreting Infertility—A View from the Social Sciences." In *Infertility around the Globe: New Thinking on Childlessness, Gender, and Reproductive Technologies*, edited by Marcia C. Inhorn and Frank van Balen, 3–23. Berkeley: University of California Press, 2002.

van der Ploeg, Irma. "Hermaphrodite Patients: In Vitro Fertilization and the Transformation of Male Infertility." *Science, Technology, and Human Values* 20 (1995):460–81.

van Wolputte, Steven. "Hang onto Yourself: Of Bodies, Embodiment, and Selves." *Annual Review of Anthropology* 33 (2004):251–69.

van Zyl, J. A. "Sex and Infertility: Part I. Prevalence of Psychosexual Problems and Subjacent Factors." *South African Medical Journal* 72 (1987a):482–84.

———. "Sex and Infertility: Part II. Influence of Psychogenic Factors and Psychosexual Problems." *South African Medical Journal* 72 (1987b):485–87.

Vayena, Effy, Herbert B. Peterson, David Adamson, and Karl-G. Nygren. "Assisted Reproductive Technologies in Developing Countries: Are We Caring Yet?" *Fertility and Sterility* 92 (2009):413–16.

Vayena, Effy, Patrick J. Rowe, and P. David Griffin, eds. *Current Practices and Controversies in Assisted Reproduction.* Geneva: World Health Organization, 2002.

Wajahat, Ali."'Sex and the City 2's' Stunning Muslim Cliches."*Salon,* May 26, 2010. http://www.salon.com/entertainment/movies/film_salon/2010/05/26.

Webb, Russell E., and Judith C. Daniluk. "The End of the Line: Infertile Men's Experiences of Being Unable to Produce a Child."*Men and Masculinities* 2 (1999):6–25.

Wentzell, Emily A."Composite Masculinities: Aging, Illness, Erectile Dysfunction and Mexican Manhood."PhD dissertation, University of Michigan, 2009.

Wentzell, Emily A., and Jorge Salmerón."You'll'Get Viagraed': Mexican Men's Preference for Alternative Erectile Dysfunction Treatment."*Social Science and Medicine* 68 (2009):1759–65.

White, Jenny. *Islamist Mobilization in Turkey: A Study in Vernacular Politics.* Seattle: University of Washington Press, 2003.

Wikan, Unni. *In Honor of Fadime: Murder and Shame.* Chicago, IL: University of Chicago Press, 2008.

Williams, Raymond. *Marxism and Literature.* Oxford, UK: Oxford University Press, 1978.

World Health Organization."The Influence of Varicocele on Parameters of Fertility in a Large Group of Men Presenting to Infertility Clinics." *Fertility and Sterility* 57 (1992):1289–93.

———. *WHO Laboratory Manual for the Examination and Processing of Human Semen.* Geneva: World Health Organization, 2010.

Yount, Katherine, and Hoda Rashad, eds. *Family in the Middle East: Ideational Change in Egypt, Iran and Tunisia.* New York: Routledge, 2008.

Zegers-Hochschild, F., J.-E. Schwarze, and V. Galdames. "Assisted Reproductive Technology in Latin America: An Example of Regional Cooperation and Development."*ESHRE Monographs* 1 (2008):42–47.

Zlotogora, J. "Genetic Disorders among Palestinian Arabs." *American Journal of Medical Genetics* 68 (1997):472–75.

Zuhur, Sherifa. *Revealing Reveiling: Islamist Gender Ideology in Contemporary Egypt.* Albany: State University of New York Press, 1992a.

———. "Of Milk-Mothers and Sacred Bonds: Islam, Patriarchy, and New Reproductive Technologies."*Creighton Law Review* 25 (1992b):1725–38.

Index

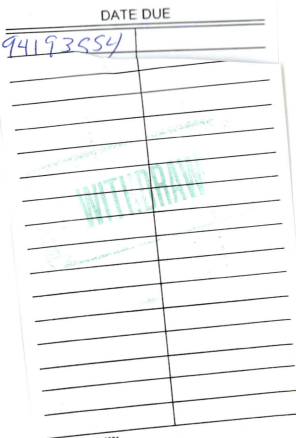